Textbook of
GENERAL ANATOMY

Textbook of
GENERAL ANATOMY
with Case Scenarios & Clinical Applications

As per the Competency Based Medical Education Curriculum (NMC)

SECOND EDITION

V Subhadra Devi MS (Anatomy)
Professor
Department of Anatomy
Apollo Institute of Medical Sciences and Research (AIMSR)
Chittoor, Andhra Pradesh, India

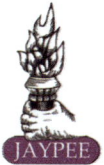

JAYPEE BROTHERS MEDICAL PUBLISHERS
The Health Sciences Publisher
New Delhi | London

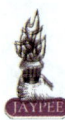 **Jaypee Brothers Medical Publishers (P) Ltd**

Headquarters
Jaypee Brothers Medical Publishers (P) Ltd.
EMCA House
23/23-B, Ansari Road, Daryaganj
New Delhi 110 002, India
Landline: +91-11-23272143, +91-11-23272703
+91-11-23282021, +91-11-23245672
E-mail: jaypee@jaypeebrothers.com

Corporate Office
Jaypee Brothers Medical Publishers (P) Ltd.
4838/24, Ansari Road, Daryaganj
New Delhi 110 002, India
Phone: +91-11-43574357
Fax: +91-11-43574314
E-mail: jaypee@jaypeebrothers.com

Overseas Office
JP Medical Ltd.
83, Victoria Street, London
SW1H 0HW (UK)
Phone: +44-20 3170 8910
Fax: +44(0)20 3008 6180
E-mail: info@jpmedpub.com

Website: www.jaypeebrothers.com
Website: www.jaypeedigital.com

© 2023, Jaypee Brothers Medical Publishers

The views and opinions expressed in this book are solely those of the original contributor(s)/author(s) and do not necessarily represent those of editor(s) and publishers of the book.

All rights reserved by the author. No part of this publication may be reproduced, stored or transmitted in any form or by any means, electronic, mechanical, photocopying, recording or otherwise, without the prior permission in writing of the publishers.

All brand names and product names used in this book are trade names, service marks, trademarks or registered trademarks of their respective owners. The publisher is not associated with any product or vendor mentioned in this book.

Medical knowledge and practice change constantly. This book is designed to provide accurate, authoritative information about the subject matter in question. However, readers are advised to check the most current information available on procedures included and check information from the manufacturer of each product to be administered, to verify the recommended dose, formula, method and duration of administration, adverse effects and contraindications. It is the responsibility of the practitioner to take all appropriate safety precautions. Neither the publisher nor the author(s)/editor(s) assume any liability for any injury and/or damage to persons or property arising from or related to use of material in this book.

This book is sold on the understanding that the publisher is not engaged in providing professional medical services. If such advice or services are required, the services of a competent medical professional should be sought.

Every effort has been made where necessary to contact holders of copyright to obtain permission to reproduce copyright material. If any have been inadvertently overlooked, the publisher will be pleased to make the necessary arrangements at the first opportunity.

Inquiries for bulk sales may be solicited at: jaypee@jaypeebrothers.com

Textbook of General Anatomy

First Edition: 2019
  Revised Reprint: 2022
Second Edition: **2023**

ISBN: 978-93-5465-169-4

Printed at: Sterling Graphics Pvt. Ltd. India.

Dedicated to

My husband Dr VH Rao
who has been my inspiration and motivator

PREFACE TO THE SECOND EDITION

The prerequisite for understanding a patient is comprehension of fundamental concepts in basic medical sciences and their clinical application. Integration of basic and clinical sciences leads to contextual and active learning, which in turn, improves problem-solving skills among doctors.

The *Textbook of General Anatomy* is conceived to inspire the new entrants into the medical schools to acquire basic skills and knowledge.

This book provides basic knowledge required for understanding the dissection of cadaver and study of various regions of the body adopting integrated approach. This book was prepared as per the competencies prescribed by National Medical Council (NMC) and other medical education-related boards in Asia.

All possible care was taken to ensure that the information provided facilitates understanding of importance of each of the systems in the body and their clinical relevance to motivate the students of medicine.

A simple language, easy-to-understand illustrations, flowcharts, tables, presentation of clinical application in boxes, case scenarios, and a take home message of key concepts are the unique features incorporated to facilitate learning among the new generation of students. These are highly useful to recall and for competitive examination preparation.

The additional components that are included in this book to enrich the knowledge are gross anatomical, developmental, microscopic, radiological and clinical case insights in the form of images from the authors personal collection and collection from clinicians/practitioners.

This book can be used as a self-study guide by students of medical, dental and allied health courses (nursing, physiotherapy, laboratory technology) and by students of alternate systems of medicine (ayurveda, homeopathy, etc.) to understand the basic concepts of human anatomy.

As this is a single person's effort, there is every possibility of omissions and commissions. Therefore, feedback from the anatomists, medical and allied specialists of all generations and above all the students for whose benefit this book is envisioned is solicited.

V Subhadra Devi

PREFACE TO THE FIRST EDITION

The prerequisite for understanding the patient is the strong basic fundamental concepts in the medical curriculum followed by its clinical application. Integration of basic and clinical sciences leads to contextual learning, active rather than passive involvement in the process of learning, which in turn, improves problem-solving skills of medical professionals, which is the single best approach to alleviate the suffering in the diseased.

The *Textbook of General Anatomy* is conceived with a strong belief to inspire the new entrants into the portals of medicine about the importance of learning basic skills, knowledge and attitude before they embark on reading the important branch of medicine the anatomy, that requires in-depth region-wise knowledge and skills.

This book provides basic knowledge required for understanding the dissection of cadaver and study of various regions of the body adopting integrated approach. This book was prepared as per the syllabus of anatomy recommended by the Medical Council of India (MCI) and other medical-related boards in Asia.

All possible care was taken to ensure that the information provided facilitates understanding of importance of each of the systems in the body and their clinical relevance to motivate the students of medicine on the importance of basics and its application in practicing the profession.

A simple language, easy-to-understand illustrations, flowcharts, tables and presentation in boxes are the unique adoptions in this book to drive the new age generation of students to make it student friendly. These are highly useful for the readers to recall and for competitive examination preparation.

The additional components that are included in this book to enrich the knowledge of readers is the gross anatomical, developmental, microscopic, radiological and clinical case insights in the form of author's own images, personal collections and collection from several clinicians/practitioners.

This book can be used as a self-study guide by students of medical, dental and allied health courses to understand the basic concepts of human anatomy.

As this is a single person's effort, there is every possibility of omissions and commissions that needs the feedback from the anatomists, medical and allied specialists of all generations and above all the students for whose benefit writing of this book is envisioned.

V Subhadra Devi

ACKNOWLEDGMENTS

This book is prepared with the support of several organizations and individuals who were associated with me for a long time in my career. I am thankful to the management of Apollo Institute of Medical Sciences and Research (AIMSR), for encouraging me to continue my academic work. I am thankful to staff and students in the Department of Anatomy, SV Medical College, SPMCW (SVIMS), Tirupati and Apollo Institute of Medical Sciences and Research (AIMSR), Chittoor, Andhra Pradesh, India, for their continuous support and constructive feedback.

I thank the radiologists at Sapthagiri Scan Center, Tirupati and Dr M Sreenivasulu, for facilitating me to obtain several radiological images. I am thankful to Dr T Ram Sharan, Professor, Department of Dermatology, SPMCW, for providing the images of several dermatological conditions. I am extremely thankful to Dr Ranadheer Gupta, Ex-Associate Professor, Department of Nuclear Medicine and Radiology, SVIMS, Tirupati, for providing the necessary images.

I am thankful to Mr K Thyagaraju, Assistant Professor, SPMCW-SVIMS, for his continuous help and innovative views in preparing and labeling the figures and photographs. I am exceptionally thankful to Mr Ravindra Kumar Boddeti and Mr Kishore Naick, for their support in correcting the manuscript and for extending their views.

I am also thankful to Shri Jitendar P Vij (Group Chairman), Mr Ankit Vij (Managing Director), and MS Mani (Group President), for kindly agreeing to publish this book and the production team, especially Dr Madhu Choudhary (Director–Educational Publishing), Ms Pooja Bhandari (Production Head), Ms Sunita Katla (Executive Assistant to Group Chairman and Publishing Manager), Dr Aditya Tayal (Development Editor), Mr Rajesh Sharma (Production Coordinator), Ms Seema Dogra (Cover Visualizer), Ms Geeta Srivastava (Proofreader), Ms Uma Adhikari (Typesetter), and Mr Ankush Sharma (Graphic Designer), for their dedicated work.

I thank all my students who are my continuous source of inspiration to organize the content that will be beneficial for them.

CONTENTS

1. **Introduction to Anatomy**   1
   - ☐ Definition of Anatomy   1
   - ☐ Structure Contributing to Function   1
   - ☐ Evolutionary Revolutions in Anatomy   1
   - ☐ Importance of Anatomy   2
   - ☐ Subdivisions of Anatomy   2
   - ☐ Approaches for Studying Anatomy   5
   - ☐ Anatomical Position and Planes   5
   - ☐ Anatomical Terminology   8
   - ☐ History of Anatomy   10

2. **Levels of Organization and Tissues of the Body**   16
   - ☐ Levels of Organization of the Human Body   16
   - ☐ Cell   16
   - ☐ Development of a Human Being   16
   - ☐ Tissues of the Body   20
   - ☐ Epithelial Tissue   20
   - ☐ Connective Tissue   26

3. **Introduction to Skin and Fascia**   34
   - ☐ Skin   34
   - ☐ Fascia   43
   - ☐ Cavities of the Body   46

4. **Skeletal System**   52
   - ☐ Skeletal System   52
   - ☐ Cartilage   53
   - ☐ Bone   55

5. **Introduction to Muscular System**   76
   - ☐ General Features of Muscular Tissue   76
   - ☐ Types of Muscle   77
   - ☐ Structure of Skeletal Muscle   78
   - ☐ Structural Components of a Skeletal Muscle   82
   - ☐ Microscopic Appearance of Skeletal Muscle   83
   - ☐ Blood Supply of Skeletal Muscle   85
   - ☐ Innervation of Skeletal Muscle   87
   - ☐ Importance of Skeletal Muscle   90
   - ☐ Functions   90
   - ☐ Structures Associated with Skeletal Muscle   90
   - ☐ Classification of Skeletal Muscles   90
   - ☐ Actions of Skeletal Muscles   93
   - ☐ Naming of Muscles   95

6. **Introduction to Arthrology/Joints**   100
   - ☐ Definition   100
   - ☐ Classification of Joints   100

- ☐ Synovial Joints 106
- ☐ Basic Terms Used for Describing Movements in Joints 114
- ☐ Terminology of Body Movements 117

7. Introduction to Blood Vascular System 125
- ☐ Purpose and Functions 125
- ☐ Types of Circulation of Blood 130
- ☐ Classification of Blood Vessels 131
- ☐ Structure of Vascular Tree from Center to Periphery 131
- ☐ Anastomoses 135
- ☐ Collateral Circulation 135
- ☐ End-arteries 137
- ☐ Vasa Vasorum 137

8. Introduction to Lymphatic System 143
- ☐ Defense Mechanisms of the Body 145
- ☐ Functions of Lymphatic System 145
- ☐ Components of Lymphatic System and Lymph Flow 146

9. Introduction to Nervous System 157
- ☐ Subdivisions of Nervous System 157
- ☐ Nervous Tissue 158
- ☐ Spinal Cord and Spinal Segments 168
- ☐ Dermatomes 170
- ☐ Receptors 171
- ☐ Reflex Arc 173
- ☐ Nerve Fibers and their Myelination 175
- ☐ Autonomic Nervous System 179

10. Introduction to Splanchnology 185
- ☐ Respiratory System 186
- ☐ Digestive System 190
- ☐ Urinary System 195
- ☐ Reproductive System 197
- ☐ Male Reproductive System 197
- ☐ Female Reproductive System 198
- ☐ Endocrine System 200

11. Introduction to Radiological Anatomy 206
- ☐ Classification of Radiological Procedures 206

12. Introduction to Surface Anatomy 219
- ☐ Importance 219
- ☐ Techniques Used 219

13. Introduction to Dissection of Cadaver 228
- ☐ Dissection 228
- ☐ Cadaver Respect 228
- ☐ Care of Cadaver 229
- ☐ Dissection Safety Measures 230

Index 243

COMPETENCY TABLE

Number	The student should be able to	Core (Y/N)	Chapter No.	Page No.
AN1.1	Demonstrate normal anatomical position, various planes, relation, comparison, laterality and movement in our body	Y	1	5
AN1.2	Describe composition of bone and bone marrow	Y	4	59, 61
AN2.1	Describe parts, blood and nerve supply of a long bone	Y	4	55, 60
AN2.2	Enumerate laws of ossification	N	4	69
AN2.3	Enumerate special features of a sesamoid bone	N	4	65
AN2.4	Describe various types of cartilage with its structure and distribution in body	Y	4	53
AN2.5	Describe various joints with subtypes and examples	Y	6	100
AN2.6	Explain the concept of nerve supply of joints and Hilton's law	Y	6	120
AN3.1	Classify muscle tissue according to structure and action	Y	5	77
AN3.2	Enumerate parts of skeletal muscle and differentiate between tendons and aponeuroses with examples	Y	5	78
AN3.3	Explain shunt and spurt muscles	N	5	93
AN4.1	Describe different types of skin and dermatomes in body	N	3	34, 38
			9	170
AN4.2	Describe structure and function of skin with its appendages	Y	3	34
AN4.3	Describe superficial fascia along with fat distribution in body	Y	3	43
AN4.4	Describe modifications of deep fascia with its functions	Y	3	43
AN4.5	Explain principles of skin incisions	N	3	34
			12	219
AN5.1	Differentiate between blood vascular and lymphatic system	Y	7	125
AN5.2	Differentiate between pulmonary and systemic circulation	Y	7	130
AN5.3	List general differences between arteries and veins	Y	7	128
AN5.4	Explain functional difference between elastic, muscular arteries and arterioles	Y	7	131
AN5.5	Describe portal system giving examples	Y	7	134
AN5.6	Describe the concept of anastomoses and collateral circulation with significance of end-arteries	Y	7	135, 137
AN5.7	Explain function of meta-arterioles, precapillary sphincters, arterio-venous anastomoses	N	7	136
AN5.8	Define thrombosis, infarction and aneurysm	N	7	139
AN6.1	List the components and functions of the lymphatic system	N	8	146
AN6.2	Describe structure of lymph capillaries and mechanism of lymph circulation	N	8	146
AN6.3	Explain the concept of lymphoedema and spread of tumors via lymphatics and venous system	N	8	153
AN7.1	Describe general plan of nervous system with components of central, peripheral and autonomic nervous systems	Y	9	157
AN7.2	List components of nervous tissue and their functions	Y	9	158
AN7.3	Describe parts of a neuron and classify them based on number of neurites, size and function	Y	9	158

Competency Table

Number	The student should be able to	Core (Y/N)	Chapter No.	Page No.
AN7.4	Describe structure of a typical spinal nerve	Y	9	169
AN7.5	Describe principles of sensory and motor innervation of muscles	N	5	87
			9	180
AN7.6	Describe concept of loss of innervation of a muscle with its applied anatomy	Y	5	87
			9	180
AN7.7	Describe various type of synapse	N	9	164
AN7.8	Describe differences between sympathetic and spinal ganglia	N	9	165
AN13.5	Identify the bones and joints of upper limb seen in anteroposterior and lateral view radiographs of shoulder region, arm, elbow, forearm and hand	Y	11	206
AN13.6	Identify and demonstrate important bony landmarks of upper limb: Jugular notch, sternal angle, acromial angle, spine of the scapula, vertebral level of the medial end, Inferior angle of the scapula	Y	12	219
AN13.7	Identify and demonstrate surface projection of: Cephalic and basilic vein, Palpation of Brachial artery, Radial artery, Testing of muscles: Trapezius, pectoralis major, serratus anterior, latissimus dorsi, deltoid, biceps brachii, Brachioradialis	Y	12	219
AN20.6	Identify the bones and joints of lower limb seen in anteroposterior and lateral view radiographs of various regions of lower limb	Y	11	206
AN20.7	Identify and demonstrate important bony landmarks of lower limb: Vertebral levels of highest point of iliac crest, posterior superior iliac spines, iliac tubercle, pubic tubercle, ischial tuberosity, adductor tubercle, Tibial tuberosity, head of fibula, Medial and lateral malleoli, Condyles of femur and tibia, sustentaculum tali, tuberosity of fifth metatarsal, tuberosity of the navicular	Y	12	219
AN20.8	Identify and demonstrate palpation of femoral, popliteal, post tibial, anti-tibial and dorsalis pedis blood vessels in a simulated environment	Y	12	219
AN20.9	Identify and demonstrate: Palpation of vessels (femoral, popliteal, dorsalis pedis, post-tibial), Mid-inguinal point, Surface projection of: femoral nerve, Saphenous opening, Sciatic, tibial, common peroneal and deep peroneal nerve, Great and small saphenous veins	Y	12	219
AN43.7	Identify the anatomical structures in 1) Plain X-ray of skull, 2) AP view and lateral view, 3) Plain X-ray cervical spine-AP and lateral view, 4) Plain X-ray of paranasal sinuses	Y	11	206
AN54.1	Describe and identify features of plain X-ray abdomen	Y	11	206
AN54.2	Describe and identify the special radiographs of abdominopelvic region (contrast X-ray, Barium swallow, Barium meal, Barium enema, Cholecystography, Intravenous pyelography and Hysterosalpingography)	Y	11	206
AN54.3	Describe role of ERCP, CT abdomen, MRI, Arteriography in radiodiagnosis of abdomen	N	11	206
AN55.1	Demonstrate the surface marking of; Regions and planes of abdomen, Superficial inguinal ring, Deep inguinal ring, McBurney's point, Renal angle and Murphy's point	Y	12	219

Competency Table

Number	The student should be able to	Core (Y/N)	Chapter No.	Page No.
AN55.2	Demonstrate the surface projections of: Stomach, Liver, Fundus of gallbladder, Spleen, Duodenum, Pancreas, Ileocaecal junction, Kidneys and Root of mesentery	Y	12	219
AN65.1	Identify epithelium under the microscope and describe the various types that correlate to its function	Y	2	20
AN66.1	Describe and identify various types of connective tissue with functional correlation	Y	2	26
AN72.1	Identify the skin and its appendages under the microscope and correlate the structure and function	Y	3	34
AN 82.1	Demonstrate respect and follow the correct procedure when handling cadavers and other biologic tissue	Y	13	228

ANATOMICAL TERMS—HISTORICAL DERIVATION AND MEANING

There are approximately 170,000 medical terms that include names of medicines, medical investigations, medical conditions, medical examination, surgical procedures, body parts, body functions, etc. There are about 8000 frequently used terms.

Learning anatomy is not memorizing the facts. It has to be learnt by understanding the underlying development, evolution, function, and its clinical application. The complexities in learning can be reduced if one understands the meaning of the terms used in describing the various parts, their actions, shapes and relations.

Most of the anatomical terms we use have their roots from Latin or Greek. Memorization without understanding the meaning can lead to stress for the new learners. To facilitate the students certain of the terms are given in alphabetical order.

Anatomical term and its origin L–Latin G–Greek Fr–French	Meaning	Example
Abdomen (L)	*Abdere = to hide*, Belly	Part of trunk between thorax and perineum
Abducent nerve (L)	*Ab = from; ducere = lead (movement)*	6th cranial nerve that moves a muscle of eyeball (lateral rectus) that moves it away from midline
Abductor (L)	*Ab = from; ducere = lead (movement)*	A muscle that moves the part of body/limb away from midline
Aberrant (L)	*Ab = from* *Errare = to wander* *Deviation from normal*	Aberrant epiphysis
Accessory (L)	*Accedere = to be added to*	Accessory nerve: The 11th cranial nerve, functionally added to the vagus nerve (10th cranial nerve)
Acetabulum	*Acetum = vinegar* *-bulum—suffix signifying instrument*	Acetabulum of hip bone cup-shaped part of hip bone
Acromion (G)	*Akron = tip or extremity* *omos = shoulder*	Acromion process of scapula
Afferent (L)	Bringing towards	Afferent nerves bring information from the peripheral parts of the body to the central nervous system
Ala (L)	*Wing*	Ala of sacrum
Alba (L)	*Albicare = white*	Linea alba: The white linear fibrous structure that runs in the midline of the abdomen
Allantois (G)	*Allas = a sausage* *Edios = resemblance*	Foetal membrane

Contd…

Anatomical Terms—Historical Derivation and Meaning

Contd...

Anatomical term and its origin L–Latin G–Greek Fr–French	Meaning	Example
Alveolus (L)	Alveus—hollowed out structure	Alveoli of lung
Amygdala (G)	Amygdale = almond	A structure in the temporal lobe of brain
Angio (G)	Angeion = a vessel	Angiography, angioplasty
Artery (G)	Aer = air, terein = to keep	Various arteries of the body
Articulation (L)	Articulus = joint, -atio, a suffix originally denoting action	Various joints between bones
Arytenoid (G)	Arytaina = a pitcher, eidos = resemblance	Arytenoid cartilage of larynx
Atavistic (L)	Atavus = 'forefather' + suffix -istic Reversion to something ancestral	Atavistic epiphysis
Atlas (G)	Atlas—the mythological Titan who supported the world on his shoulders	First cervical vertebra, that supports the head
Atrium (L)	Atrium = a hall, or an entrance	Right and left atria of heart
Auditory (L)	Audire = to hear	Auditory tube
Autonomic (G)	Autos = self, nomos = law	Autonomic nervous system which is self-controlled
Autopsy (G)	Autos = self, opsi = seen observations on the patient made by the physician himself	A postmortem examination to find out the cause of death
Axilla (L)	Axilla = armpit	A region in the upper limb
Axis (L)	Axis = axle or pivot	Second cervical vertebra
Azygos (G)	a = not, zygos = a yoke (paired) Any unpaired or unyoked structure	Azygos vein or azygos lobe of lung
Basilic (G)	Basileus, Basilikē = king, royal	Basilic vein—inner vein of forearm
Bipennate (L)	Bis = two, pinna = feather	Bipennate muscle
Brachial (L)	Belonging to arm	Brachialis—a muscle in the arm
Branchia (G)	Gills	Branchial arches
Bregma (G)	Bregma = front of the head	Junction of sagittal and coronal sutures of skull
Bronchus (G)	Bronchos = windpipe	Respiratory passage
Buccinator (L)	Buccinare = 'blow a trumpet'	A muscle in the cheek
Bulla (L)	Bubble	Ethmoid bulla—a convex bulge beneath the concha of middle meatus of nose
Bunion (Fr)	Buignon, from buigne = 'bump on the head'	A bony bump at the base of great toe. Also called hallux valgus
Bursa (L)	Bursa = a purse Any closed sac	Synovial bursa
Cadaver (L)	Cadere = to fall dead body	Cadaveric donor
Calcaneus (L)	Calcaneus = relating to the heel	A bone of the foot

Contd...

Anatomical Terms—Historical Derivation and Meaning

Contd...

Anatomical term and its origin L–Latin G–Greek Fr–French	Meaning	Example
Calcar (L)	Spur	Calcarine fissure on the medial surface of brain
Calyx (G)	*Kalyx* = husk or cup	Major and minor calyces of kidney—recesses in the pelvis of kidney.
Cancellous (L)	*Cancelli* = latticework	Cancellous bone
Canthus (G)	*Kanthos* = corner of the eye	Medial/lateral canthus
Capillary (L)	Capillaries = pertaining to hair	Capillaries—fine branching blood vessels that form a network between arterioles and venules
Capitulum (L)	*Caput* = head	Capitulum of humerus Caput succedaneum
Carina (L)	Keel	Carina of trachea—a point where the trachea divides into the two bronchi
Carotid (G)	*Karoun* = stupefy, drowsiness	Carotid arteries
Carpus (G)	*Karpos* = wrist	Carpal bones
Cauda (L)	*Cauda* = a tail, equina or "horse's tail"—spinal cord	Cauda equina
Cauda, caudal (L)	Tail	Cauda equina
Caudate (L)	*Caudatus* = tail	Caudate nucleus in brain
Cerumen (L)	Wax	Ceruminous glands
Cervix (L)	*Cervix* = neck	Cervix of uterus
Chiasma (G)	*Chiasma* = two crossing lines	Optic chiasma
Chondral (L)	*Chondros* = cartilage	Endochondral ossification
Choroid (G)	*Chorion* = skin, *eidos* = resemblance	Layer of eyeball
Cingulum (L)	Belt, gird	Curved bundle of nerve fibers in each hemisphere of the brain
Circumflex (L)	*Circum* = around + *flexere* = to bend	Circumflex humeral arteries, circumflex nerve
Cistern (L)	*Cisterna* = a reservoir or cistern	Subarachnoid cistern
Claustrum (L)	Lock, enclosed place	A layer of gray matter in cerebrum
Clavicle (L)	*Clavis* = a key. Resemblance to the shape	Collar bone
Clivus (L)	Slope	A slopping bony part at the skull base
Coccyx (G)	*Kokkux* = 'cuckoo' Resemblance to cuckoo's bill	Small triangular bone at the end of sacrum, formed of fused vestigial vertebrae
Cochlea (G)	Snail	A part of inner ear
Comitans (plural—comitantes) (L)	*Comitari* = to accompany	Venae comitantes
Commissure (L)	*Commissura* (*cum* + *mittere*) = connection	Commissures of brain

Contd...

Anatomical Terms—Historical Derivation and Meaning

Contd…

Anatomical term and its origin L–Latin G–Greek Fr–French	Meaning	Example
Condyle (G)	*Kondulos* = 'knuckle' Rounded protuberances at the ends of bones	Condyles of tibia/femur
Conjunctiva (L)	Join together	The white of the eye
Conus (L)	Cone	Conus medullaris
Coracoid (G)	*Korax* = Raven (Crow) *Korakoeidēs* = 'raven-like' Resemblance to Raven's beak	Coracoid process of scapula
Corona (L)	Crown	Coronal suture
Corpus (plural—corpora) (L)	Body	Corpus callosum Corpora cavernosa Corpus spongiosum
Corrugator (L)	*Corrugare* = to wrinkle very much	Corrugator supercilia muscle of the eye Corrugator cutis ani—a thin involuntary muscle around the anus
Costal (L)	*Costa* = rib	Costal cartilage Costal chondritis—inflammation of costal cartilage
Cranium (G), cranial	*Kranion* = skull, head	Cranial end
Cremaster (G)	*Krema* = hang	Cremaster muscle of spermatic cord
Cribriform (L)	*Cribrum* = a sieve	Cribriform plate of ethmoid bone Cribriform fascia in thigh
Cricoid (G)	*Krikos* = ring + *eidos* = form, likeness	Cricoid cartilage of larynx
Crista (L)	*Crista* = crest	Crista terminalis
Crista galli (L)	*Crista* = crest + *gallus* = cock, cock's comb appearance, crest of the rooster	Crista galli—part of ethmoid bone
Cruciate (L)	*Crux* = cross	Cruciate anastomosis Cruciate ligaments
Crypt (G)	Hidden, deep invagination	Tonsillar crypt
Cuboid (G)	*Kuboeides* = cube-shaped	Cuboid bone of tarsus
Cuneiform (L)	*Cuneus* = wedge, + *forma* = shape, likeness	Cuneiform bone of tarsus
Cyst (G)	*Kystis* = bag, bladder, pouch	Cholecystitis—inflammation of gallbladder
Dacryon (G)	*Dacryon* = tear	Dacryocystitis—inflammation of tear sac
Dartos (G)	*Dartos* = skinned	Dartos muscle of scrotum
Decidua, deciduous (L)	*Deciduus* (de + cado) = falling off	Deciduous teeth
Decussate, decussation (L)	*Decussation* = intersection of two lines	Pyramidal decussation
Deltoid (G)	*Delta* = letter in Greek alphabet, triangular-shaped	Deltoid muscle

Contd…

Anatomical Terms—Historical Derivation and Meaning

Contd…

Anatomical term and its origin L–Latin G–Greek Fr–French	Meaning	Example
Demilune (Fr)	Half-moon	Serous demilunes
Dendrite (G)	*Dendros* = tree	Dendrites—short processes of neuron
Dens (L)	Tooth	Dens of the axis vertebra
Dentate (L)	Tooth like or serrated edge	Dentate gyrus
Dentine (L)	Dense bony tissue of tooth	Tooth
Dermis (G)	*Derma* = skin	Dermatology
Detrusor (L)	*Detrudere* = to push down	Detrusor muscle of urinary bladder
Diaphragm (G)	*Dia* = through + *phragma* = wall	Diaphragm—dome shaped muscular partition separating thoracic and abdominal cavities
Diaphysis (G)	*Dia* = between + *physis* = growth	Diaphysis of long bone
Diarthrosis (G)	*Dia* = through + *arthroun* = to fasten by a joint	Joint that permits free movement
Digastric (G)	*Dis* = double + *gaster* = belly	Digastric muscle
Diploe, diploid, diplopia (G)	*Diploë* = fold *Diploos* = two-fold *Diploos* = double + *opsis* + vision	Diploe of skull—two tables of compact bone with intervening spongy bone. Diploid number of chromosomes
Diverticulum (L)	*Devertere* = to turn aside	An abnormal pouch opening from a hollow organ like intestine or bladder like Meckel's diverticulum
Duct (L)	To lead or draw	Parotid duct
Duodenum (L)	*Duodeni* = twelve (twelve Finger breadths)	Part of small intestine
Ectoderm (G)	Ecto = outside + derma = skin	A germ layer
Ectopia (G)	*Ektopos* = distant	Ectopia vesicae
Efferent (L)	Going away	Efferent nerves send information from the central nervous system to the peripheral structures for producing the desired effects
Effusion (L)	*Effundere* = 'pour out'	Effusion in knee
Emboliformis (G)	*Embolus* = wedge + *forma* = shape	Emboliform nucleus of cerebellum
Emissary (L)	E = out + *mittere* = to send escape channels	Emissary veins connect intracranial dural venous sinuses with extracranial veins
Endo (prefix) (G)	Within	Endoneurium, endoderm, endometrium
Ependyma (G)	*Ependuein* = 'put on over'	Ependymal covering of neural tube
Epicondyle (G)	Upon a knob	Epicondyles of femur
Epidermis (G)	Upon dermis	Epidermis in relation to skin
Epididymis (G)	Upon testis	Epididymis is a male reproductive organ
Epigastrium (G)	Upon belly	Over the region of stomach

Contd…

Anatomical Terms—Historical Derivation and Meaning

Contd...

Anatomical term and its origin L–Latin G–Greek Fr–French	Meaning	Example
Epiglottis (G)	Upon tongue	Epiglottis is a cartilage of larynx
Epiphysis (G)	*epi* = 'upon, in addition' + *phusis* = 'growth'	Epiphyseal plate of cartilage
Epithelium (G)	Upon nipple	Epithelial tissue
Erector (L)	To stand up	Erector spinae muscle
Ethmoid (G)	Sieve-like	Ethmoid bone
Falciform (L)	Sickle shape	Falciform ligament
Fasciculus (L)	A passage	Fasciculus gracilis
Femur (L)	Thigh	Femur is a thigh bone
Fenestra (L)	Window	Fenestra vestibuli
Fetus (L)	Offspring	Fetal medicine
Fibula (L)	Needle of brooch	A bone of the leg
Fimbria (L)	A fringe or border	Fimbria of uterine tube
Fissure (L)	A cleft	Fissures of cerebellum
Fistula (L)	A pipe	Anal fistula
Flocculus (L)	A tuft of wool	Flocculonodular lobe of cerebellum
Folium (L)	Leaf	Cerebellar folia
Fontanelle (L)	Small fountain	Fontanelle of skull
Foramen (L)	Hole	Foramina of skull
Fornix (L)	Arch	Fornices of cerebrum
Fossa (L)	Ditch	Cranial fossa
Fovea (L)	*Fovea* = small pit	Fovea centralis
Frenulum (L)	*Fraenum* = a little bridge	Frenulum of tongue
Frontal (L)	*Frons, frontis* = forehead, brow	Frontalis muscles, frontal bone
Fundus (L)	*Fundus* = bottom	Fundus of stomach, fundus of gallbladder, fundus of uterus
Funiculus (L)	Rope	Funiculus is a bundle of nerve fibers enclosed in connective tissue sheath and forming tracts of spinal cord
Fusiform (L)	Spindle shaped	Fusiform shaped muscle
Genu (L)	*Genu* = knee	Genu valgus (knock knee), genu varum (bowing at the knee)
Glottis (G)	Tongue	Part of larynx between vocal cords
Glenoid (G)	*Glene* = socket + *eidos* = form, likeness	Glenoid cavity of scapula
Gracilis (L)	*Gracilis* = thin	Gracilis muscle
Glomerulus (L)	*Glomus* = a ball	Tuft of capillaries in relation to Bowman's capsule of nephron
Hepatic (L)	*Hepar* = liver	Hepatitis (inflammation of liver)

Contd...

Contd...

Anatomical term and its origin L–Latin G–Greek Fr–French	Meaning	Example
Hernia (L)	Protrusion	Inguinal hernia
Hydrocele (G)	*Hydor* = water + *koilos* = hollow	Fluid-filled sac around testis
Hymen (G)	*Hymen* = membrane	Membrane covering the vaginal orifice partially
Ileum (L)	Final part of small intestine	Ileal arteries
Ilium (L)	Flank	Hip bone
Indusium (L)	A tunic	Indusium griseum—a gray tunic covering the corpus callosum of brain
Inguinal (L)	Groin	Inguinal canal, inguinal lymph nodes
Inion (G)	Nape of neck	Projecting part of occipital bone
Innominate (L)	*In* = 'not' + *nominatus* = 'named' Un named	Innominate bone—hip bone
Isthmus	Narrow	Isthmus of fallopian tube
Jejunum (L)	Empty or fasting	Part of small intestine
Joint (L)	To join	Hip joint, knee joint
Jugular (L)	Throat	Jugular vein
Latissimus (L)	Broadest	Latissimus dorsi—broadest muscle of the back
Lumbricals (L)	A worm (muscle)	Lumbrical muscles
Limbus (L)	Border	Limbus fossa ovalis
Limen (L)	Threshold	Limen insula
Lingual (L)	*Lingua* = tongue	Lingual tonsil
Lingula (L)	Small tongue	Lingula of cerebellum
Locus (L)	Place	Locus ceruleus
Lunate (L)	*Luna* = moon	Lunate bone of carpus
Luteum (L)	*Luteus* = yellow	Corpus luteum—yellow body
Macula (L)	*Macula* = spot	Macular degeneration
Malleus (L)	Hammer	Malleus—an ear ossicle
Mammary (L)	*Mamma* = breast	Mammary gland
Mammillary (L)	Mammillaris (*mamma*, -*ae*), little breast	Mammillary bodies
Mandible (L)	*Mando* = I chew	Mandible—bone of the chin
Manubrium (L)	Handle or hilt of a weapon	Manubrium of sternum
Meniscus (L)	*Menis* = crescent, half-moon	Menisci of knee joint
Merocrine (G)	*Meros* = portion + *krinein* = to separate	Merocrine gland
Mesentery (G)	*Mesos* = midway between + *enteron* = gut	Fold of peritoneum in relation with small intestine
Mesocolon (G)	*Mesos* = middle + *kolon* = great gut	Fold of peritoneum in relation with colon

Contd...

Contd...

Anatomical term and its origin L–Latin G–Greek Fr–French	Meaning	Example
Mesosalpinx (G)	Mesos = middle + salpinx = tube	Fold of peritoneum in relation with uterine tube
Metaphysis (G)	Meta = after + physis = growth	Metaphysis of a long bone
Neurenteric (G)	Neuron = nerve + enteron = gut	Neurenteric canal
Neurilemma (L)	Neuron = nerve + lemma = husk, sheath	Covering nerve
Obturator (L)	A stopper of	Obturator nerve, obturator foramen
Occiput (L)	Back of head	Occipital bone
Oculomotor (L)	Oculus = eye + moto = mover	Oculomotor nerve
Odontoid (G)	Odous = tooth + eidos = shape, likeness	Odontoid process of axis vertebra
Olecranon (G)	Point of elbow	Olecranon process of
Oligo (G)	Few (G)	Oligodendrocyte
Operculum (L)	Lid/cover	Opercula of insula in brain
Otic (G)	Ear	Otitis (inflammation of ear)
Pachymeninx (G)	Thick covering	Dura mater covering the brain
Pallium (L)	Clock or mantle	Neopallium—cerebral cortex
Pampiniform (L)	Tendril	Pampiniform plexus of veins
Panniculus (L)	A piece of cloth, a layer of membrane	Panniculus carnosus
Perforator (L)	To bore through	Perforating veins
Portal (L)	Porta = gate	Portal vein enters the gate of the liver
Perichondrium (L and G)	Peri = 'around' + khondros = 'cartilage'	Covering of cartilage
Perineum (G)	Swim around penis	It is an area between anus and scrotum in males and between anus and vulva in females
Periosteum (G)	Peri = 'around' + osteon = 'bone'	Outer covering of bone
Phallus (G)	Phallos = penis	Male copulatory organ
Piriform (L)	Pear shaped	Piriform fossa in relation to larynx Piriformis muscle
Pisiform (L)	Pisum = a pea + forma = form	Pisiform bone—carpal bone
Platysma (G)	Flat	Subcutaneous muscle in the neck
Pons (L)	Pons = a bridge	Part of brainstem
Porta (L)	porta = gate	Porta hepatis
Proctodeum (G)	Proktos = anus + hodaios = pertaining to a way	Proctoscopy
Profundus (L)	Pro = "before" + fundus = "the bottom"	Profunda femoris muscle—deep muscle
Promontory (L)	Prominence	Sacral promontory
Pronation (L)	Pronus = leaning forwards	Pronator teres muscle

Contd...

Anatomical Terms—Historical Derivation and Meaning

Contd...

Anatomical term and its origin L–Latin G–Greek Fr–French	Meaning	Example
Prostate (G)	Pro = before, the root sta = stand, and the suffix -tes. In ancient Greece prostate means a guard or protector—one who stood before	The prostate gland is an accessory gland of male reproductive system and it stands in front of the urinary bladder
Quadratus (L)	Quadratus = a square in shape	Quadratus muscle
Quadriceps (L)	Quattuor = four + caput = head	Quadriceps muscle
Retroversion (L)	Retro = backward + versio = turning	Turning backward
Rima (L)	Rima = cleft	Rima glottides
Risorius (L)	Risus = laughter	Muscle of face
Rotator (L)	Rotare = to whirl about	Rotator cuff of shoulder
Rugae (L)	Ruga = wrinkle	Gastric rugae
Saphenous (L)	Saphenes = clear or manifest	Saphenous vein
Sartorius (L)	Sartor = a tailor	Muscle: It is used in squatting position by old fashioned tailors, with the legs crossed
Scapula (L)	Scapula = shoulder blade. In ancient times it was used in the plural to mean "the back"	A bone at the back of shoulder
Sella turcica (L)	Sella = saddle and turcica = Turkish	Sella turcica of sphenoid bone—saddle-shaped prominence of the sphenoid bone
Sigmoid (G)	Sigma = the Greek letter S + eidos = resemblance. In earlier times the letter sigma was written as a single curve (now the letter C)	Sigmoid colon—curved part of large intestine Sigmoid venous sinus—in skull
Sesamoid (L)	Sesamen = sesame plant, or seed + eidos = shape, likeness	Sesamoid bone—patella
Sphenoid (G)	Sphen = wedge, and eidos = resemblance	Sphenoid bone
Styloid (G)	Stylos = pillar + eidos = resemblance	Styloid process of temporal bone
Subcutaneous (L)	Adjacent to skin	Subcutaneous fat
Sural (L)	Calf	Sural nerve
Synarthrosis (G)	Sun=together+ arthrosis = joining	Immovable, fixed joints
Syndesmosis (G)	Sundesmos = binding, fastening	Tibiofibular syndesmosis
Taenia, Tenia (L)	Taenia = band, ribbon	Taenia coli
Talipes (L)	Talipes = club foot; from talus = ankle, and pes = foot	Talipes equinovarus of foot
Tarsus (G)	Tarsos = sole of the foot	Tarsal bones
Tegmen, Tegmentum (L)	Tegmen = covering	Tegmen tympani, tegmentum of midbrain
Tendon (L)	Tendere = to stretch	Biceps tendon

Contd...

Contd...

Anatomical term and its origin L–Latin G–Greek Fr–French	Meaning	Example
Tentorium (L)	*Tentorium* = tent	Tentorium cerebelli
Teres (L)	*Tero* = I grind, rub	Teres major muscle
Terminalis (L)	*Terminare* = to limit	Laminal terminalis
Theca (L)	*Theca* = envelope, sheath	Theca interna, theca externa in relation with ovarian follicle
Thyroid (G)	*Thyreos* = a shield+ *eidos* = resemblance	Thyroid gland
Trachea (G)	*Tracheia* = windpipe	Airway
Triceps (L)	*Tres* = three + *caput* = head	A muscle of arm with three heads
Trigeminus (L)	*Trigeminus* = born three together	Trigeminal nerve is the 5th cranial nerve
Triquetrum (L)	*Triquetrus* = three-cornered, triangular.	Bone of the hand
Trochanter (G)	*Trochanter* = a runner; derived from *trochos* = a wheel	A process below the neck of femur
Trochlea (L)	*Trochlea* = pulley	Trochlea of humerus Trochlear nerve—4th cranial nerve that supplies the muscle that traverses through a pulley
Tuberosity (L)	*Tuber* = knob or localized collection + *osity* = condition	Tuberosity of tibia
Tunica (L)	Undergarment	Tunics of eye, blood vessel
Tympanic (L)	*Tympanum* = drum	Tympanic membrane
Umbilicus (L)	Navel	Umbilical hernia
Uncus (L)	*Uncus* = a hook	A structure in brain
Uterus (L)	*Uterus* = womb	Female reproductive organ
Uvea, Uvula (L)	*Uva* = grape	Uveal tract Uvula
Vagina (L)	*Vagina* = sheath	A muscular tube extending from the external genitalia to the cervix of the uterus
Vagus (L)	*Vagus* = wandering	Vagus nerve—the 10th cranial nerve
Vallate (L)	*Vallum* = rampart, walled.	Circumvallate papillae
Vallecula (L)	*Vallus* = fossa	Vallecula
Vas (L)	Vessel	Blood vessels/lymph vessels Vas deferens—male reproductive tube
Vasa vasorum (L)	Vessels of the vessels	Seen in the walls of aorta and inferior vena cava
Vermiform	*vermis* = worm, *forma* = form	Vermiform appendix
Vitelline (L)	*Vitellus* = yolk of egg	Vitelline arteries

Contd...

Contd...

Anatomical term and its origin L–Latin G–Greek Fr–French	Meaning	Example
Vitreous (L)	*Vitreus* = glassy/transparent	Vitreous humor of the eye in vitro, meaning in a glass receptacle, in contrast to in vivo, meaning in the living body
Volar (L)	*Vola* = palm	Palm of hand
Xiphoid (G)	*Xiphos* = sword, *eidos* = resemblance	Xiphoid process of sternum
Zona, zonula (L)	*Zona* = belt, girdle.	Zona pellucida
Zygoma *(G)*	*Zygoma* = bolt or bar	Zygomatic bone—cheek bone
Zygote (G)	*Zugōtos* = 'yoked'	A fertilized ovum

RAPID REVIEW

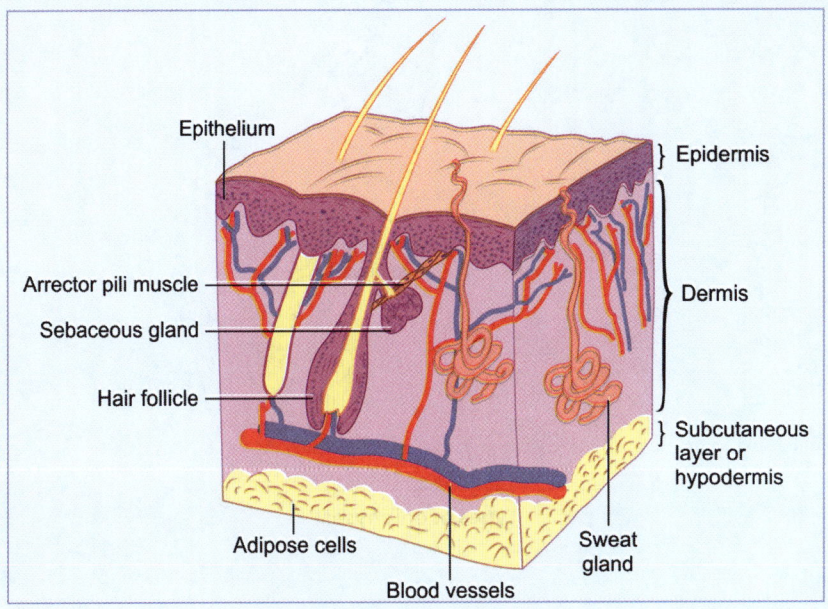

Skin and appendages

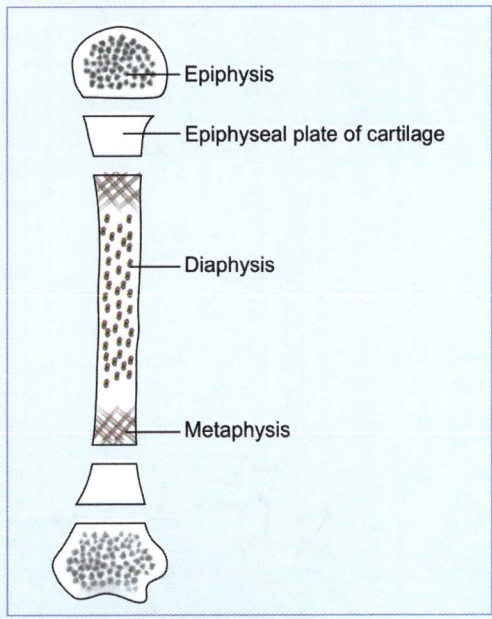

Parts of a long bone

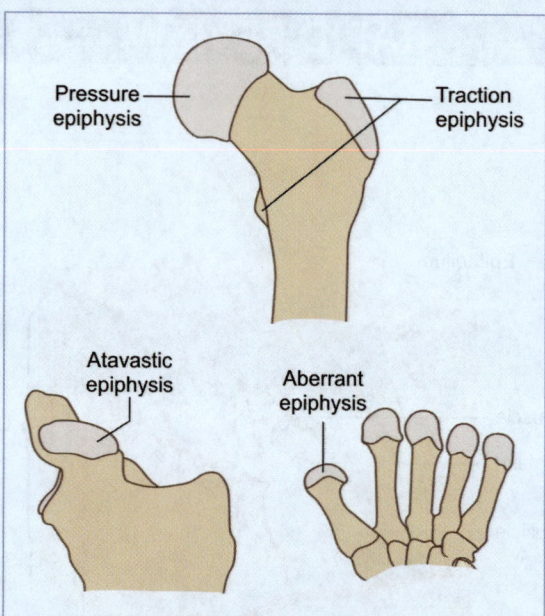

Types of epiphyses

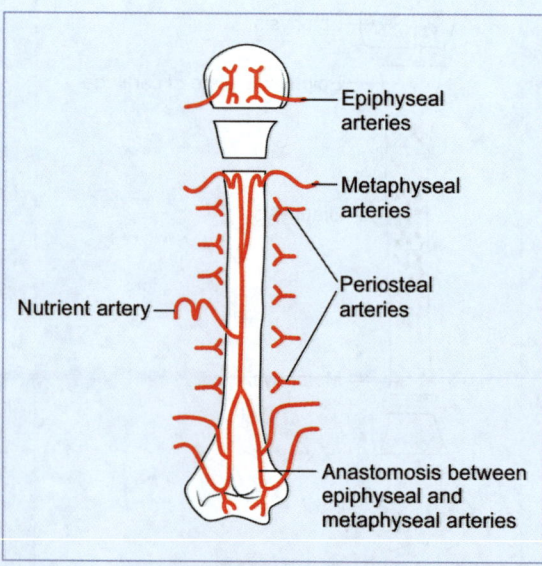

Blood supply of a long bone

Rapid Review

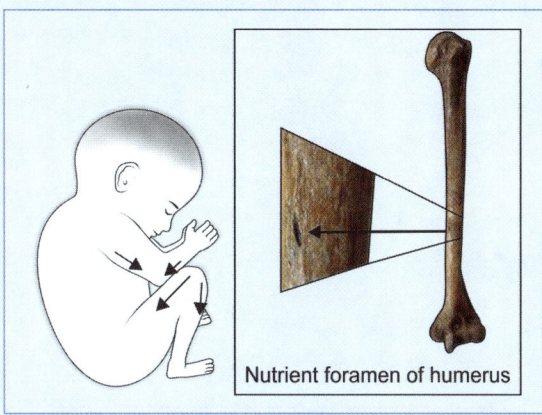

Direction of nutrient foramen in a long bone

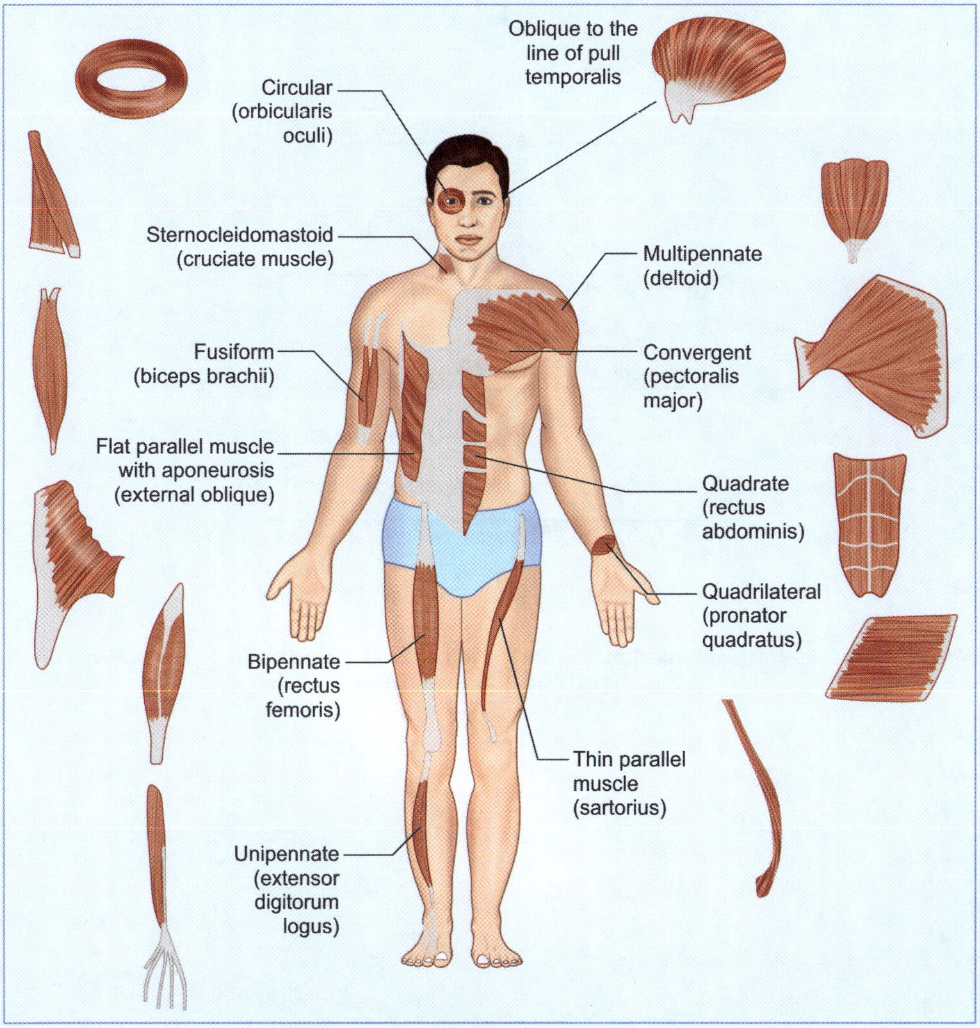

Classification of muscles according to direction of muscle fibers

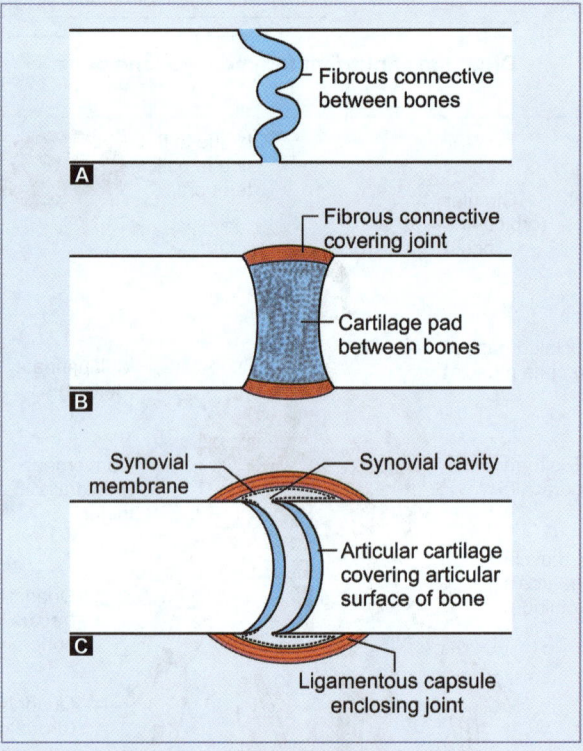

Classification of joints: (A) Synarthrosis—fibrous joint; (B) Amphiarthrosis—cartilaginous joint; (C) Diarthrosis—synovial joint

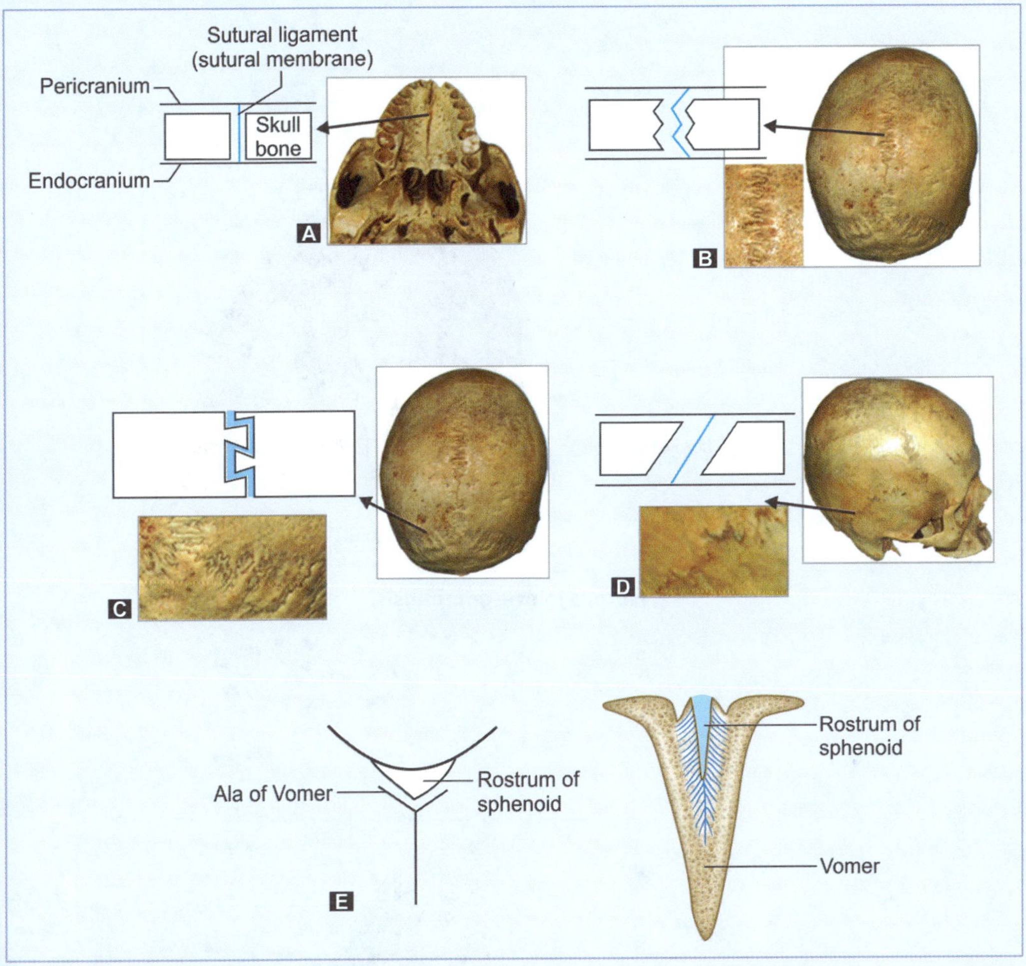

Rapid Review

Fibrous joint—sutures: (A) Plane suture (palatine process of two maxilla); (B) Serrate suture (sagittal suture); (C) Denticulate suture (lambdoid suture); (D) Squamous suture (between parietal and squamous part of temporal bone); (E) Schindylesis (wedge and groove suture)

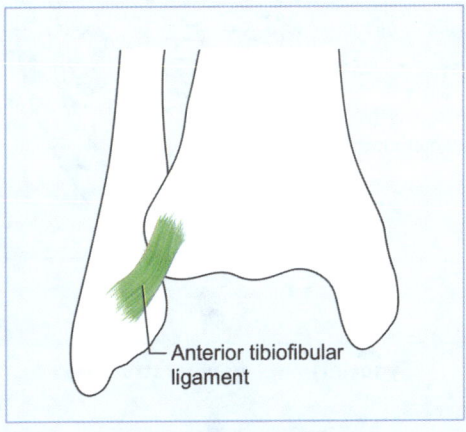

Fibrous joint—syndesmosis

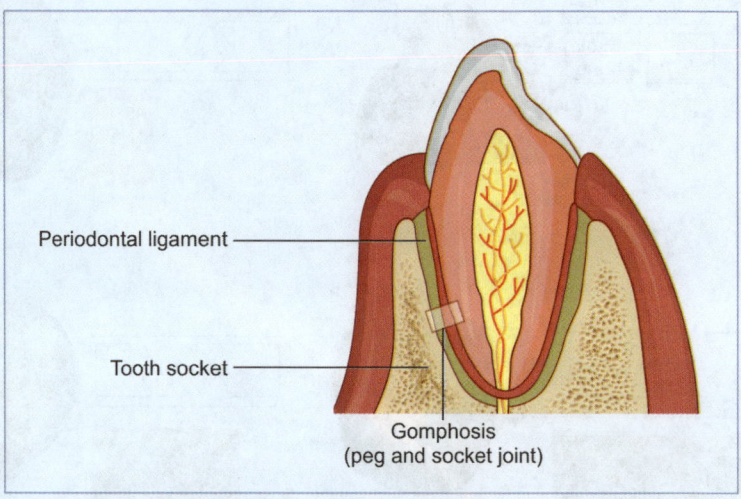

Fibrous joint—gomphosis.

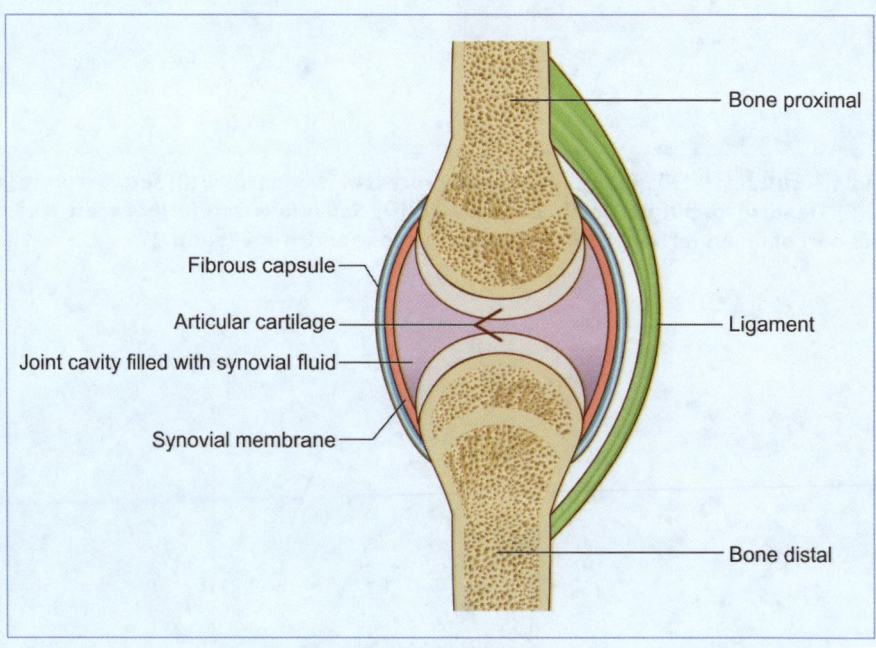

Synovial joint—general structure

Rapid Review

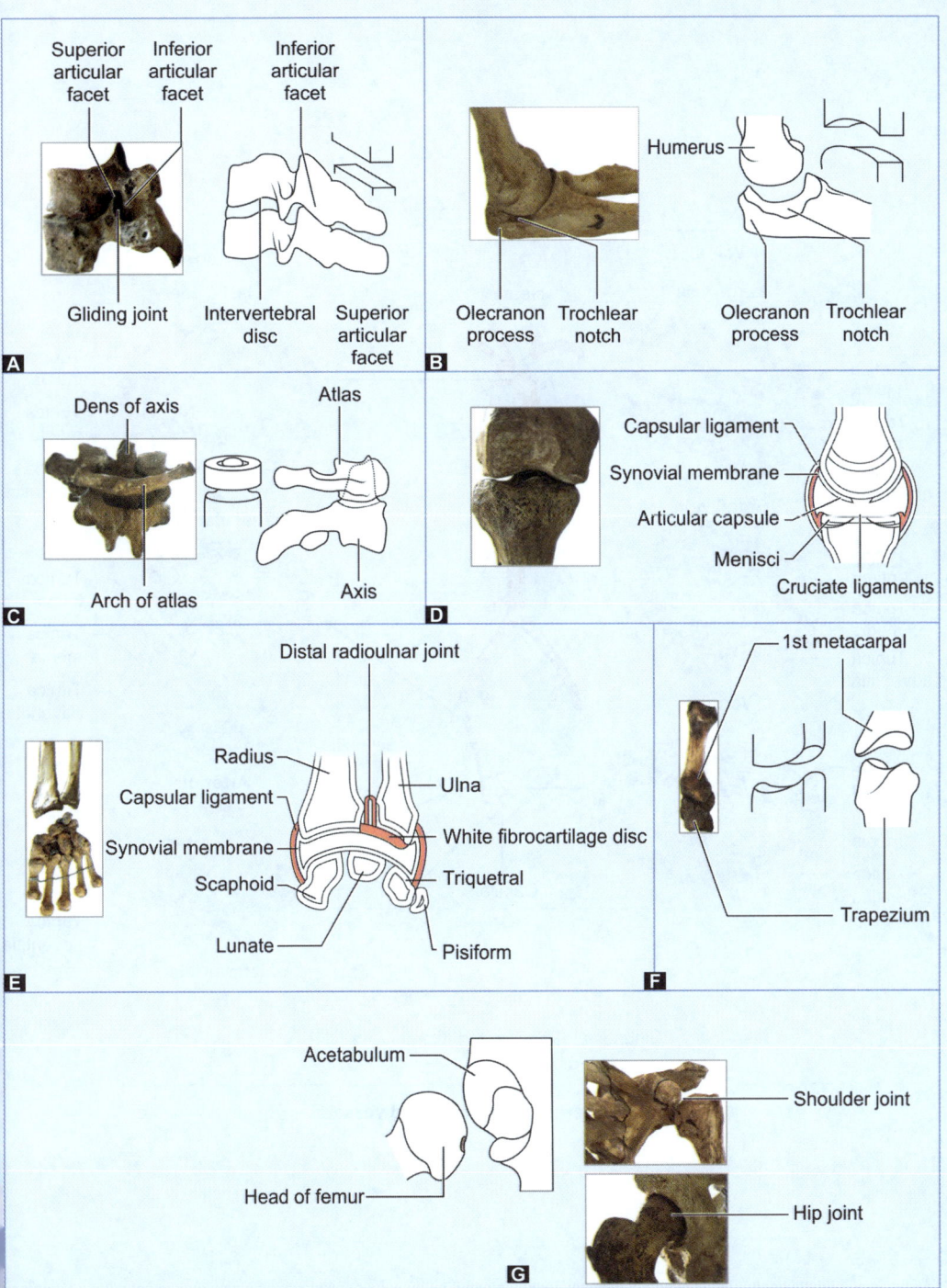

Synovial joint—subtypes. (A) Planner or gliding joint; (B) Hinge joint; (C) Pivot joint; (D) Condylar joint; (E) Ellipsoid joint; (F) Saddle joint; (G) Ball and socket joint

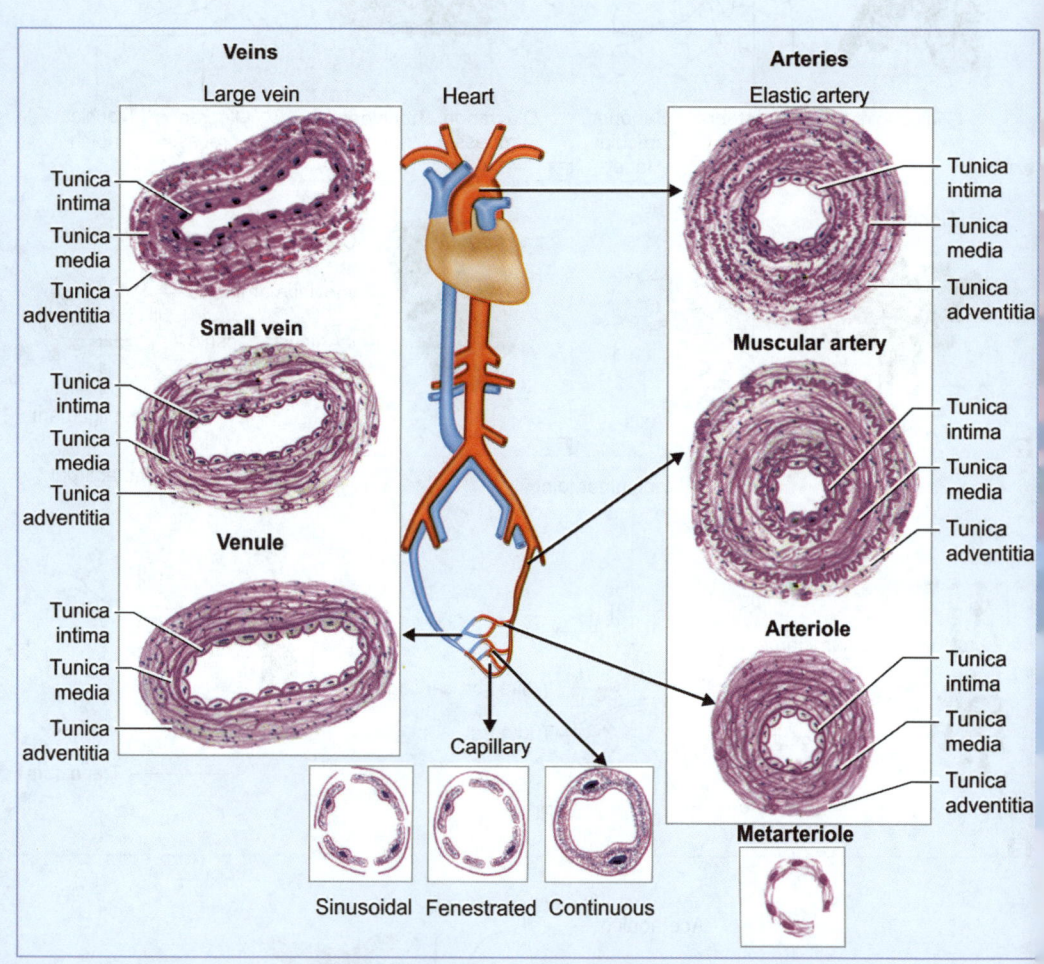

Different types of blood vessels

Rapid Review

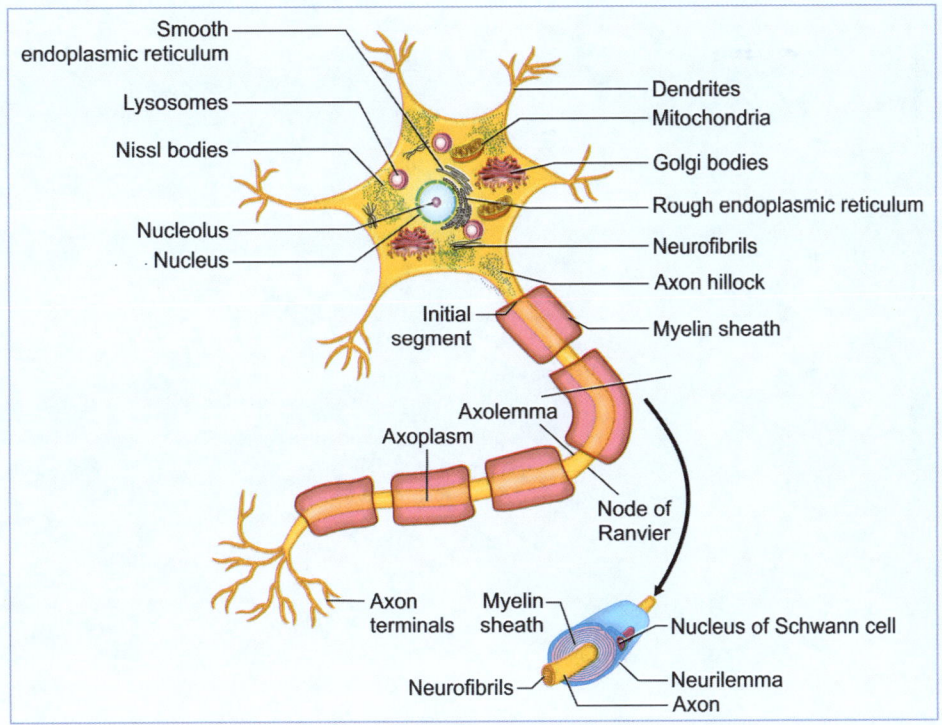

Structure of neuron

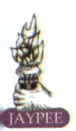

TOP DOC BANE WOHI
JISKA GUIDE HO SAHI

diginerve
A Jaypee Initiative

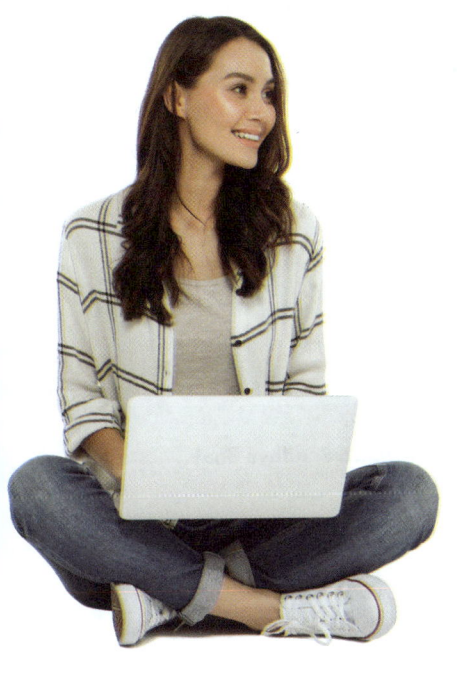

YOUR GUIDE AT EVERY STEP

Expert Knowledge Anytime, Anywhere

SCAN QR CODE
FOR MORE DETAILS

WHY CHOOSE US

Video Lectures

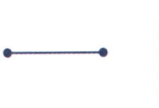

Self-Assessment Questions

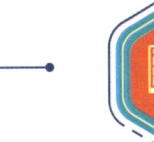

Top Faculty

New CBME Curriculum

Clinical Case Based Approach

NEET Preparation

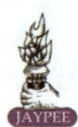 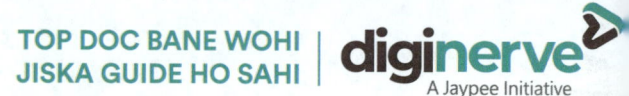

TOP DOC BANE WOHI JISKA GUIDE HO SAHI

Video Lectures | Notes | Self-Assessment
UnderGrad Courses Available

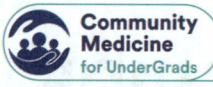 — by Dr. Bratati Banerjee

 Forensic Medicine & Toxicology for UnderGrads — by Dr. Gautam Biswas

 Medicine for UnderGrads — by Dr. Archith Boloor

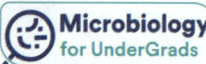 **Microbiology** for UnderGrads — by Dr. Apurba S Sastry, Dr. Sandhya Bhat & Dr. Deepashree R

 OBGYN for UnderGrads — by Dr. K. Srinivas

 Ophthalmology for UnderGrads — by Dr. Parul Ichhpujani & Dr. Talvir Sidhu

 Orthopaedics for UnderGrads — by Dr. Vivek Pandey

 Pathology for UnderGrads — by Prof. Harsh Mohan, Prof. Ramadas Nayak & Dr. Debasis Gochhait

 Pediatrics for UnderGrads — by Dr. Santosh Soans & Dr. Soundarya M

 Pharmacology for UnderGrads — by Dr. Sandeep Kaushal & Dr. Nirmal George

 Surgery for UnderGrads — by Dr. Sriram Bhat M (SRB)

*T&C Apply

Contact
+91 8800 418 418
marketing@diginerve.com

CHAPTER 1

Introduction to Anatomy

LEARNING OBJECTIVES

- ❖ Definition of anatomy
- ❖ Importance of anatomy
- ❖ Subdivisions of anatomy
- ❖ Approaches for learning anatomy
- ❖ Anatomical position
- ❖ Anatomical planes
- ❖ Anatomical terminology
- ❖ History of anatomy
- ❖ Clinical case with anatomical explanation

DEFINITION OF ANATOMY

Anatomy is the science that deals with structural (morphological) arrangement of various components of an organ, tissue or part of the body and its correlation with function. The word *morphology* is derived from Greek which means structure.

The word *anatomy* is derived from Greek "anatome" which means cutting up; ana = up, tome = cutting. Latin equivalent for anatomy is *dissection*. Dis = as under, secare = to cut. Cutting up of *cadaver* (dead body) is the method by which study of structure of living things is made possible.

Physiology is the study of functions of the body. Functions include digestion, respiration, circulation, reproduction, movement of lower limbs for walking and upper limbs for holding an object, etc. Structure and function are inseparable. Structural arrangement is based on function, and functional requirement decides the structural arrangement.

Biochemistry is the study of chemical processes involved in performing a function by the structure in a living organism.

STRUCTURE CONTRIBUTING TO FUNCTION

Structure plays an important role in function. For example, a building or a bridge is constructed keeping in mind its weight-bearing function (People, goods, etc.). Similarly, the structure of bones of skull and face differs from that of limb bones as their functions are different. The bones of skull and face are for lightening the head. The bones of limbs are for weight bearing.

EVOLUTIONARY REVOLUTIONS IN ANATOMY

From time immemorial, anatomy has been studied by methodically dissecting and observing the *cadavers* (dead bodies) that are preserved by injecting chemicals. The anatomical dissections are done region-wise and the various structures, their positions and relations are observed. *Gross anatomy*, *microscopic anatomy* (histology) and *developmental anatomy* (embryology) are the major subdivisions of such a study. Embryology is also studied by dissecting dead fetuses.

In the earlier times, the teaching and learning of anatomy was more of descriptive in nature. New breakthroughs in the field of medicine (imaging techniques, invasive procedures) have brought revolution in the teaching and learning of anatomy. At present, the descriptive anatomy needs to be learnt with a functional orientation and should form the basis for clinical application in the patient care. It is now possible to visualize internal structure without cutting open the body, even in a living individual. In fact, such techniques can be done properly if only there is sound knowledge of anatomy. Lacunae in anatomical knowledge while performing such techniques can lead to damage of structures and in turn, other complications. On the other hand, by using such techniques, knowledge of anatomy can be refined and intricate details can be added.

IMPORTANCE OF ANATOMY

- *Foundation for understanding health-related fields:* Human anatomy is the foundation for students of health-related fields like medicine, nursing, dentistry, laboratory technology, and physician assistant courses. It can be better understood by visual observation of cadaveric dissections and pictures or photographs or colorful illustrations.
- *Basis and clinical application:* Anatomy is the basis for understanding structure and function of human body. Application of anatomical knowledge is required for understanding the clinical conditions, for planning and interpreting laboratory investigations and for planning and undertaking treatment procedures.

SUBDIVISIONS OF ANATOMY

For understanding the structure and its function in health and disease, the subject of anatomy can be studied under the following subdivisions.
- *Gross anatomy or macroscopic anatomy:* (Macro = large). A branch of anatomy for

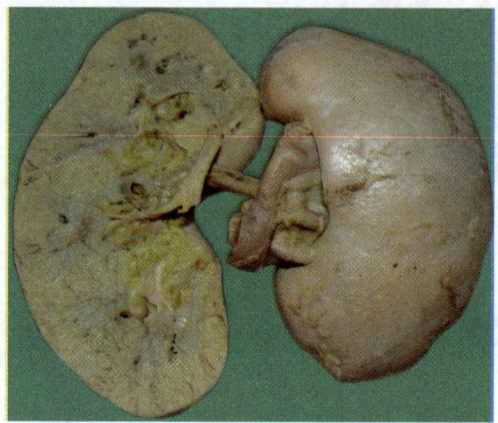

Fig. 1.1A: Macroscopic anatomy of kidney.

understanding the appearance of parts or organs and their relations with unaided eye. It is the study of organ systems, such as the nervous system, respiratory system, digestive system, etc. **(Fig. 1.1A)**.
- *Histology or microscopic anatomy:* (Micro = small; histo = tissue). Study of structures that cannot be seen with the unaided eye. It requires the use of microscope **(Fig. 1.1B)**.
- *Embryology or developmental anatomy:* Study of early developmental stages of an organism. Knowledge of embryology provides the basis for certain of the clinical conditions that might have resulted from errors during early developmental period of an organism. Embryology provides the basis for location and relations of the structure, e.g., location and relations of heart, liver, stomach, spleen, kidney, etc. **(Fig. 1.1C)**.
- *Radiographic anatomy or living anatomy:* With the advancements in medicine, it is now possible to visualize internal structures in a living individual without opening the body. Various parts of body and organ systems can be visualized by X-rays, ultrasound, computed tomography (CT), magnetic resonance imaging (MRI), bronchoscopy, intravenous pyelography, etc. for understanding the normal appearance in health and for

Chapter 1: Introduction to Anatomy

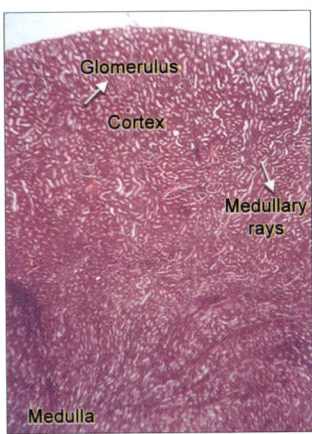

Fig. 1.1B: Microscopic anatomy of kidney.

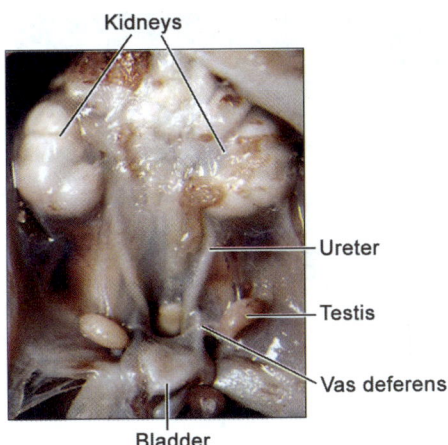

Fig. 1.1C: Developmental anatomy of urinary system.

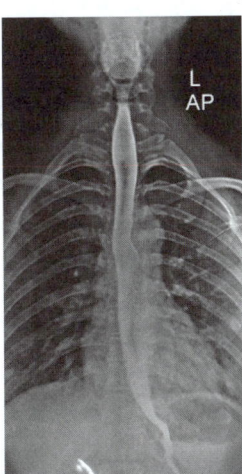

Fig. 1.1D: Radiological anatomy—contrast X-ray of esophagus.

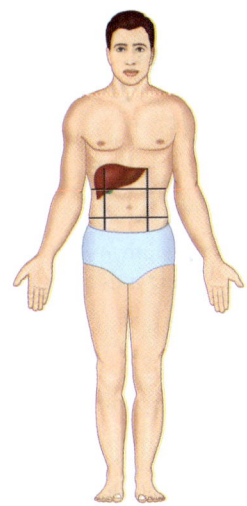

Fig. 1.1E: Topographic anatomy of liver.

identifying the abnormality in disease. Sound anatomical knowledge is required for performing the technique and for interpretation of the structures visualized (**Fig. 1.1D**).

- *Surface or topographic anatomy:* This method can be used both on the cadavers and on the living individuals. This forms the basis for physical examination of a patient and for performing surgical procedures in clinical practice. In this method, internal structures of the body were studied by marking them on the surface of the cadaver or palpating them on the surface of the body like the liver, kidney, heart, etc. (**Fig. 1.1E**).
- *Living anatomy:* Study of anatomy in a living individual by using simple techniques like (**Figs. 1.2A to D**):
  - *Inspection:* By visual observation, e.g., observing the movement of thyroid gland by asking a person to swallow wherein it moves up and down (**Fig. 1.2A**); observing the apex beat of the heart in a person with naked chest.
  - *Palpation:* By feeling with the hand, e.g., feeling the apex beat of heart with your hand placed on the

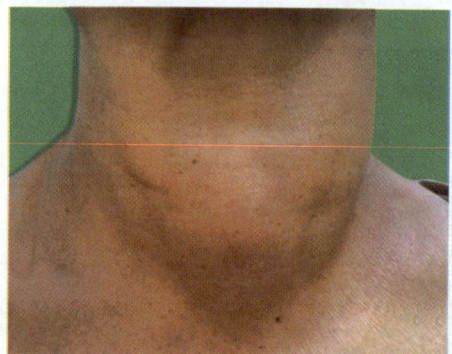

Fig. 1.2A: Living anatomy—inspection—enlarged thyroid gland.

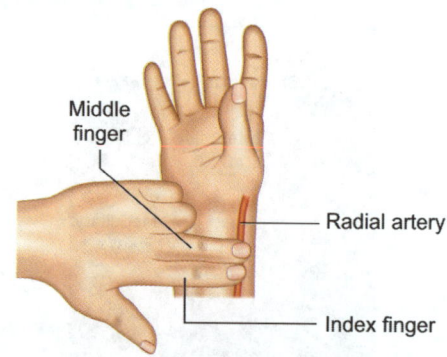

Fig. 1.2B: Living anatomy—palpation—feeling the radial artery pulsations.

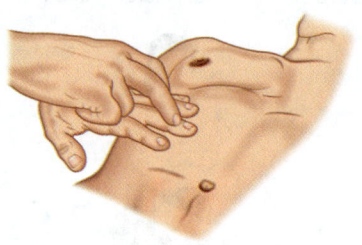

Fig. 1.2C: Living anatomy—percussion—thorax for boundaries of heart.

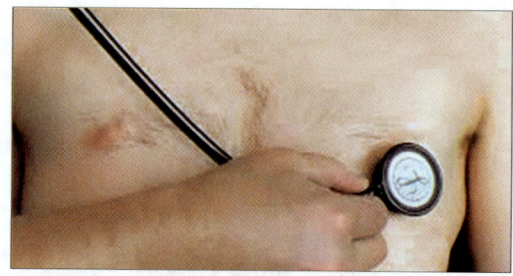

Fig. 1.2D: Living anatomy—auscultation—listening to heart beat with stethoscope.

topographical location of apex of heart or feeling the radial pulse with your fingers by appropriately holding the topographical area where it can be felt near the wrist **(Fig. 1.2B)**.
- *Percussion:* By tapping the surface of a body part with middle finger of one hand on the middle finger of other hand that was kept in contact with the body surface. Interpretation is by the resulting sound, i.e., a resonant note or a dull note. By this method, collection of fluid in the lung (pleural effusion) can be identified **(Fig. 1.2C)**.
- *Auscultation:* By listening to the sounds arising within organs by using stethoscope, e.g., heart sounds, breath sounds and bowel sounds that aid in diagnosis and treatment **(Fig. 1.2D)**.

♦ *Clinical anatomy:* Application of anatomical knowledge in the diagnosis and treatment of patients either by medical or by surgical methods. *Surgical anatomy* is the study of structures giving emphasis on its direct practical significance in the practice of surgery **(Fig. 1.3)**.

♦ *Comparative anatomy:* Comparison of changes in the morphology and function of different organs and organ systems of the human body that has occurred during evolution from the stage of fish to that of mammalian.

♦ *Physical or biological anthropology:* A discipline that deals with physical, biological and behavioral aspects of human beings, their related nonhuman primates and their hominoid ancestors those are extinct. It is the study of human evolution. It focuses on origin, evolution and diversity of people of different race, ethnicity and sociocultural background.

♦ *Human genetics:* It is the study of heredity, the process of transmission of genes (characters or traits) from parents to offspring and associated variations that can

Chapter 1: Introduction to Anatomy

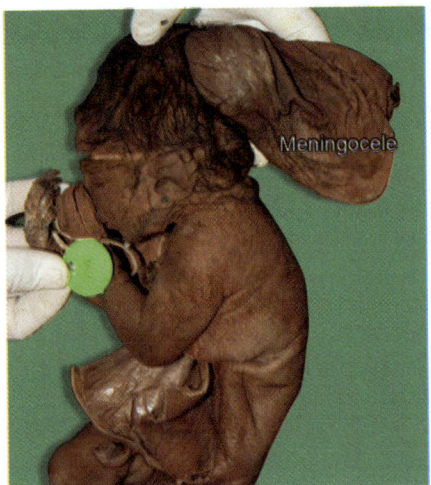

Fig. 1.3: Clinical anatomy—abnormal fetus with meningocele.

play a role in the causation of defects or diseases.

APPROACHES FOR STUDYING ANATOMY

The human body can be studied region-wise or system-wise for a logical understanding.
- *Region-wise or regional anatomy:* It is the study of one region of the body at a time and learning everything about that region. The regions of the body from head to foot are as shown in **Table 1.1**.
- *System-wise or systemic anatomy:* It is the study of one system at a time. For convenience of description and for easy understanding, it is divided into various systems as shown in **Table 1.2**.

Table 1.1: Region-wise subdivisions of anatomy.	
Region	Organs/structures/subdivisions present
Head and neck	Face, neck, brain, eyes, ears, mouth, pharynx, larynx, and trachea
Trunk a. Thorax b. Abdomen c. Pelvis	Heart, lungs, digestive system, urinary system, and reproductive system
Limbs	Bones, joints, muscles, nerves, and vessels
a. Upper	Shoulder, arm, forearm, wrist and hand
b. Lower	Hip, thigh, leg, ankle and foot

Note: For a medical graduate, region-wise approach with a correlation of related systems and subdivisions is followed for a comprehensive understanding of the subject. For other branches of medical field, a system-wise approach is followed giving emphasis on structures of importance for practicing their profession.

ANATOMICAL POSITION AND PLANES

> **AN 1.1:** Demonstrate normal anatomical position, various planes, anatomical terms, relation, comparison, laterality and movement in our body.

For visual orientation and for understanding of various structural arrangements of organs, the body has to be sectioned and studied along three fundamental planes, viz. sagittal, coronal and transverse. These descriptive planes and terms of direction are standardized with reference to anatomical position for maintaining uniformity in description, understanding and interpretation throughout the world by medical professionals. Adopting uniform medical terminology avoids confusion and ambiguity. Hence, all descriptions of the human body are made with reference to a standard position called the *normal anatomical position* (**Fig. 1.4**).

Anatomical Position

For understanding and for describing the relationship of body parts and organs to one another the human body is described by imagining as if the person is standing in an artificial posture known as anatomical position.

In anatomical position, the body is imagined as described in **Table 1.3 and Figure 1.4**. The anatomical position is used as a standard reference in medical profession in:
- Describing the cadaver
- For positioning and in examination of a patient
- Positioning a patient for radiological or surgical procedure

Table 1.2: System-wise subdivisions of anatomy.

System	Components	Functions
Integumentary	Skin, hair and nails	Protection, excretion, thermoregulation
Musculoskeletal	Muscles, bones, joints, tendons and ligaments	Bodily movements, support for the body, protection of various organ systems
Nervous	Brain, spinal cord, peripheral nerves and cranial nerves	Receiving, modifying and transmitting the information for appropriate action
Cardiovascular	Heart and blood vessels	Pumps and circulates blood from heart to various parts of body and receives blood from the lungs
Lymphatic	Contains structures like tonsils, thymus, spleen, lymph nodes and lymph vessels	Involved in transfer of lymph between tissues and the bloodstream. It transports cells of immune system that defends disease-causing agents
Respiratory	Pharynx, larynx, trachea, bronchi, lungs, and diaphragm	Breathing Purification of blood
Digestive	Salivary glands, esophagus, stomach, intestines, rectum, anal canal, liver and pancreas	Digestion of food and excretion of undigested food
Urinary	Kidneys, ureters, bladder and urethra	Maintenance of fluid, electrolyte balance and excretion of urine
Reproductive a. *Males* b. *Females*	Differs in sexes Testes, vas deferens, seminal vesicles, prostate, and penis Ovaries, fallopian tubes, uterus, vagina and mammary glands	Formation of gametes by ovary and testis. Fusion of gametes in uterine tube is called fertilization. Attachment of fertilized ovum and its growth in uterus as embryo and fetus. Growth of fertilized embryo in uterus. Secretion of milk by mammary glands in females
Endocrine	Hypothalamus, pituitary, pineal, thyroid, parathyroid and adrenal glands	Production of hormones that maintain the internal environment constant

Table 1.3: Description of anatomical position.

Description of body

Always imagine that the person is:
- Standing erect
- Both the feet close, parallel to each other, flat on the ground
- Toes directed forwards
- Arms hanging by the side of the trunk with the palms of hands facing forwards
- Fingers facing straight downwards
- Head facing forwards
- Eyes fixed on a distant point

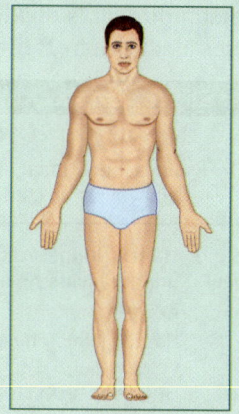

Fig. 1.4: Anatomical position.

- Interpreting the radiological images
- Sectioning a tissue for histological examination
- Communicating the observations on the patient with medical professionals globally.

Various Positions of the Body of Clinical Importance

*For examination or for treatment purposes, certain positions are adopted in clinical practice. They are right or left lateral, Trendelenburg, Fowler, Sims, etc. (**Table 1.4 and Fig. 1.5**).*

Anatomical Planes

Anatomical planes describe the sectional views of a part of body or an organ. They help in understanding the relationship of one organ with the other and structural orientation of tissue. These are useful in radiology

Table 1.4: Clinically important positions of the body.	
Position and description	Figs. 1.5A to D: Clinically important positions.
Supine position: A position where the individual will be lying down on his back on a flat surface, upper limbs placed by the side of trunk, palms facing up and the person looking upward. *Prone position:* It is opposite to that of supine position with the individual lying down with the face, chest and belly touching the surface, upper limbs on the side of the trunk.	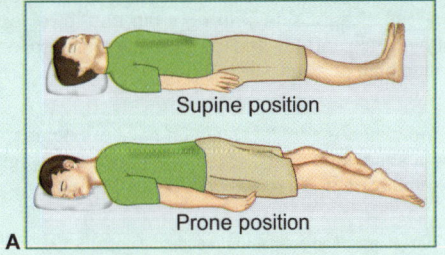 A
Right/left lateral recumbent position: Patient lying on right/left side with right/left side of body touching the surface.	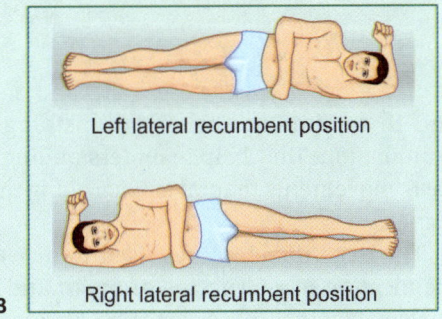 B
Trendelenburg position: Lying supine with feet higher than head by 15–30°. This is the common position preferred for laparoscopic surgeries of lower abdomen and pelvis. If a person is having hypotension and shock, this position is adopted to increase blood flow to the brain.	C
Reverse Trendelenburg position: The head is elevated higher about 15–30° in the air. The patient is kept in this position to expose the prostate and upper abdominal region during surgery. This position is good for performing procedures in head and neck. This position also helps respiration for overweight and obese individuals during surgery by relieving the pressure on the head. But, there is risk of hypotension, hypothermia. Hence, a constant monitoring is required.	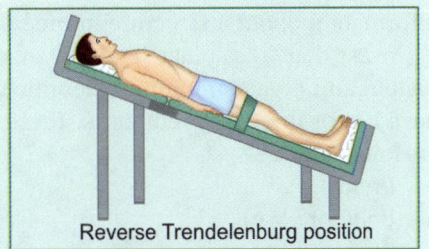 D

Contd...

Contd...

Position and description	Figs. 1.5E to G: Clinically important positions.
Fowler's position: It is sitting straight up or leaning slightly backwards. It is the standard patient position to relax tension of abdominal muscles, improve breathing in immobile patients and for increasing the comfort during eating.	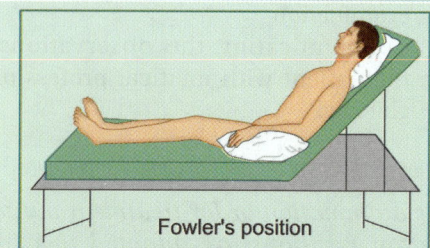 E — Fowler's position
Sims' position: This position is used for rectal examination, therapies for rectal conditions and for giving enemas. Upper part of patient is in prone position and lower part in lateral (right/left) position. Patient can lie, for example, on his/her right side with right hip and lower extremity straight, and left hip and knee bent. It is also called lateral recumbent position.	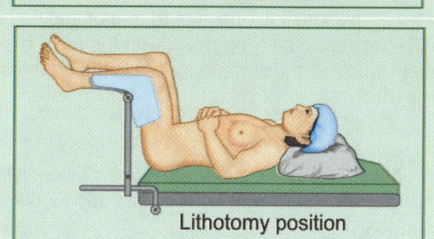 F — Sims' position
Lithotomy position: It is lying on back with knees bent and thighs apart. This is the position for vaginal examination and vaginal delivery of the fetus.	G — Lithotomy position

and in sectioning tissues for histological examination. They help in understanding the basic movements that take place along these planes.

The descriptive planes used to describe the location of a structure or organ and the movements along these planes are represented in **Table 1.5** and **Figures 1.6A to D**.

ANATOMICAL TERMINOLOGY

The importance of language of medical field to the students of that profession is for communicating with their professional colleagues and for understanding the subject. Scientific medical term is a word that gives information about a structure in the body or a process that takes place in an organ, organ system and organism. Some scientific terms have two or three different parts. These parts are known as:
- Prefix
- Root (or base)
- Suffix

Examples:
- Subcutaneous
  - Sub = below (prefix)
  - Cutis = skin (root)
  - Subcutaneous = below the skin
- Myocardium
  - Myo = muscle (prefix)
  - Cardio = heart (root)
  - Myocardium = muscular wall of the heart
- Appendicitis
  - Appendix = appendix (a specific organ) (root)
  - Itis = inflammation (suffix)

Naming of Structures

Names identify structures according to:
- *Shape:* Trapezius muscle—trapezius= trapezoid in shape
- *Size:* Palmaris longus—long tendon extending to palm
- *Color:* Erythrocyte—erythro = red (color), cyte = cell

Chapter 1: Introduction to Anatomy

Table 1.5: Anatomical planes.

Plane	Description	Figs. 1.6A to C: Anatomical planes.
Sagittal plane	<ul><li>It is an imaginary vertical plane</li><li>It passes through the center of the body</li><li>By cutting along this plane, the body can be divided into two identical halves, i.e., right and left half</li><li>Basic movements along this plane are flexion and extension</li></ul>	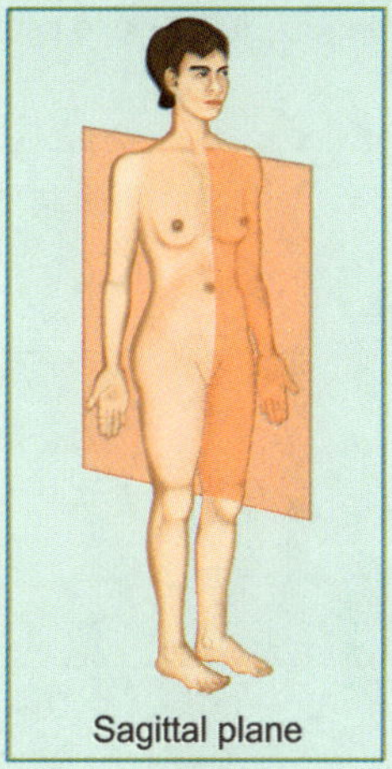 A — Sagittal plane
Coronal plane	<ul><li>It is an imaginary vertical plane</li><li>It is at right angles to the sagittal plane</li><li>This plane divides the body into an anterior/ventral part and a posterior/dorsal part</li><li>Basic movements along this plane are abduction and adduction</li></ul>	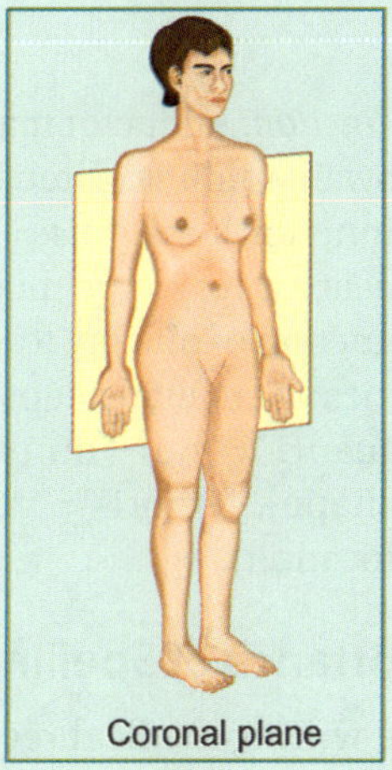 B — Coronal plane
Transverse plane	<ul><li>It is at right angles to both the sagittal and frontal planes</li><li>This plane divides the body/limb into an upper part and a lower part</li><li>Basic movements along this plane are rotations</li></ul>	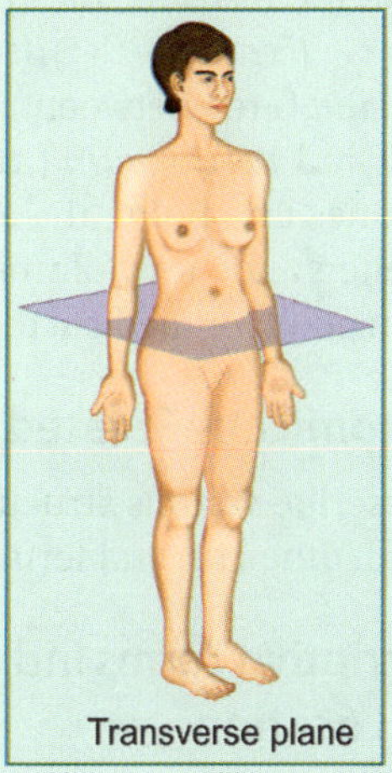 C — Transverse plane

Contd…

Contd...

Plane	Description
Oblique plane	It is a plane perpendicular to all the above planes 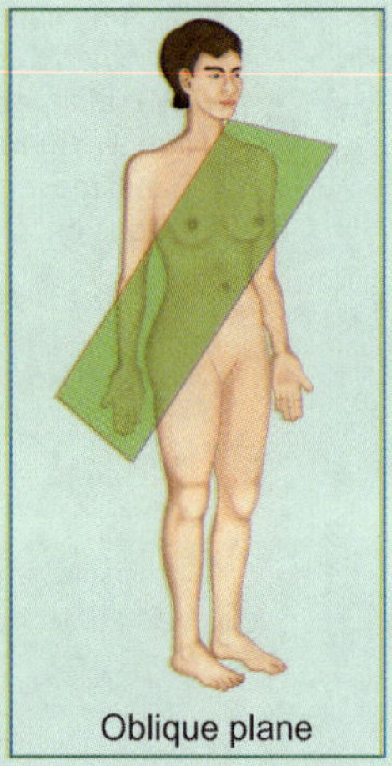

Fig. 1.6D: Anatomical planes.

- *Function:* Adductor magnus muscle—Ad = toward midline (direction), duct = to carry (function), magnus = very large (size). It means a very large muscle that carries the function of moving towards midline.
- Location: Quadriceps femoris muscle—Quadri = four (number), ceps = head (shape), femoris = in relation to femur (location).

Importance of Spelling

While writing medical records, mis-spellings can be the basis for life-threatening medical errors. *Example:* Difference between *perineum* (area between the genitals and the anus) and *peritoneum* (membrane covering intestines and lining the abdomen). Just two (*to*) letters and the whole meaning of a sentence or paragraph or medical record is changed.

Anatomically Related Terms

To describe various structures with reference to each other, several terms are required.

Descriptive Terms Indicating Direction and Location

- For understanding and explaining the location of various structures and their relation with each other and for eliciting and interpreting the movements of body parts several terms of location, relation and movement are required.
- These are described along the midsagittal and transverse planes. These are pair of words with meaning in opposite direction. These are used for expressing the relationship of a given structure to another structure. They are presented in **Table 1.6** and **Figures 1.7A to I**.

HISTORY OF ANATOMY

Herophilus (335–280 BC)

- *Greek physician—Father of Anatomy*
- Made a twist in medicine.
- Introduced human experimentation.
- He started the practice of making incisions on human beings and doing public dissections on human corpses.
- Described the eye, liver, salivary glands, pancreas, genitals, duodenum, prostate gland, and measuring of pulse.
- First to distinguish nerves from tendons.
- He discovered parts of brain.
- Described a part of the cerebellum and called it *calamus scriptorius*, because it looked like a writing pen.

Chapter 1: Introduction to Anatomy

Table 1.6: Pair of related terms used for describing direction and location of a part.

Pair of terms	Description	Figs. 1.7A to D: Direction and location terms.
A. Superior/cranial/rostral B. Inferior/caudal	Above/towards head end of the body, e.g., heart superior to liver. Below/towards foot end of the body, e.g., stomach is inferior to lungs.	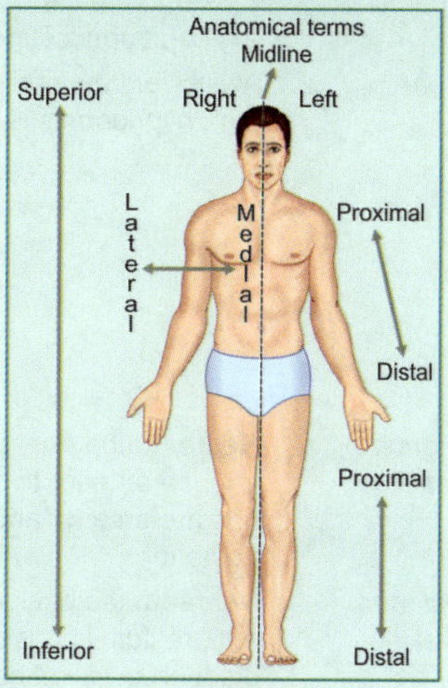 A (Anatomical terms: Midline, Superior, Right, Left, Lateral, Medial, Proximal, Distal, Inferior)
A. Medial B. Lateral	Towards/nearer to the midline of the body, e.g., heart medial to lungs Away from the midline/towards one side (right/left) of the body, e.g., kidneys are situated lateral to vertebrae.	
A. Proximal (applied to limbs) B. Distal (applied to limbs)	Nearer to shoulder joint/hip joint, i.e., trunk, e.g., scapula is proximal to the humerus. Further away from the shoulder joint or the hip joint, i.e., trunk, e.g., wrist is distal to the elbow.	
A. Medial border/ (applied to limbs) B. Lateral border (applied to limbs)	Border close to the trunk. Ulnar border in upper limb and tibial border in lower limb Border away from the trunk. Radial border in upper limb and fibular border in lower limb.	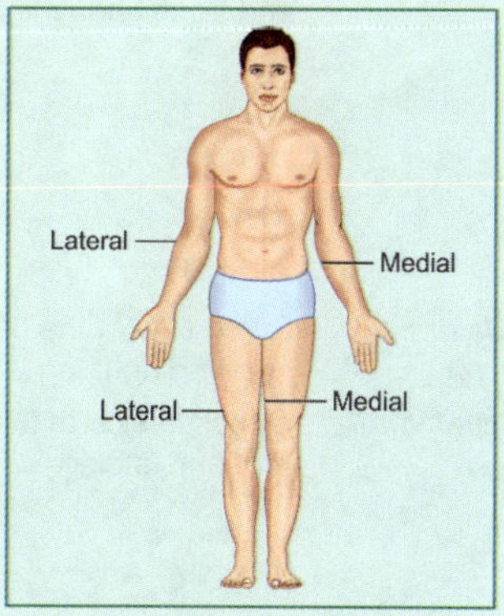 B (Lateral, Medial, Lateral, Medial)
A. Palmar surface (hand)/plantar surface (foot)	Anterior surface of hand or inferior/plantar surface of foot.	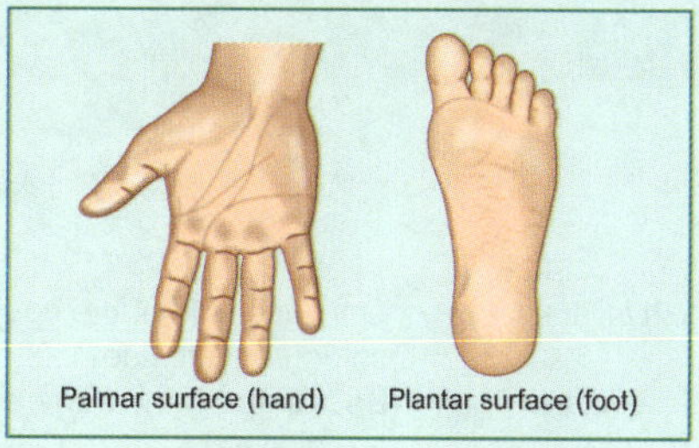 C (Palmar surface (hand), Plantar surface (foot))
B. Dorsal surface (hand and foot)	Posterior surface of hand and upper/dorsal surface foot.	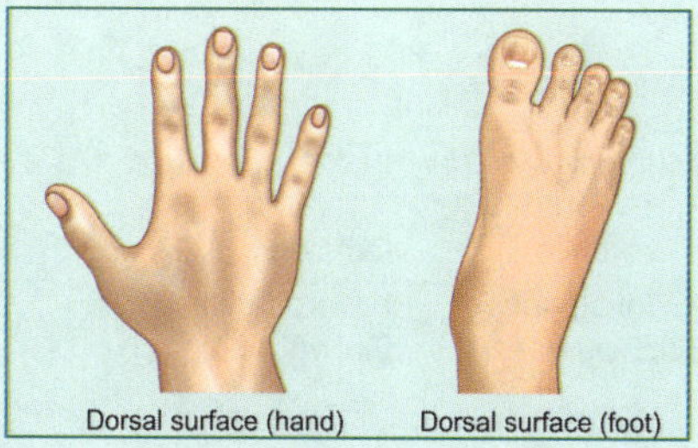 D (Dorsal surface (hand), Dorsal surface (foot))

Contd...

Contd...

Pair of terms	Description	Figs. 1.7E to I: Direction and location terms.
A. *Superficial*	Closer to the surface of the body, e.g., epidermis superficial to dermis.	E
B. *Deep*	Away from the surface of the body, e.g., hypodermis is deep dermis.	
A. *Anterior/ ventral*	Nearer to the front of the body, e.g., trachea anterior to esophagus; ribs are anterior and vertebrae are posterior	F
B. *Posterior/ dorsal*	Nearer to the back of the body, e.g., rectum is posterior to urinary bladder; occipital bone is posterior and frontal bone is anterior	
A. *Ipsilateral*	Same side of the body, e.g., right arm and right leg	G
B. *Contralateral*	Opposite side of the body, e.g., right arm and left leg	
A. *Unilateral*	Only one side of the body, e.g., spleen on left side	H
B. *Bilateral*	Both sides of the body, e.g., lungs are bilateral	
A. *Internal/interior*	Inside	I
B. *External/ exterior*	Outside	
A. *Invagination*	Inward bulging	
B. *Evagination*	Outward bulging	

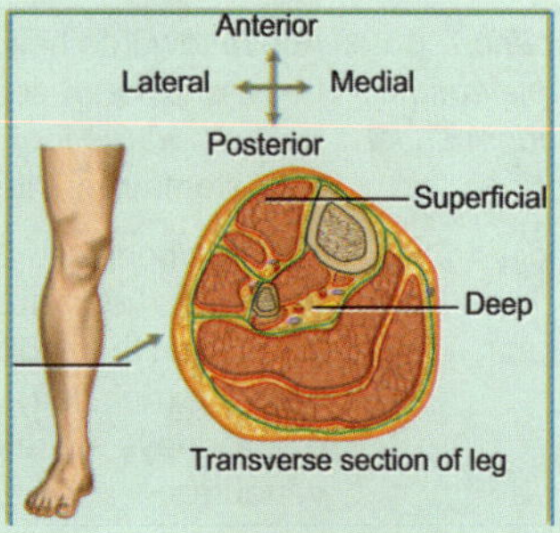

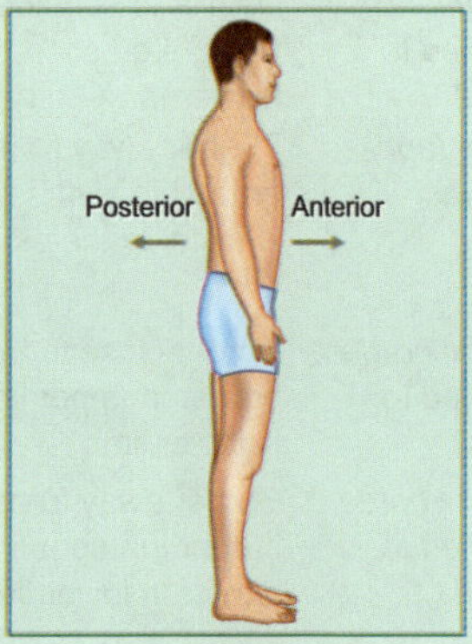

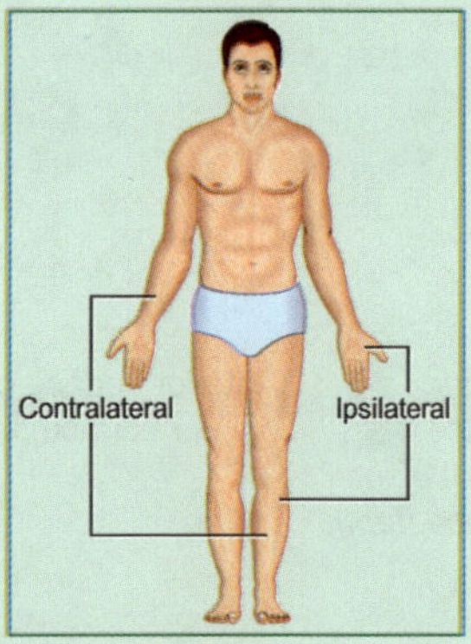

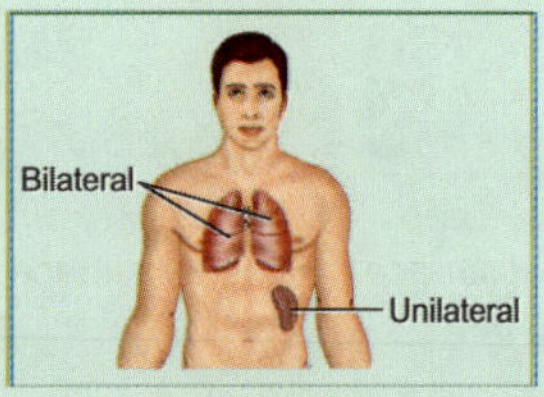

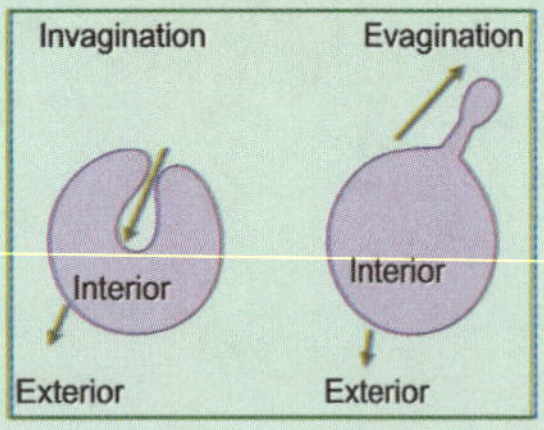

Chapter 1: Introduction to Anatomy

"When health is absent, wisdom cannot reveal itself, art cannot manifest, strength cannot fight, wealth becomes useless, and intelligence cannot be applied."
—**Herophilus**

Galen of Pergamum (130–210 AD)

- Ancient Roman physician.
- Conducted dissections of monkeys, pigs.

"The best physician is also a philosopher."
—**Galen**

Mondino de Liuzzi–Mundinus (1270–1326)

- Italian physician and anatomist—restorer of anatomy.
- First to incorporate a systematic study of anatomy and dissection into a medical curriculum.
- Written first dissection manual and true anatomy text.
- Stated that the purpose of anatomy is the verification or demonstration of the text.

Leonardo da Vinci (1452–1519)

- A Master of Arts, Mathematics, Engineering and Science.
- He is known for his anatomical sketches which he used to draw by dissecting human corpses though he is not a medical person and dissection was not legal.
- He was remembered for the perfect drawing of things he observed, e.g., Mona Lisa painting in Louvre Museum of Paris.
- His work is the basis for cross-sectional anatomy.

Andreas Vesalius (1514–1564)

- Belgian reformer of anatomy—founder of modern anatomy.
- He is the first medical student to dissect human body who continued as professor of anatomy in Padua in Italy.
- He emphasized that anatomy can be learnt only through dissection.
- He wrote 7 volumes *De humani corporis fabrica* (*On the Fabric of the Human Body*).
- His drawings were like a 3D view of anatomy.

"I am not accustomed to saying anything with certainty after only one or two observations."
—**Andreas Vesalius**

William Hunter (1718–1783)

- Scottish anatomist and obstetrician.
- He started the procedure of embalming of the cadaver.
- He worked till he dropped and lectured when he was dying.
- His head was preserved in the Hunterian Museum, Glasgow, Scotland.

Henry Gray (1827–1861)

- English anatomist.
- He is recipient of Astley Cooper Prize for his work "On the Structure and Use of Spleen".
- In 1858, his first edition of *Anatomy*, with 750 pages and 363 figures was published.

20th and 21st Century

- The cadaveric dissections were made compulsory in learning anatomy.
- There is increased zeal to learn anatomy. This lead to stealing of cadavers from grave yards. The scandal of Burke the butcher, Hare the thief and Knox the person who buys the cadavers was brought to light. Warburton Anatomy Act came into effect taking the legal aspects into consideration for cadaveric dissections.
- Anatomy was recognized as a science and the chemical formalin was used as a preservative to preserve the dead bodies.
- Formation of anatomical societies was encouraged.
- Anatomy acts—United Kingdom (UK) Murder Act (1752) permitted use of corpses of executed criminals for dissection. Anatomy Act of UK (1832) permitted donation of the body of the deceased by his kin for dissection purpose. Bombay Anatomy Act (1949) modified in 1975 was formulated for use of unclaimed body in an approved institution for anatomy dissection or for similar medical education uses.

- *Body donation awareness:* With increasing awareness of organ and body donation, several voluntary organizations are encouraging body donation to overcome the shortage of cadavers.

Anatomical Basis for Clinical Condition

Case Scenario

Problem: For doing laparoscopic surgery for the removal of uterus (*hysterectomy*), the patient was kept on the operating table with the body lying down with the back touching the surface of the table and face up. Further the foot end is 15–30° higher than head end.

Questions:

1. What do you call the position in which the patient was lying on the bed?
2. What do you call the position in which the patient was kept with foot end elevated for surgery?
3. Why the foot end was elevated?

Anatomical explanation:

1. The position in which the patient was lying on the table with the body lying down, back touching the surface of the table and face up is called *supine position*. This position is ideal for some of the abdominal and gynecological surgeries.
2. For performing the surgical procedure, the patient was kept in supine position with the foot end elevated by 15–30°. This position is called *Trendelenburg's position*.
3. This position allows better access to the pelvic organs (uterus in the present case) as the intestines move away because of gravity, thus facilitate access to the uterus.

☞ Key Concept

Take Home Message—For Life Long Learning of Anatomy

Approach to Learning Anatomy

Learning anatomy is an art which requires well-dissected cadaver, good anatomical models, radiological images, well-equipped laboratory and above all experienced and motivated teachers who will guide and inspire the student towards self-directed learning. The best place to learn anatomy is at the dissection table.

Mastering the subject of anatomy with diverse fields (Gross, histology, development, radiological, etc.) is a formidable task. The purpose of learning anatomy is to apply the knowledge gained in anatomy to the context of individual patient and relate it to the clinical condition.

Tips for Learning the Subject are:

- *Not to memorize*: Anatomy should not be learnt by memorizing the topics. Mere memorization will lead to quickly forgetting the subject and feeling of boredom.

Contd...

Contd...

- *Careful observation*: It should be learnt by careful observation of the spatial relation between various structures of the body, by understanding their functions and by correlating the structural details with the function.
- *Systematic approach*: The student must approach the subject in a systematic manner. For example, by studying the skeletal relations of a certain region of the body, the joints, the muscular system, the cardiovascular system (arteries and veins), the nervous system (sensory and motor nerves), etc.
- *Application of knowledge to clinical case scenarios*: Application of knowledge of anatomy requires a collection of clinical cases that are designed to simulate a patient, clinical approach for arriving at the diagnosis and stressing the lead role of basic knowledge of anatomy. Explanation for the clinical condition should be thought provoking emphasizing the underlying mechanisms and their relation to the structure and function. The student should try to apply the knowledge of structure (anatomy) to its clinical importance. For example, imagine one of the following situations:
  - Two nerves are travelling closely in an area or a nerve and a vessel are closely placed during their travel.
  - Two organs are closely related because of their locational or structural or neurovascular closeness.
  - In such situations, one with the basic knowledge of anatomy could speculate that an injury or a tumor might affect the related structures. Because of damage to the structure, their function would be affected and the deficits expected on physical examination can be correlated.

QUESTIONS

1. Define anatomy.
2. Describe anatomical position.
3. Define terms used to describe anatomical directions and planes of the body.

MULTIPLE CHOICE QUESTIONS

1. **Regarding anatomical position which one of the following statements is not correct?**
   A. Imagine the person in a lying down position
   B. Toes directed forwards
   C. Head facing forwards
   D. Eyes fixed on a distant point

2. **Which of the following terms and their meaning are wrongly presented?**
   A. Dorsum of foot—upper surface of foot
   B. Ipsilateral—same side
   C. Recumbent position—the back of body touches flat surface
   D. Invagination—inward bulging

ANSWERS

1. A   2. C

CHAPTER 2

Levels of Organization and Tissues of the Body

LEARNING OBJECTIVES

- ❖ Levels of organization
- ❖ Cell and intracellular organelles
- ❖ Development of various tissues and organs
- ❖ Definition of tissue and classification of tissues
- ❖ Epithelia—classification of different epithelia
- ❖ Connective tissue—structural components, classification
- ❖ Clinical case with anatomical explanation

LEVELS OF ORGANIZATION OF THE HUMAN BODY

Human body is a complex organization of smaller invisible (chemical) components to those visible under a microscope (micro) and to those visible to the unaided eye (macro). The various levels of organization of the human body are presented in **Table 2.1** and **Figure 2.1**.

CELL

Cell is the basic functional unit of structure. Some organisms, such as bacteria are unicellular and consist of a single cell. Other organisms, such as human beings are multicellular. Humans have about 100 trillion or 10^{14} cells. A typical cell is 10 μm in size.

Parts of a Cell

The cells are covered by *cell membrane* and filled with *cytoplasm*. The cytoplasm contains organelles for performing various functions of a cell. The intracellular organelles of the cell are broadly divided into the *nucleus* and *cytoplasmic organelles*. Various functional components of a cell and their structure are described in **Table 2.2** and **Figure 2.2**.

DEVELOPMENT OF A HUMAN BEING (FIG. 2.3)

Development of a human being begins with the fusion of male (spermatozoon) and female (ovum) gametes at fertilization to form single-celled *zygote*. The zygote undergoes series of mitotic divisions (*cleavage*) to form a mass of cells, the *morula*. The cells of morula reorganize to from a structure called blastocyst with an outer single layer of cells (*trophoblast*) and an inner mass of cells (*embryoblast*) with a fluid-filled *blastocyst cavity* (*blastocoel*). At this stage the developing embryo is implanted in the uterine endometrium. The cells of trophoblast contribute for the formation of placenta along with the uterine endometrium (*decidua*). The cells of inner cell mass contribute for the formation of the three *primitive germ layers*, i.e., (1) Ectoderm, (2) Endoderm, and (3) Mesoderm from which develops the various tissues and organs of the body (**Figs. 2.4A and B**).

Chapter 2: Levels of Organization and Tissues of the Body

Table 2.1: Levels of organization of the human body.			
Levels	Name	Description	Examples
I	Atoms	Minute particles	Carbon, hydrogen, and oxygen
II	Molecules	Units of two or more atoms	Water
III	Macromolecules	Molecules grouped in a specific pattern to form functional organelle like mitochondria, Golgi apparatus to perform a specific function in a cell	Deoxyribonucleic acid (DNA) which carries the genetic information from parent to offspring
IV	Organelles	Groups of molecules arranged in a particular pattern to form a specific structure for a specific function	Mitochondria, lysosomes, endoplasmic reticulum, and Golgi apparatus
V	Cells	Structural and functional units of a living organism. Required for carrying out the functions of growth, repair, and metabolic functions by the cell	Ovum, sperms, lymphocyte, neuron, and muscle cell
VI	Tissue	Arrangement of groups of cells of similar structure to perform a specific function	Epithelial tissue, connective tissue, and lymphoid tissue
VII	Organ	Two or more tissues combine to form the organ	Liver, stomach, kidney, and lung
VIII	Organ system	Contains combination of various organs that has similar function	Digestive, respiratory, nervous, etc.
IX	Organism	Contains various systems, viz. digestive, respiratory, circulatory, etc.	Human being

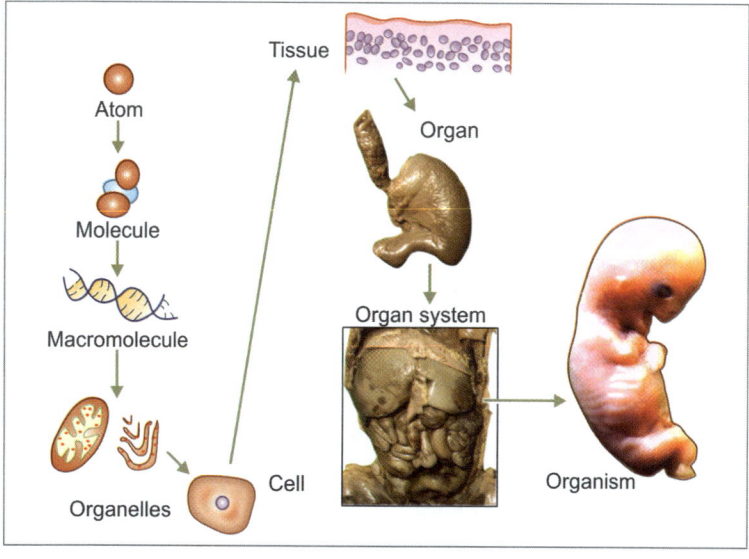

Fig. 2.1: Levels of organization.

Table 2.2: Description of organelles and their functions in the cell.

Components of cell	Description of structure	Functions
Cell membrane/plasma membrane	❑ 8–10 nm in width ❑ Trilaminar containing proteins, carbohydrates, and lipids	❑ Maintains shape of cell ❑ Controls passage of substances to and from the cell
Nucleus	❑ Bilaminar nuclear membrane with pores ❑ It has nuclear sap rich in deoxyribonucleic acid (DNA)—the genetic material	❑ Contains hereditary material ❑ Genetic code in the DNA is required for protein synthesis
Cytoplasm—cytosol	❑ Fluid component ❑ Contains water, dissolved and suspended components like glucose, carbohydrates, proteins, and ions	Site of many chemical reactions required for the survival of the cell like glycolysis
Cytoplasm—organelle		
Rough endoplasmic reticulum (RER)	It has connections with nuclear membrane. Its surface is studded with ribosomes. Hence, called RER	Rough endoplasmic reticulum is more in protein synthesizing cells
Smooth/agranular endoplasmic reticulum (SER)	❑ It extends from RER ❑ Smooth membrane not studded with ribosomes. Hence, called SER	Concerned with the: ❑ Synthesis of steroids, lipids ❑ Detoxification of toxic substances
Ribosomes	Small particles	Concerned with protein synthesis
Mitochondria	❑ Elliptical in shape ❑ Double layered ❑ Outer membrane smooth. Inner membrane folded called cristae	Power houses of energy and more in number in muscle cells and liver cells
Golgi apparatus	❑ Contains 5–20 cup-shaped membranous sacs stacked one over the other ❑ It presents a convex surface to which secretory vesicles are attached and a concave surface through which the vesicles are released	Protein synthesis, storage, and secretion and are more in secretory cells
Lysosomes	Membrane bound vesicles containing hydrolytic enzymes	Breaking down of unwanted material, i.e., phagocytic activity
Centrioles	Two rod shaped structures. Each contains nine groups of three microtubules each arranged in a circular fashion	❑ Spindle formation in mitosis and meiosis ❑ Movement of cilia, flagella, and tail of spermatozoon
Cytoskeletal framework	Complex network of protein fibers	Concerned with cell shape, movement, and cell division
Inclusions	❑ Nonliving components of cell ❑ Not bounded by membrane ❑ These include glycogen, lipids, crystals, and pigments	Not included in metabolic activities of cell

Chapter 2: Levels of Organization and Tissues of the Body

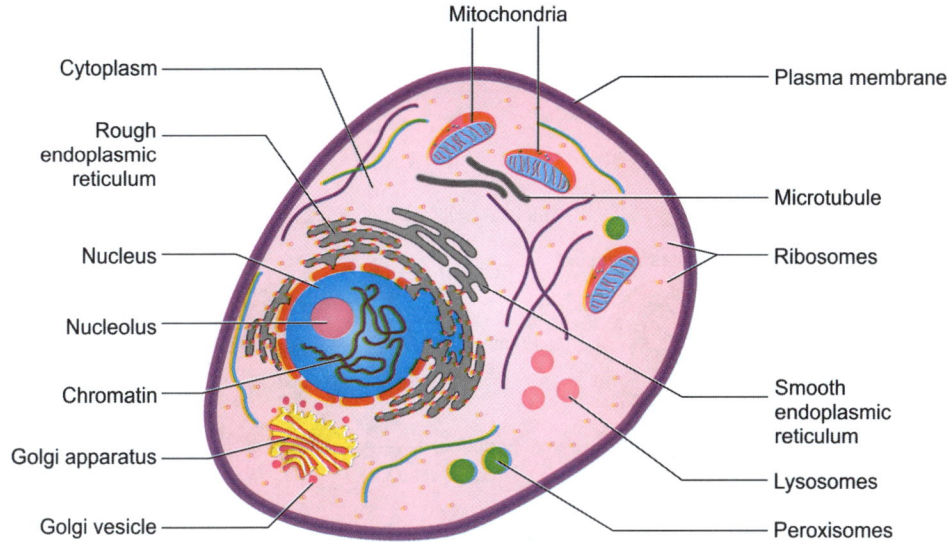

Fig. 2.2: Cell and intracellular organelles.

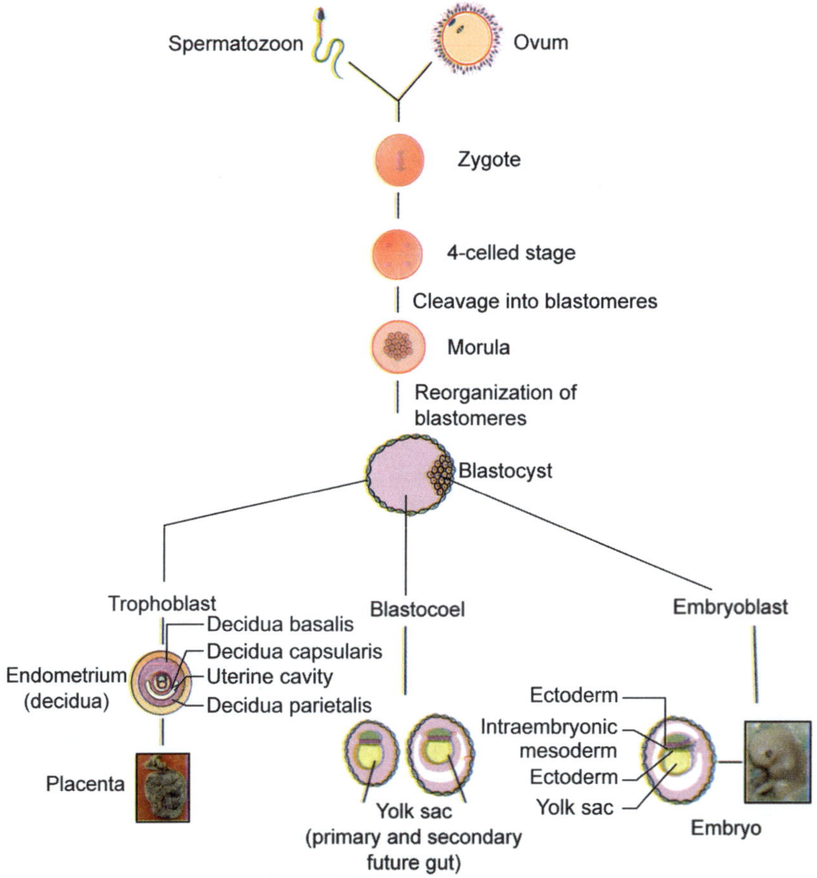

Fig. 2.3: Development of a human being.

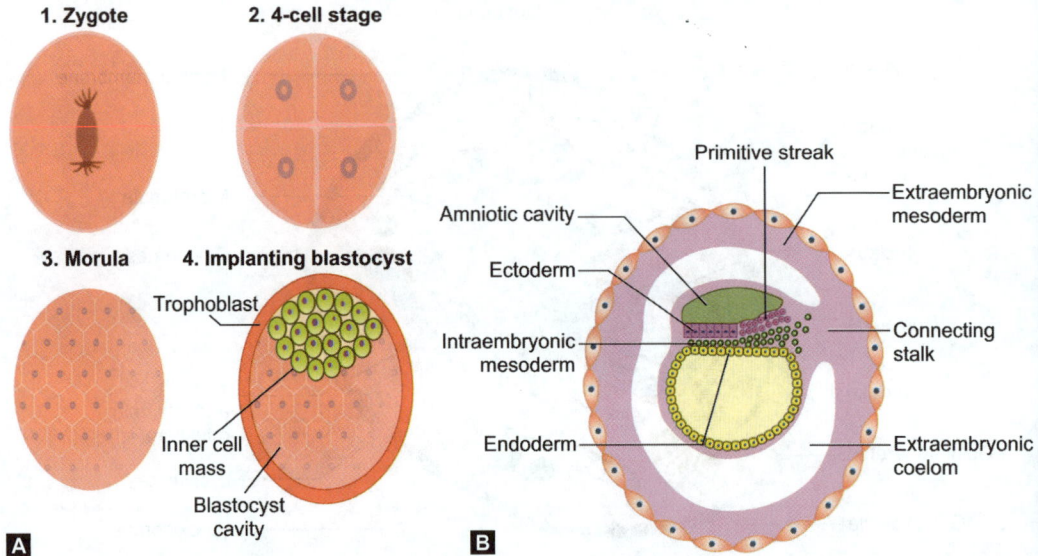

Figs. 2.4A and B: Development of primitive germ layers.

TISSUES OF THE BODY

Tissues are the building blocks of an organism. Various structures of the body starting from bones, muscles, vessels, and nerves to organs like kidney, heart, brain, etc. are made up of tissues.

Definition

Cells and extracellular components having certain morphological characters and organized in different proportions and patterns to perform specific function are called tissue.

Classification

Based on morphology and function the tissues are classified:
- *Epithelial tissue:* Covers the surface of the body (skin), lines the cavities inside the body (pleural, pericardial, peritoneal) and inner aspect of tubular structures with a lumen (blood vessels, digestive tract).
- *Connective tissue:* It joins and supports other tissues. It stores substances required for the maintenance of homeostasis like calcium, lipids, proteins, etc.
- *Muscular tissue:* Its cells are capable of contraction to move the parts of the body, movement of solids, fluids and air along the digestive, circulatory, and respiratory systems, respectively.
- *Nervous tissue:* It receives, conducts, and integrates information from outside and inside the body and transports neurotransmitter substances.

EPITHELIAL TISSUE

AN65.1: Identify epithelium under the microscope and describe the various types that correlate to its function.

- One of the basic tissues of the body.
- Consists of closely attached cells with very little intercellular substance between them.
- Covers the surface of the body, lines the cavities of the body, and forms glands.
- Its functions are protection, secretion, absorption, excretion, barrier, and diffusion.

Classification

The epithelia are broadly classified into covering and lining epithelia and glandular epithelia.

Chapter 2: Levels of Organization and Tissues of the Body

- *Covering and lining epithelia:* Sheets of cells covering the surface of a solid structure or lining internal surface of a hollow tubular structure, e.g., skin, digestive tube.
    - Largest epithelial tissue in the body is the skin.
- *Glandular epithelia:* Secretory parts and ducts of glands, e.g., salivary glands, pancreas.

Classification of Covering and Lining Epithelia

Covering and lining epithelia are classified on the basis of number of cell layers, shape of cells in the surface layer, and surface specializations.
- Based on number of cell layers or thickness:
    - *Simple:* Only one layer of cells, e.g., stomach
    - *Stratified:* Two or more layers of cells, e.g., urinary bladder.
- Based on the shape of cells in the surface layer: The shape of cell is described according to its height.
    - *Squamous (scale or plate-like):* Width of cell more than length/height, e.g., endothelium of blood vessels
    - *Cuboidal:* Length and width are equal, e.g., thyroid follicles
    - *Columnar:* Length of cell is more than the width, e.g., gallbladder.
- Based on surface specialization at free surface:
    - *Microvilli:* Intestine
    - *Cilia:* Trachea
    - *Stereocilia:* Epididymis.

The structure of different types of simple epithelia and their identification features with examples are presented in **Table 2.3** and **Figures 2.5A to E**.

Table 2.3: Different types of simple epithelia and their structure.	
Simple epithelia	Structure (Figs. 2.5A to C)

Simple squamous (pavement) epithelium:
☐ Most common epithelium in the body
☐ Consists of single layer of thin and flattened cells forming a membrane
☐ Nuclei are flat, located close to the center of the cells
☐ *Examples:*
  ➢ Lining the pleural, pericardial, and peritoneal cavities where it is called mesothelium
  ➢ Lining heart, blood vessels, and lymph vessels where it is called endothelium
  ➢ Parietal layer of Bowman's capsule in kidney
  ➢ Alveoli of lung
☐ *Functions:* Rapid transport of substances, filtration of fluids, diffusion of gases, and osmosis
	A
	
	Simple squamous epithelium

Simple cuboidal epithelium:
☐ Cells are cuboidal in shape
☐ Nuclei are round and centrally placed
☐ *Examples:*
  ➢ Follicles of thyroid gland
  ➢ Tubules of kidney
☐ *Functions:* Secretion and absorption
	B
	
	Simple cuboidal epithelium

Simple columnar epithelium: ☐ Cells are cylindrical or rod shaped ☐ Nuclei are oval in shape ☐ Free surface of cells may show modifications like microvilli or cilia	C Simple columnar epithelium

Contd...

Contd...

Simple epithelia
- In between the cells goblet cells are present that secrete mucus which protects the epithelium.
- *Examples*:
  - Cells lining the internal surface of the gastrointestinal tract—simple columnar
  - Small bronchi of lungs—ciliated columnar
  - The cells lining intestine contain microvilli that give the appearance of striated border.
- *Functions*: Secretion, absorption, and ciliary action to move mucus in respiratory tract

Structure (Figs. 2.5D and E)

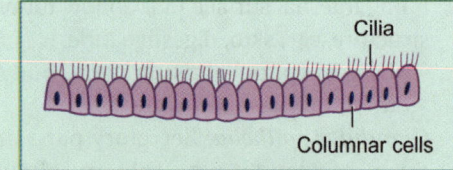

D
Ciliated columnar epithelium

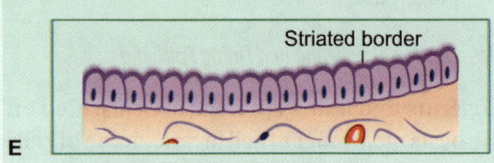

E
Columnar epithelium with microvilli

Stratified Epithelia

These are found at places that are subjected to friction.

General Features of Stratified Epithelium

- Consists of several layers of cells.
- Close to the basement membrane the cells are columnar.
- In middle layers they are polyhedral cells.
- Depending on the shape of superficial cells they are further classified into different types.

The structure of different types of stratified epithelia and their identification features with examples were presented in **Table 2.4** and **Figures 2.6A to F**.

Mucosa/Mucous Membrane

- Layer of epithelial tissue lining an area of the body which comes into contact with air is called mucous membrane.
- It is moist because of the presence of glands that secrete a thick fluid known as mucus.
- Mucus is important for a number of bodily functions.
- *Location:* Urogenital tract, digestive tract, respiratory tract, and lining of the interior of the nose.

Serosa/Serous Membrane

- Layer of mesothelium attached to a surface by a thin layer of connective tissue.
- Covering membranes which line body cavities that do not open to the exterior.
- Found around organs that move a lot, such as the heart and lungs.
- It consists of two layers, one covering the wall of the cavity known as parietal layer and the other covering the surface of the viscera known as visceral layer.
- *Location*: Peritoneum (surrounding the intestines), *pleura* (surrounding the lungs), and *pericardium* (surrounding the heart).

Surface Specializations of Epithelial Cells

Free or apical surface modifications of epithelial cells are cilia, microvilli, and stereocilia. They are described in **Table 2.5** and in **Figures 2.7A to C**.

Glands and Glandular Epithelia

A gland is an organ made up of multiple epithelial cells that are specialized in synthesizing and secreting complex molecules. The characteristic features of glands are:
- They can be seen as discrete organs like liver, pancreas, or are seen in the layers of viscera.
- They consist of secretory units, duct system (exocrine glands).
- Secretions of glands can be:
  - *Enzymes:* Exocrine glands
  - *Hormones:* Endocrine glands
  - *Mucus:* Goblet cells
  - *Fat:* Sebaceous glands.

Table 2.4: Different types of stratified epithelia and their structure.

Stratified epithelia	Structure (Figs. 2.6A to E)

Stratified squamous: The surface cells are flattened. There are two types:
1. *Stratified squamous epithelium (keratinized)*:
  • Present at dry surfaces where the superficial cells at surface lay down the protein keratin and lose their nuclei
  • Superficial cells are dead, dehydrated, non-nucleated, and scale like in appearance
  • Dead cells become hard or cornified
  • *Location*: Epidermis of skin
  • *Functions*: Protection of underlying tissues, prevents absorption of water, and keratin prevents dehydration of underlying tissues
2. *Stratified squamous epithelium (nonkeratinized)*:
  • Present on surfaces that are kept moist or wet
  • The deepest cells are columnar in shape. The intermediate cells are polyhedral and the surface cells are flattened
  • Shapes of nuclei of deepest cells are elongated, intermediate cells are rounded, and surface cells are flat
  • *Examples*: Lining epithelium of:
    – Oral cavity
    – Tongue
    – Esophagus
    – Vagina
    – Cornea
  • *Function*: Protection of deeper tissues
	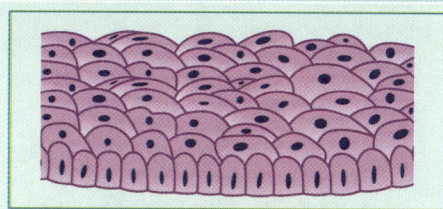
	A
	Stratified squamous keratinized epithelium
	
	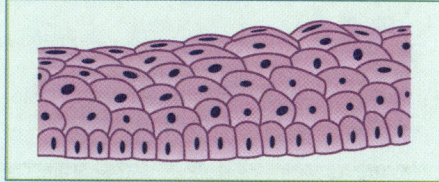
	B
	Stratified squamous nonkeratinized epithelium

Stratified cuboidal: ☐ Cells of superficial layer are cuboidal. This is not a common epithelium ☐ *Example*: Ducts of sweat glands	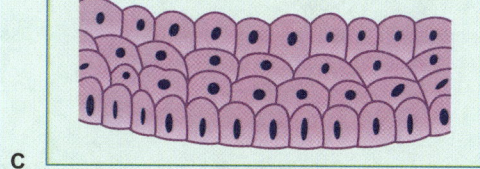 C Stratified cuboidal
Stratified columnar: ☐ Cells of superficial layer are columnar ☐ *Examples*: Major ducts of the mammary gland and large salivary glands	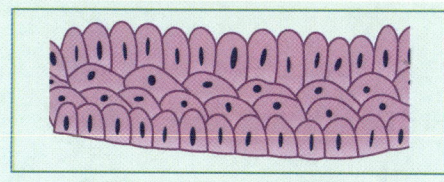 D Stratified columnar epithelium
Transitional epithelium (urothelium): ☐ It is found lining hollow organs which are subject to great mechanical changes due to contraction and distension ☐ The shapes of cells in the surface layer of a transitional epithelium are convex, dome-shaped/umbrella shaped ☐ *Examples*: Ureter, urinary bladder ☐ *Functions*: Acts as a barrier and prevents absorption of toxic substances from urine and facilitates distension of urinary bladder	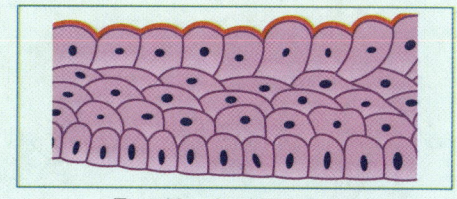 E Transitional epithelium

Contd...

Chapter 2: Levels of Organization and Tissues of the Body

Contd...

Stratified epithelia	Structure (Fig. 2.6F)

Pseudostratifed columnar epithelium:
❑ Simple columnar epithelium in which regular arrangement of cells is distorted so that their nuclei lie at different levels
❑ All cells are in contact with the basement membrane, but not all of them reach the surface of the epithelium
❑ Nuclei of cells are located at different heights and give the epithelium a stratified appearance
❑ The epithelium may be ciliated or nonciliated and may contain goblet cells
❑ Examples:
  ➤ *Pseudostratified ciliated columnar epithelium*: Upper respiratory tract, epididymis
  ➤ *Pseudostratified nonciliated epithelium*: Excretory ducts of many glands
	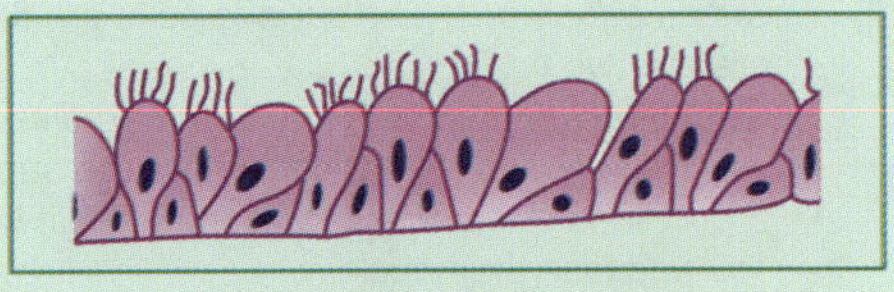 F
	Pseudostratified columnar epithelium

Table 2.5: Surface specializations of epithelial cells.

Features	Cilia	Microvilli	Stereocilia
Description	Fine hair-like projections on apical plasma membrane	❑ Minute brush-like projections of apical plasma membrane. ❑ Give striated or brush border appearance to the surface of cells	Very long and thick microvilli on apical surface
Length	5–10 μ	0.5–1.0 μ	5–10 μ
Number per cell	300 and visible under light microscope	3,000 but not visible under light microscope	Visible under light microscope
Motility	Motile	Nonmotile	Nonmotile
Internal arrangement	One central and nine peripheral pairs of microtubules	Cross-linkage of actin filaments with certain proteins and myosin filaments	Rigid cross-linked actin filaments with positive ends at the tips and negative ends at the bases of stereocilia
Function	Rapid back and forth movements	Absorption	❑ Absorption in vas deferens and epididymis. ❑ Hearing and balance in inner ear
Location	Respiratory tract, uterine tube	Intestine, proximal convoluted tubules of kidney	Vas deferens, epididymis, and inner ear

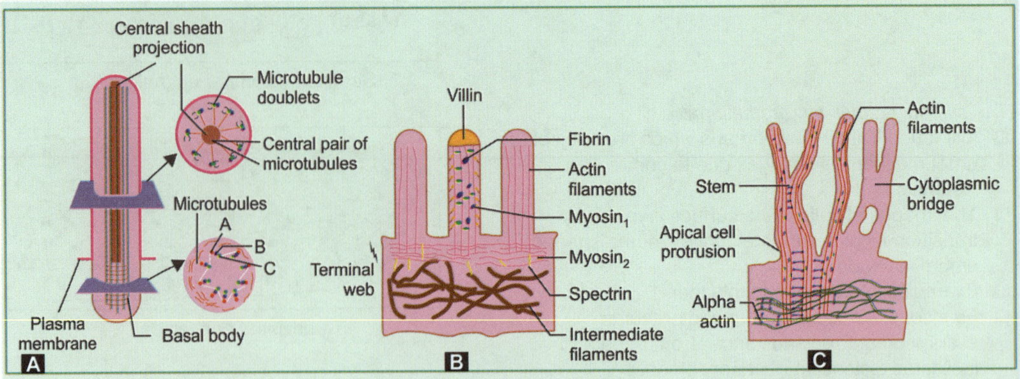

Figs. 2.7A to C: Surface specializations of epithelial cells. (A) Cilia; (B) Microvilli; (C) Stereocilia.

Classification of Glands

The glands are broadly classified based on site of release of secretions into:

- *Exocrine glands:* Release their secretions on to the outside by means of a duct system. Examples: Salivary glands, isolated glands in the walls of viscera.
- *Endocrine glands:* Release their secretions into the adjacent blood vessels through which they will be transported to distant places in the body. Examples: Pituitary, thyroid, parathyroid, and adrenal glands.
- *Paracrine:* They send their secretions adjacent to them. Example: In the gastrointestinal tract (GIT).

Classification of exocrine glands: They are classified based on:

- *Number of cells*:
  - *Unicellular gland:* Single-celled gland. Its secretions have lubricative and protective function, e.g., goblet cell.
    - Goblet (chalice) cells **(Fig. 2.8)**:
      » These are modified columnar cells.
      » Cytoplasm contains mucinogen in its apical part.
      » Nucleus is pushed to the basal part of the cell.
      » *Location:* Seen in intestines, trachea.
  - *Multicellular gland*: Majority of the glands are multicellular. Their function is lubrication, protection, cooling the body surface, digestion, and homeostasis, e.g., sweat glands, sebaceous glands, liver, and mammary gland.

- *Based on mode of secretion*:
  - *Merocrine:* The secretions are wrapped in membrane bound vesicles internal to the cell. These are moved to the apical surface where the vesicles coalesce with the membrane on the apical surface to release the product. *Example:* Salivary glands.
  - *Apocrine:* Apical portions of cells are pinched off and lost during secretory process. *Example:* Mammary glands.
  - *Holocrine:* Secretory cell is released as it breaks apart. Contents of the cell become secretory product. *Examples:* Sweat glands located in the axilla, pubic areas, and sebaceous glands.
- *Based on nature of secretion*:
  - *Serous glands* **(Fig. 2.9A)**:
    - The cells lining serous secretory units (acini) are pyramidal in shape.
    - The nuclei are round in shape and centrally placed.
    - Base of the cell is intensely basophilic due to the presence of large amounts of rough endoplasmic reticulum (RER).
    - Apical region contains prominent Golgi apparatus and numerous rounded, protein-rich, membrane-bound vesicles containing zymogen granules.
    - Lumen of acinus is small.
    - *Example:* Parotid salivary gland.
  - *Mucus glands* **(Fig. 2.9B)**:
    - The cells lining mucus secretory units (acini) are columnar in shape.
    - The nuclei are flat and placed close to the base of the cell.
    - Apical cytoplasm contains mucinogen granules.
    - Lumen of acinus is large.
    - *Examples:* Isolated glands in the wall of duodenum, esophagus.
- *Mixed glands*:
  - Contain mixture of serous and mucus acini.
  - *Examples:* Submandibular and sublingual salivary glands.

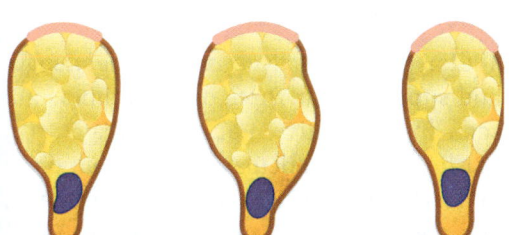

Fig. 2.8: Goblet cell.

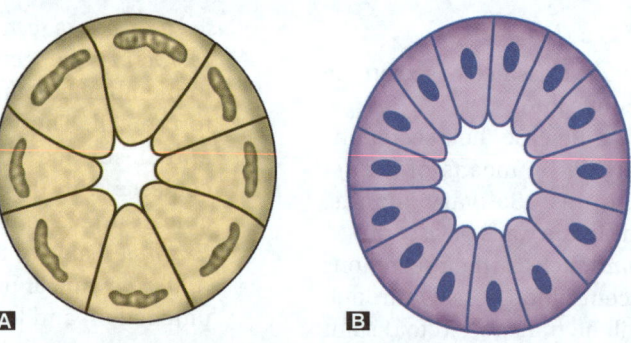

Figs. 2.9A and B: (A) Mucus acinus; (B) Serous acinus.

> **Clinical Application of Epithelia**
>
> *Epithelial tumors*: Excessive erratic growth of epithelium causes epithelial tumors. These can be benign (noncancerous) or malignant (cancerous).
> - *Benign*: For example, papilloma—tumors of cutaneous or mucous membrane origin.
> - *Malignant*: Cancer
> - *Adenoma*: Tumors of secreting glandular origin.

CONNECTIVE TISSUE

> **AN66.1:** Describe and identify various types of connective tissue with functional correlation.

Connective tissue connects all the other tissues together and fills the interstices between other specialized elements in a tissue.

Functions

- Binding other tissues.
- Supportive.
- Strengthening.
- Protection and insulation of internal organs: Capsules, septa, and sheaths.
- Transport: Blood.
- Storage of fat: Superficial fascia—insulation and prevention of heat loss.

Components of Connective Tissue

- *Cells:* They are few and widely separated by intercellular substance. They are categorized into two types:
  1. *Fixed cells:* These are intrinsic components of connective tissue, e.g., fibroblasts, undifferentiated mesenchymal cells, pigment cells, and fat cells.
  2. *Free cells:* These will be circulating in the blood and reach the connective tissue, e.g., macrophages, plasma cells, mast cells, lymphocytes, neutrophils, eosinophils, and leukocytes.
- *Intercellular substance:* The two components of it are:
  1. *Ground substance* in which is embedded numerous fibers.
  2. *Fibers:* These are of three types: (1) Collagen, (2) Reticular, and (3) Elastic.

The fibers and ground substance are synthesized by connective tissue cells. The relative abundance of various kinds of fibers, cells, and ground substance varies greatly from one type of connective tissue to another. The different types of cells of connective tissue, their structure, and their functions were presented in **Table 2.6** and **Figures 2.10A to H**.

Fibers of Connective Tissue

The fibers of connective tissue provide strength and support to it. Three different fibers are seen in the matrix, i.e., (1) Collagen, (2) Elastic, and (3) Reticular. The different types of fibers of connective tissue, their structure, and their functions were presented in **Table 2.7** and **Figures 2.11A to C**.

Chapter 2: Levels of Organization and Tissues of the Body

Table 2.6: Description of different cells of connective tissue.

Cells and description	Structure (Figs. 2.10A to E)
Fibroblasts: ❑ Most common cells of connective tissue ❑ Cells are large and flat with branching processes ❑ Appear fusiform in profile view ❑ Functions: ➢ Synthesize proteins, collagen, and elastin that forms collagen, reticular, and elastic fibers ➢ Secrete "ground substance" ➢ Help in wound healing	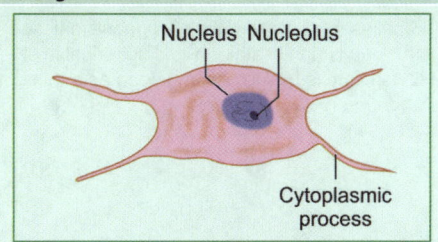 A

Macrophages (histiocytes):
❑ Most abundant in highly vascular areas
❑ They are of two types, i.e., (1) Fixed/resting and (2) Free/wandering macrophages
  1. Resting cells are irregular in shape with number of processes. The nucleus is round in shape. The cytoplasm is darkly stained
  2. The wandering cells are active cells and are larger containing cytoplasm filled with granules. The nucleus is kidney shaped and eccentrically located
❑ Function: Concerned with immunity
	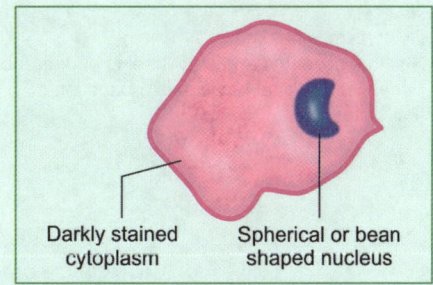
	B

Adipose cells: ❑ They are also called fat cells because of accumulation of fat droplets in their cytoplasm ❑ They occur singly or in groups ❑ The cells are rounded in shape. Cytoplasm is displaced peripherally by a single large fat droplet ❑ The nucleus is oval in shape and pushed against cell membrane giving signet ring appearance ❑ Functions: ➢ Store house of energy ➢ Provides insulation ➢ Protection and support to adjacent viscera	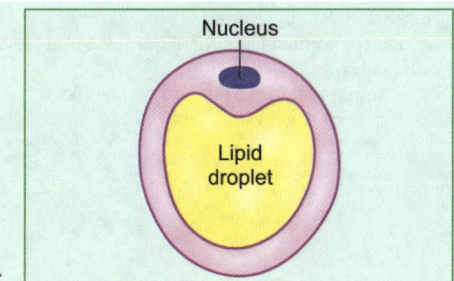 C
Mast cells: ❑ They are seen in small groups around blood vessels ❑ They are irregular in shape with short pseudopodia ❑ Nucleus is small and cytoplasm is crowded by large number of prominent secretory granules ❑ The granules contain heparin (anticoagulant) and histamine (vasodilator) ❑ Function: They are responsible for allergic reaction known as hypersensitivity reaction	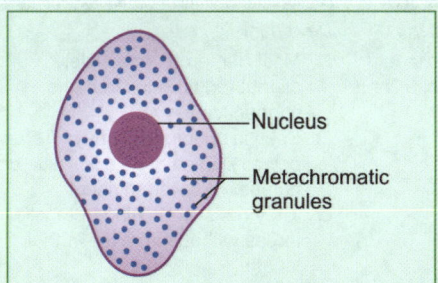 D
Pericytes: ❑ These are cells that are seen external to endothelium of capillaries and small venules ❑ Cytoplasm is pale staining and possesses long processes ❑ They can differentiate into fibroblasts, smooth muscle cells, and myofibroblasts during wound healing	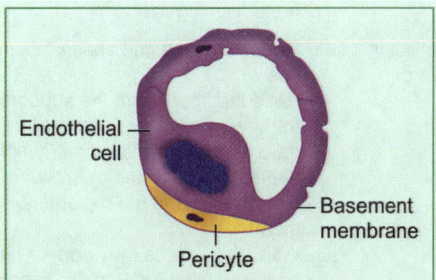 E

Contd...

Contd...

Cells and description	Structure (Figs. 2.10F to H)
Lymphocytes: ❑ Smallest of the free cells of connective tissue ❑ Nucleus is darkly stained and spherical in shape ❑ Cytoplasm is basophilic and seen as a thin rim	F — Nucleus, Agranular cytoplasm
Plasma cells: ❑ Cytoplasm is basophilic ❑ Nucleus eccentric and cartwheel in appearance ❑ *Function*: Principal function is production of antibodies	G — Nucleus cartwheel appearance
Eosinophils: ❑ Nucleus is usually bilobed ❑ Cytoplasm contains spherical granules that stain with acid dyes ❑ Their number increases in certain allergic inflammatory conditions	H — Bilobed nucleus, Acidophilic cytoplasm with granules

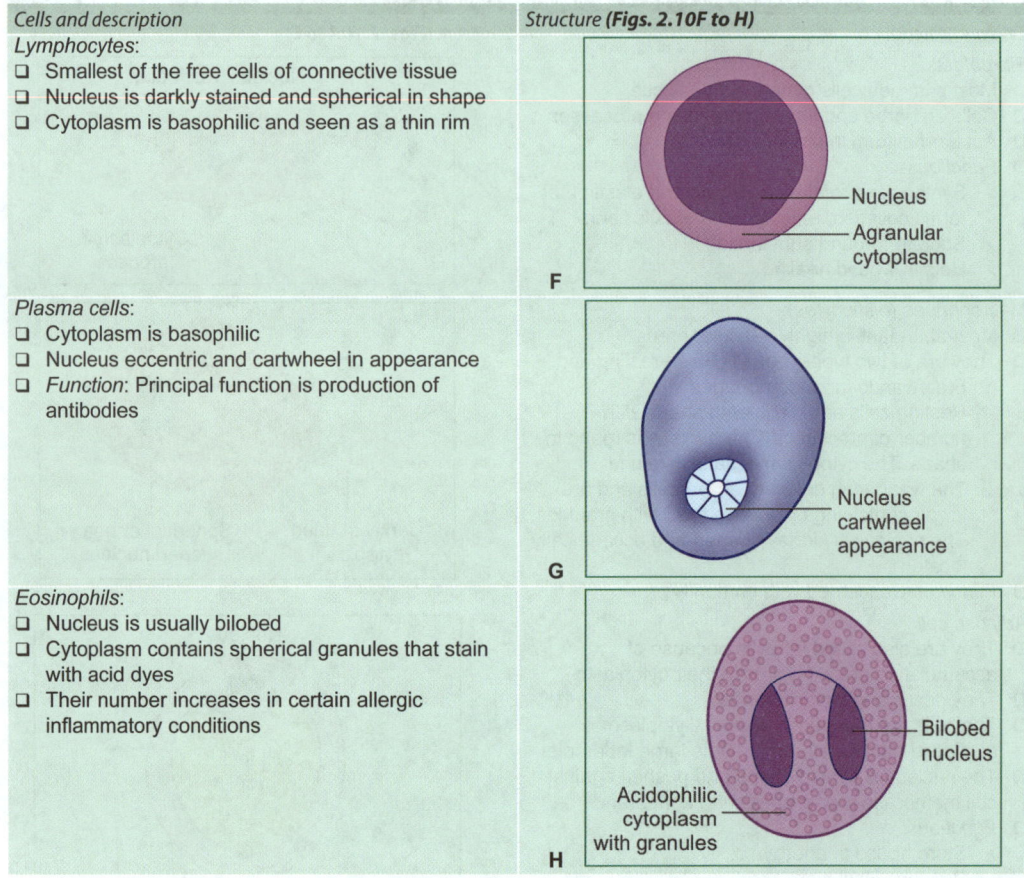

Table 2.7: Description of different fibers of connective tissue.

Fibers	Description	Structure (Figs. 2.11A and B)
Collagen/white fibers	❑ Most numerous and widely distributed fibrous elements of connective tissue ❑ Seen in bundles that may be straight or wavy. Each bundle is made up of number of collagen fibers ❑ They resist stretching or tensile forces without increase in their length ❑ Collagen fibers are made up of protein collagen	A — Nucleus, Fibroblast, Collagen fibers
Reticular fibers	❑ Fine branching and anastomosing fibers ❑ Reticular fibers form the supporting framework of many glands of reticuloendothelial tissues (lymph nodes, spleen, bone marrow, and liver) and in the basement membrane ❑ With silver stains they appear black and are called argyrophilic fibers	B — Reticular fibers

Contd...

Chapter 2: Levels of Organization and Tissues of the Body

Contd...

Fibers	Description	Structure (Fig. 2.11C)
Elastic fibers	❏ They are thinner than collagen fibers and are yellowish in color ❏ They are seen singly, branch, and rejoin freely with other fibers ❏ They are present in skin, blood vessels, and lung tissue ❏ The fibers are chiefly composed of the protein elastin together with some glycoprotein	Elastic fibers C

Ground Substance

It is a viscous colorless gel containing mostly water, mucopolysaccharides and glycoproteins. It supports cells and acts as a medium for exchange of substances between blood and cells.

Classification of Connective Tissue

AN66.1: Describe and identify various types of connective tissue with functional correlation.

The connective tissue is broadly classified into the following types and subtypes:

- *Connective tissue proper:*
  - *Loose areolar tissue:* Subcutaneous tissue.
  - *Dense regular connective tissue:* Tendon.
  - *Dense irregular connective tissue:* Capsules of organs.
- *Specialized connective tissue:*
  - Adipose tissue.
  - *Elastic tissue:* Ligamentum nuchae, lungs, and walls of arteries.
  - *Hemopoietic:* Blood.
  - *Embryonic/mucoid connective tissue:* Seen as Wharton's jelly or mucoid connective tissue in umbilical cord.
- *Supportive connective tissue:*
  - Cartilage
  - Bone.

Detailed description of major types of proper and specialized connective tissue was presented in **Table 2.8** and in **Figures 2.12A to D**.

The supportive connective tissue, i.e., cartilage and bone will be discussed in the chapter of skeletal system.

Muscular tissue and nervous tissue will be dealt in the respective chapters (5 and 9).

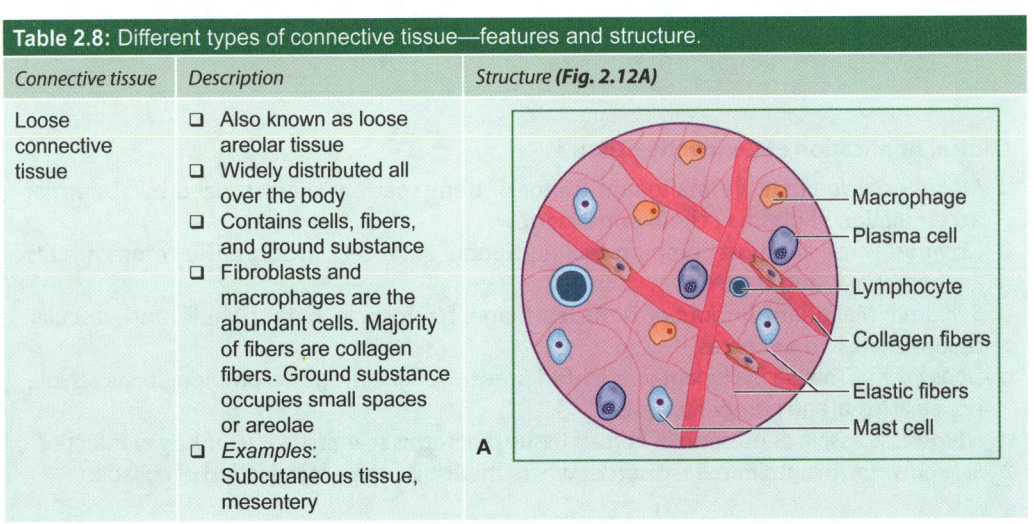

Table 2.8: Different types of connective tissue—features and structure.

Connective tissue	Description	Structure (Fig. 2.12A)
Loose connective tissue	❏ Also known as loose areolar tissue ❏ Widely distributed all over the body ❏ Contains cells, fibers, and ground substance ❏ Fibroblasts and macrophages are the abundant cells. Majority of fibers are collagen fibers. Ground substance occupies small spaces or areolae ❏ Examples: Subcutaneous tissue, mesentery	Macrophage, Plasma cell, Lymphocyte, Collagen fibers, Elastic fibers, Mast cell A

Contd...

Contd...

Connective tissue	Description	Structure (Figs. 2.12B to D)
Dense regular connective tissue	❑ Dense bundles of collagen fibers arranged parallel to each other in the form of cords or bands ❑ *Examples*: Tendons, aponeurosis, and ligaments	
Dense irregular connective tissue	❑ Seen in the form of sheets ❑ Fibers interlace to form dense network ❑ *Examples*: Dermis of skin, periosteum, perichondrium, and capsules of some organs (liver, testis, and lymph nodes)	
Adipose tissue	❑ It is widely distributed ❑ Fat cells are round or polyhedral ❑ Cells appear empty with the cytoplasm pushed to the rim ❑ Nucleus pushed to the periphery ❑ *Examples*: Subcutaneous tissue, hypodermis, and around kidney	

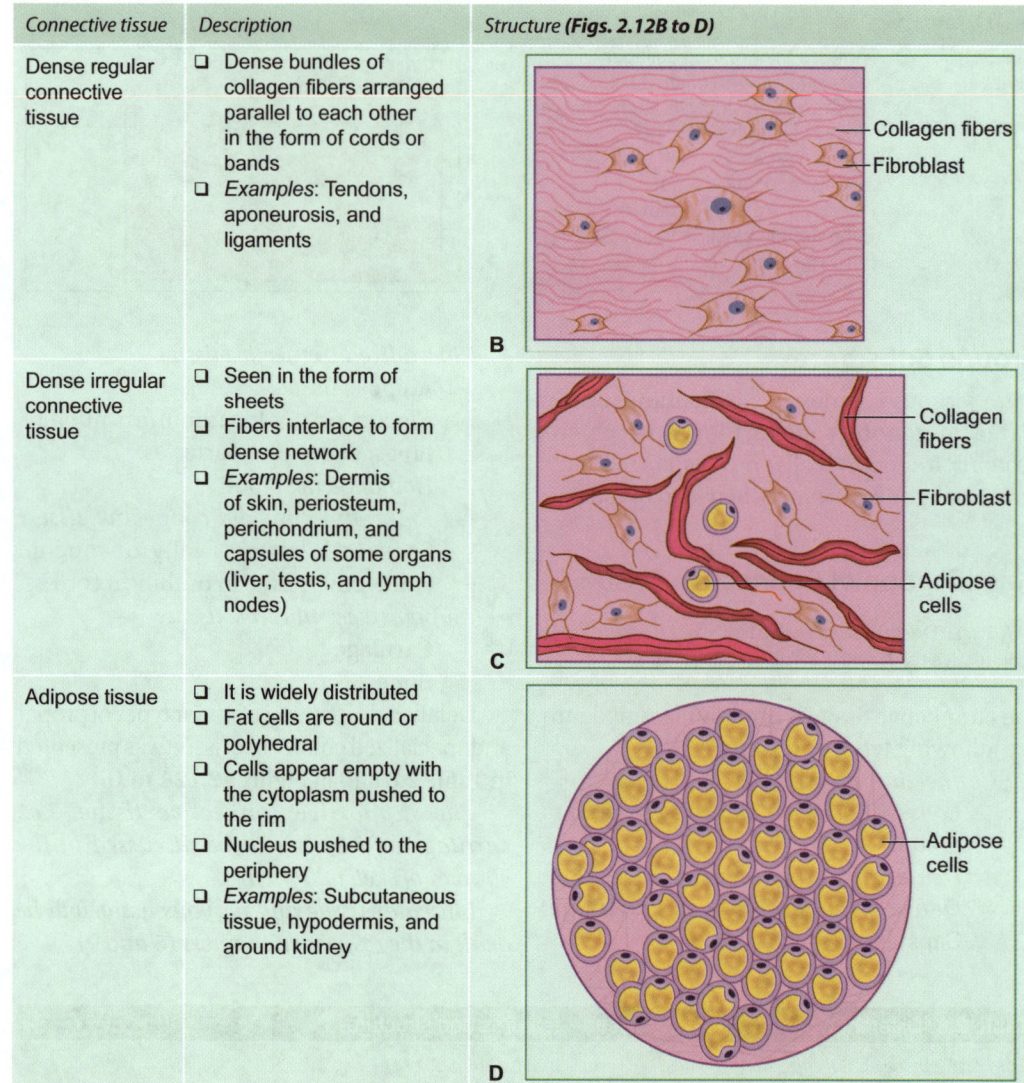

Clinical Application of Connective Tissue

- *Multiple myeloma*: It is a malignant tumor of bone marrow characterized by abnormal accumulation of plasma cells in bone marrow.
- *Lipomas*: These are most common benign tumors of fat cells in adult. The common sites are neck, back, and shoulder.
- *Sarcoma*: Malignant tumors of bone, cartilage, fat, muscle, hemopoietic, and vascular tissues are called sarcomas.
- *Liposarcoma*: This is a malignant tumor of adipose cell origin. The most common sites are thigh, popliteal fossa, and retroperitoneal.
- *Fibrosis*: Excessive deposition of fibrous tissue that forms scar tissue after injury or infection.
- *Scleroderma*: An autoimmune disorder where there will be overproduction of collagen.

Contd...

Chapter 2: Levels of Organization and Tissues of the Body

Contd…

- *Osteogenesis imperfecta*: Improper formation of collagen fibers in bone resulting in weak and breakable bones.
- *Marfan's syndrome*: Abnormal elastic tissue in the body due to the defective fibrillin production presents abnormalities in organs that contain elastic fibers. This is an autosomal dominant disorder. This can cause:
  - Subluxation (dislocation) of lens due to weakness of suspensory ligament of lens.
  - Rupture of major blood vessels like aorta (aortic aneurysm) due to the weakness of tunica media in its wall.
  - Uncontrolled growth of long bones leading to gigantism.

Anatomical Basis for Clinical Condition

Case Scenario

Problem: A teenage male comes to the physician with a complaint of loose joints, short-sightedness (myopia), and chest pain that is referring to back.
History: On enquiry he stated that one of his maternal uncles had a similar problem and died at a premature age.
Clinical examination: On examination the teenager was found to be very thin and tall (6 ft and 5 inches) with long limbs, long hands, and depressed chest.
Investigations: The patient was advised eye examination by an ophthalmologist, chest X-ray, and an echocardiogram.

Questions:
1. What is the probable diagnosis?
2. What is the importance of family history in this case?
3. What tissue is defective in this condition?
4. What is the basis for the defects in heart or cardiovascular system, eyes, long bones, and joints? Why examination of eye, chest X-ray, and echocardiogram were advised?

Anatomical explanation:
1. It is a case of Marfan's syndrome.
2. Family history of a closely related member dying with the same defect suggests that it has a genetic basis with familial incidence.
3. Marfan's syndrome is due to abnormality in elastic tissue in the body that resulted from defective fibrillin production.
4. It presents abnormalities in organs that contain elastic fibers, i.e.,
   - Weakness of suspensory ligament of lens resulting in dislocation of lens of eye and resulting myopia. *Hence, an examination of eye was advised to find out dislocation of lens.*
   - Loose joints are due to the stretching of the ligaments containing elastic fibers in relation to joints and resultant weakness.
   - Uncontrolled growth of long bones leading to gigantism is the cause for tall stature, long arms and legs, hands, and feet. It is because of the defect in elastic fibers in periosteum of long bones. The chest bone can be depressed that shows pressure symptoms on heart. *Hence, chest X-ray was advised to rule out abnormalities in chest bones, heart, and lungs.*
   - Because the disease affects the elastic fibers in the tunica media of blood vessels especially the elastic artery or aorta near its origin from the heart the symptom of chest pain referring to back (*tearing or dissecting of tunica media of aorta*) is complained by the patient. *An echocardiogram was advised to rule our cardiac or aortic defect.*

☞ Key Concept

Take Home Message—Levels of Organization, Cell, and Tissue

- The six levels of structural organization of human body, i.e., chemical, cellular, tissue, organ, organ system, and organism coordinate and work together for maintaining the life processes.
- Structure of various intracellular organelles and their function facilitates logical interpretation of the conditions of improper function due to damage or disease of the organelles, e.g., loss of Golgi apparatus function affects the bone and cartilage cells. Defective function of mitochondria affects the cells that require high energy, i.e., muscle, brain, heart, etc.
- Epithelia have different functions at different locations, e.g., epithelial tissue of skin protects from various harmful chemicals, bacteria, excessive temperatures, etc. Cells cannot function properly when they are getting older as in cells of skin; can get damaged with wear and tear and by disease; cannot be replaced when they are shed normally as in skin and epithelia of GIT. Some of the cells cannot be replaced like the neurons as in cases of paralysis, Parkinson's disease, etc. In cancers there is uncontrolled growth of defective cells.
- Glandular epithelial are responsible for secretion of specific substances that play an important role in various functions like absorption (intestinal epithelium), excretion (epithelial of kidney) as failure of their function results in toxicity.
- Connective tissue connects all the other tissues and fills the interstices between other specialized elements in a tissue. The three important components of connective tissue are: (1) Cells, (2) Fibers, and (3) Ground substance.
- Defective formation of collagen and elastic fibers can result in defects in the function of the organ containing the fibers.
- Tumors of connective tissue can arise from various cells like fat cells, plasma cells.
- For the study of tissues and their organization light microscope is sufficient. For study of organelles electron microscope is required.
- Understanding of structure and function of different epithelia and connective tissue are required for interpreting their alterations in various disease conditions.

QUESTIONS

1. Describe the endoplasmic reticulum.
2. Classify epithelia with examples.
3. Structure of serous and mucus acini.
4. Microscopic structure of loose connective tissue.
5. Classification of connective tissue with examples.
6. Describe the cells of connective tissue.
7. Describe the fibers of connective tissue.

MULTIPLE CHOICE QUESTIONS

1. **Centrioles are present in all of the following, *except*:**
   A. Cilia
   B. Flagella
   C. Mitotic spindle
   D. Microvilli

2. **Which one of the following statements is true about rough endoplasmic reticulum?**
   A. Concerned with steroid synthesis

B. Concerned with detoxification
C. Concerned with protein synthesis
D. Concerned with storage

3. **Which one of the following combinations is correct?**

A. Microvilli—epididymis
B. Cilia—trachea
C. Microvilli—proximal convoluted tubules of kidney
D. Stereocilia—intestine

ANSWERS

1. D   2. C   3. C

CHAPTER

3　Introduction to Skin and Fascia

LEARNING OBJECTIVES

- ❖ Basic structure of skin and its appendages with their clinical importance
- ❖ Regional variations in the skin and its appendages
- ❖ Basic structure of fascia and types of fascia
- ❖ Superficial fascia and its contents
- ❖ Deep fascia and its modifications
- ❖ Cavities of the body
- ❖ Serous membranes
- ❖ Clinical case with anatomical explanation

SKIN

Skin is the largest sensory organ of the body. It is about 4 kg in weight which is 16% of body weight. It covers an area of 16–22 square feet (about 2 m^2). The skin forms an outer protective cover for the entire surface of the body. The thickness of skin varies in different parts of the body. Accordingly, there are two types of skin.

1. *Thick skin:* It covers the back of the body, palms and soles. It is hairless.
2. *Thin skin:* At other places of body, the skin is thin and hairy. Very thin skin is present on eyelids.

Mucocutaneous Junction

- It is the place where the skin is continuous with the mucous membrane.
- *Example*: Lips, anus, urethra, nostrils, vagina (in females), foreskin of prepuce (in males), and eyelids.

Functions

- *Protection:* Protects the body from chemicals, ultraviolet rays, mechanical injury and microorganisms.
- *Barrier:* Acts as a barrier and prevents water absorption.
- *Temperature regulation*: It helps in maintaining normal body temperature. In summer by secretion and evaporation of sweat. In winter due to the presence of subcutaneous fat, it maintains body temperature.
- *Sensory:* Presence of various sensory nerve endings in the skin facilitates perception of sensation of pain, temperature, touch, etc.
- *Excretory:* Excretion of urea.
- *Vitamin D:* It synthesizes vitamin D.

Structure of Skin

AN 72.1: Identify the skin and its appendages under the microscope and correlate the structure and function.
AN 4.1: Describe different types of skin and dermatomes in body.
AN 4.2: Describe structure and function of skin with its appendages.
AN 4.5: Explain principles of skin incisions (Details in Surface anatomy chapter).

There are three layers in skin (**Figs. 3.1 and 3.2** and **Table 3.1**) in which are located its four appendages.

Chapter 3: Introduction to Skin and Fascia

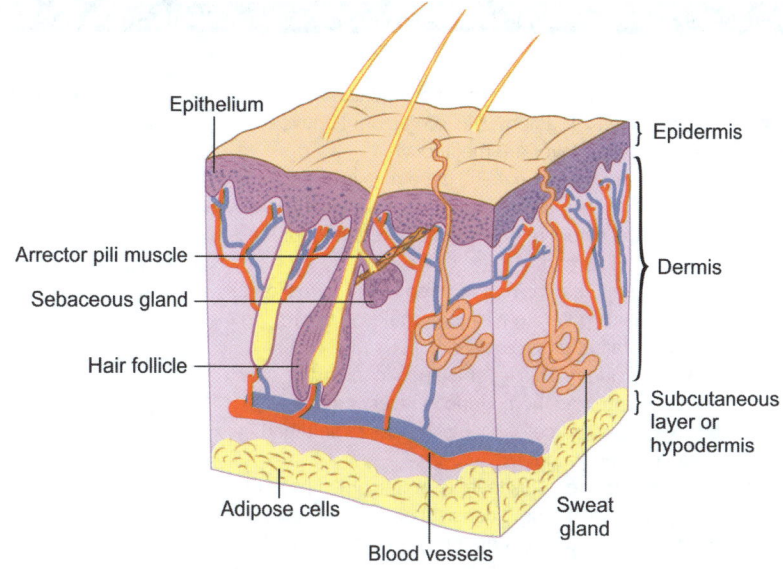

Fig. 3.1: Skin and appendages.

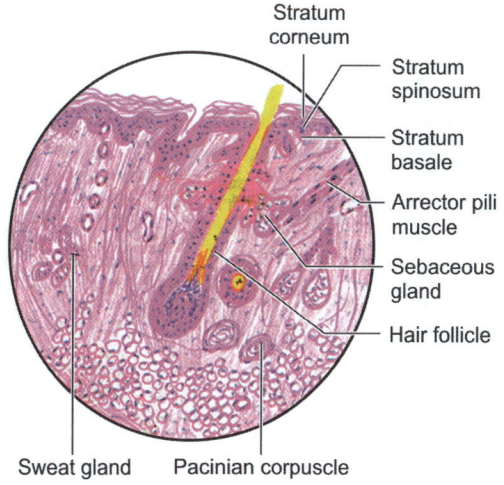

Fig. 3.2: Schematic diagram of microscopic structure of skin.

Layers of skin are as follows:
1. *Epidermis:* Surface layer of epithelium.
2. *Dermis:* Middle connective tissue layer.
3. *Hypodermis/subcutaneous layer:* It is the deeper loose connective tissue layer.

Epidermis (Fig. 3.3)
- It is the surface layer and is in contact with the external environment.
- It is lined by stratified squamous keratinized epithelium.
- It is avascular.
- It contains epithelial and nonepithelial cells.
  - *Epithelial cells*: The epithelial cells of epidermis are arranged in five layers. They are:
    1. *Stratum basale/germinativum*
    2. *Stratum spinosum*
    3. *Stratum granulosum*
    4. *Stratum lucidum*
    5. *Stratum corneum*
- *Nonepithelial cells*: There are three types of nonepithelial cells in epidermis. They are *melanocytes, Langerhans cells* and *Merkel cells*.
  1. *Melanocytes*: These are dendritic, pigmented cells that are found in stratum basale. These produce the coloring pigment melanin that is responsible for the color of skin, eyes and hair. In the eye, they are seen in the choroid layer. These protect the skin against bright sun light (UV rays). They are more in areas exposed to light, i.e., face.
  2. *Langerhans cells*: These are antigen presenting cells present in all the

Chapter 3: Introduction to Skin and Fascia

Table 3.1: Skin and its appendages—structure and regional variations (Figs. 3.1 to 3.3, 3.6 and 3.7).

Part	Structure	Regional variations
Epidermis	❑ *Stratum basale*: Single layer of cuboidal/low columnar cells. Pigment cells are present between the cells of this layer are melanocytes ❑ *Stratum spinosum*: Contains several layers of polyhedral cells, called keratinocytes as they produce the cytokeratin, the protein required for the formation of keratin ❑ *Stratum granulosum*: Two or three layers of fusiform cells containing keratohyaline granules that form the protein keratin that protects skin ❑ *Stratum lucidum*: This layer is seen in thick skin only. It is an amorphous homogenous layer composed of closely packed cells in which traces of flattened nuclei may be found ❑ *Stratum corneum*: This layer is prominent in palm of hand and sole of foot. It consists of several layers of horny/dead cell that appear flat and are without nuclei	❑ Stratum corneum/keratin layer is more prominent in palms and soles as they are subjected to friction ❑ Prominent stratum corneum in thick skin ❑ Very thin or absent of stratum corneum in thin skin
Dermis	❑ Highly vascular connective tissue in two layers ❑ Superficial papillary layer containing papillae ❑ Deep reticular layer of collagen and elastic fibers	Papillae are more prominent in palms and soles
Hypodermis	Contains adipose tissue and large vessels.	Contains: ❑ Muscles of facial expression in face ❑ Hair follicles in scalp ❑ Apocrine glands in axilla, groin
Nail	❑ *Nail plate*: Stratum corneum ❑ *Nail bed*: Stratum basale, stratum spinosum and dermis ❑ *Cuticle or eponychium*: Projecting fold of stratum corneum towards proximal part of nail ❑ *Hyponychium*: Epidermal thickening between free edge of nail and skin of finger tip ❑ *Nail matrix*: Thickened stratum germinativum. ❑ *Lunula*: White crescent shaped area	Present on dorsal aspect of terminal phalanges of fingers and toes
Hair (shaft/root)	❑ *Medulla*: It forms central axis and contains two to three layers of keratinized cuboidal cells ❑ *Cortex*: Several layers of flat keratinized cells with pigment granules ❑ *Cuticle*: Single layer of flat scale like cells	❑ Found all over the body surface ❑ *Absent* in palms, soles and lips ❑ *Absent* in labia minora, glans penis, prepuce
Hair follicle	❑ *Hair bulb*: Expanded part ❑ *Papilla*: Projection of dermis in the center of hair bulb ❑ *Medulla:* Innermost core of hair shaft ❑ *Cortex*: formed by stratum basale/germinativum ❑ *Internal root sheath*: Stratum granulosum and corneum ❑ *External root sheath*: Formed by basal layer of epidermis	

Contd...

Chapter 3: Introduction to Skin and Fascia

Contd...

Part	Structure	Regional variations
Sebaceous gland	❑ Located between hair follicle and arrectores pilorum muscle in dermis ❑ Secreting unit contains peripheral cuboidal, middle large polyhedral and central disintegrated cells ❑ Duct is lined by stratified squamous epithelium ❑ Obliquely arranged smooth muscle arrectores pilorum	❑ Modified sebaceous glands are seen in eyelid as Meibomian glands ❑ Absent in skin of palm and sole ❑ Abundant in face, scalp, ears, nostrils
Eccrine sweat glands	❑ Deep, highly coiled secretory part and superficial excretory part ❑ Secretory part is lined by cuboidal epithelium ❑ Excretory ducts open on the surface of the skin and are lined by stratified cuboidal epithelium	❑ Throughout the body ❑ More abundant in palms and soles ❑ Absent on external genitalia
Apocrine sweat gland	❑ Less coiled than eccrine glands ❑ Both secretory part and duct are lined by cuboidal epithelium The ducts open on to the hair follicle as both develop in common	❑ Present in axilla, scrotum, and perianal regions ❑ Modified apocrine sweat glands are: ➢ Ceruminous glands in ear ➢ Glands of Moll in eyelids ➢ Mammary gland

strata of epidermis with more number in stratum spinosum. These produce cell mediated immunological response in skin. Their number is increased in inflammatory skin diseases.

> **Clinical Importance of Langerhans Cells**
>
> They are responsible for skin graft rejection and they protect against epidermal tumors.

3. *Merkel cells*: These are sensory cells (Mechanoreceptors) that can recognize the sense of touch. These are seen in stratum basale. These are innervated by sensory nerves and are more in hair follicles and skin of finger tips.

Dermis
- It is highly vascular connective tissue containing collagen fibers, elastic fibers, blood vessels, lymph vessels and nerves.
- Its thickness varies in different parts of the body. It is thicker on the back of the trunk. It is thinner in women than in men.
- It is connected to the underlying deep fascia or to the bones by superficial fascia.
- The collagen, elastic and reticular fibers that provide strength, toughness, resilience and recoiling properties to the skin. Though the fibers run in different directions, in a specific location they run parallel to each other. The pattern of these fibers determines the wrinkle lines on the body.
- There are two layers in dermis. They are superficial *papillary* and deep *reticular* layers.
  1. **Papillary layer** consists of loose connective tissue with numerous highly sensitive and vascular eminences termed the papillae. These project into the pits of the epidermis. These ridges are more prominent in palm of the hand and sole of the foot. In some papillae there are tactile corpuscles. This layer provides nutrition to the epidermis.
  2. **Reticular layer** consists of strong interlacing bands of dense connective tissue composed chiefly of collagen fibers with some elastic fibers. The connective tissue bands run in parallel bundles and form *cleavage lines of Langer*.
- *Langer's line or cleavage lines:* These are the lines on the surface of skin. These are produced because of the orientation of collagen fiber bundles in the dermis.

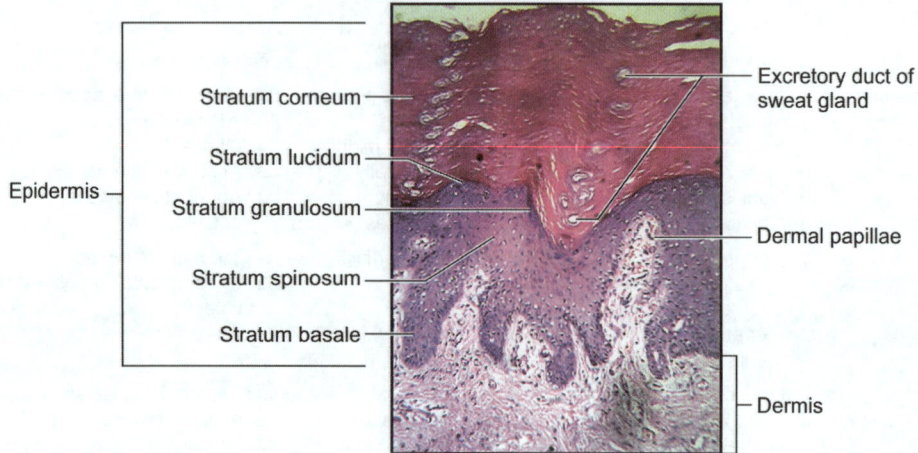

Fig. 3.3: Layers of epidermis—microscopic structure.

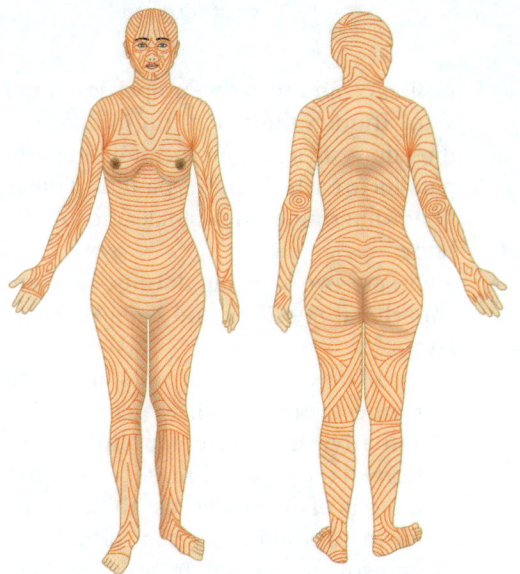

Fig. 3.4: Langer's lines—ventral and dorsal aspects of body.

The direction of these lines in different parts of the body varies as shown in **Figure 3.4**.

Clinical Importance

- The direction of Langer's lines are important in surgical procedures for cosmetic reason.
- Incisions along these lines for surgeries sever fewer collagen fibers and as a result the healing is faster and the scar is minimal.
- When incisions are made across these cleavage lines, healing is delayed and can form an ugly scar. These lines are important in surgical procedures especially cosmetic surgery.

- *Wrinkles in the skin:* Loss of collagen and elastic fibers in the dermis in old age causes senile wrinkles. Over exposure to sun also causes wrinkling of skin.
- *Dermatome:* The area of skin supplied by a single spinal segment is called dermatome. Knowledge of dermatomes is important in neurological examination to identify the involvement or localization of spinal segment of injury by testing for the loss of sensation in a conscious patient. The various dermatomes of the body are represented in **Figure 3.5**. Refer Chapter 9: Introduction to Nervous System for detailed explanation of dermatomes.

AN 4.1: Describe different types of skin and dermatomes in body.
Note: Dermatomes are described in detail in Chapter 9: Introduction to Nervous System.

Chapter 3: Introduction to Skin and Fascia

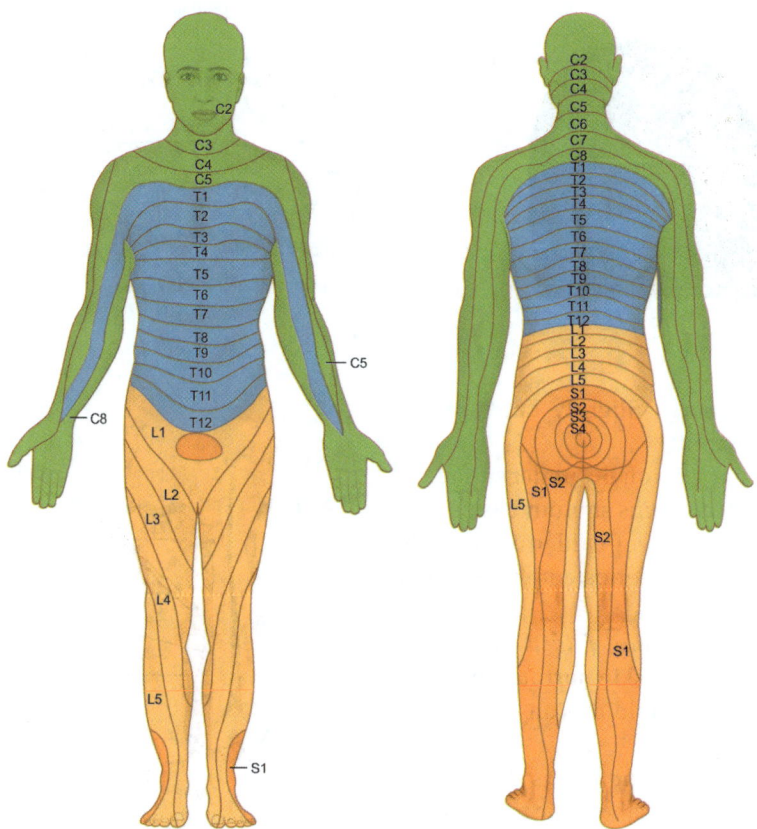

Fig. 3.5: Dermatomes of the body—ventral and dorsal aspects.

Hypodermis
- Deepest layer and contains adipose tissue and large vessels that supply and drain the dermis.
- It is divided into compartments by fibrous septa that extend from the reticular layer of dermis.
- In certain parts of the body, e.g., face it contains sheets of skeletal muscles called muscles of facial expression.
- In certain parts it contains hair follicles (scalp) or apocrine glands (axilla, groin).
- It is also called subcutaneous tissue.
- *Hypodermic needle*: This is the word used for the needle that is attached to the syringe for injecting medicines into the body by various routes (intramuscular, subcutaneous, intravenous) or for drawing fluids (blood, pleural and peritoneal, cerebrospinal, etc.). As the needle passes through the layers of skin it is called hypodermic needle.
- *Subcutaneous injection*: It is a method of administering medicine. It is a highly effective for administering vaccines, insulin, local anesthetics. The absorption of medicine is slow in this route.

Appendages of Skin

1. *Nails*
2. *Hairs and hair follicles*
3. *Sebaceous glands*
4. *Sweat glands.*

Nails **(Figs. 3.6A and B)***:* Nails are modification of stratum corneum of epidermis. They are located on the dorsal aspect of terminal phalanges of fingers and toes **(Fig. 3.6A)**. Parts of a nail are **(Fig. 3.6B)**.

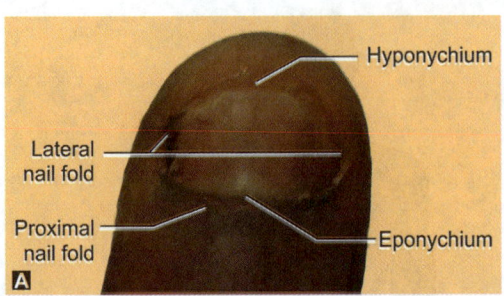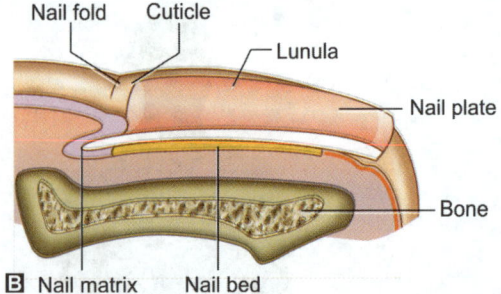

Figs. 3.6A and B: Nails.

- *Nail plate/body*: Slightly convex and semitransparent.
- *Nail bed:* It is seen on the under surface of nail plate. It contains stratum basale and stratum spinosum of epidermis, dermis and is attached to periosteum of terminal phalanx.
- *Nail groove and nail fold:* Nail groove is invagination of skin surrounded by a crescent shaped fold of skin called nail fold.
- *Cuticle or eponychium:* It is the part of skin which lies directly on the top of newly developing nail plate.
- *Hyponychium:* It is the epidermal thickening between the free edge of nail plate and skin of fingertip.
- *Nail matrix:* It is the site of active proliferation of nail located in proximal nail fold and is responsible for the growth of nail.
- *Lunula:* It is the white crescent-shaped area of nail matrix.

Hair and hair follicles (Fig. 3.7):
- The hairs are found in every part of the body surface but are absent in palm, sole, lips, labia minora, prepuce and glans penis.
- They are extensions of epidermis into the deep dermis often extending into hypodermis.
- The hair consists of:
  - *Hair follicle:* It is the deeper part containing both epidermis and dermis.

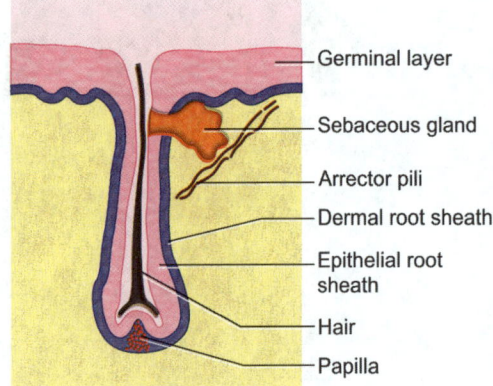

Fig. 3.7: Hair, sebaceous gland, and arrectores pilorum muscle.

- Expanded part of hair follicle at its base is called the *hair bulb*.
- In the center of hair bulb is the *hair papilla*, a projection of dermis. Hair papilla contains the blood vessels, myelinated and unmyelinated nerves.
- Duct of sebaceous gland opens into the hair follicle at the junction of dilated infundibulum and narrow isthmus region of the hair follicle.
- Minute bundles of involuntary muscle fibers, the *arrectores pilorum* are connected with the hair follicles below the level of sebaceous gland duct.
- The hair follicle is avascular and the growth of hair is due to the capillaries that form vascular plexus in the dermal papilla.

Chapter 3: Introduction to Skin and Fascia

- *Root:* It is implanted into the skin and is the extension of hair follicle.
- *Shaft:* Free part that projects from the surface.

Sebaceous glands:
- These are associated with hair follicles and located between hair follicle and arrectores pilorum muscle in dermis (**Fig. 3.7**).
- These are *holocrine glands* as their secretory products are parts of decomposed cells. It is an example for *programmed cell death* or *apoptosis* as the death of cells is normal and in a programmed or orchestrated pattern. The secretion is called *sebum* and is rich in lipids. Their secretions are transported by means of a duct into the infundibulum of hair follicle and then on to the surface of the skin.
- They are present on the slanting under surface of the follicle and lie within the dermis. They open near the neck of the follicle and pour out their secretion, the *sebum*.
- Sebum is oily and passes along the hair to reach the skin surface. It helps to preserve the flexibility of hair and also lubricates the skin surface. It collects dirt and dust and has been found to have bactericidal (bacteria killing) action.
  - *Arrectores pilorum:*
    - The muscle (or the arrector pili, Greek. Arrector = raiser, pilore = hair) runs from the under surface of the follicle to the superficial aspect of dermis (**Fig. 3.7**).
    - *Goose flesh appearance:* Contraction of this muscle causes straightening of hair (erection) and makes the skin look like that of goose skin that occurs on exposure to cold or when one is frightened.
    - Contraction of the muscle expresses the contents of sebaceous gland.

Sweat glands:
- The sweat glands (sudoriferous glands) are found in every part of the skin.
- These are of two types, i.e., eccrine and apocrine.

Pilosebaceous unit: Hair, hair follicle, sebaceous gland and arrectores pilorum muscle together form the pilosebaceous unit.

Clinical Importance

Skin and its Appendages:
- **Dermatoglyphics**: The papillary layer of dermis gives out finger-like projections called dermal papillae that project into the overlying epidermis. In the palms and soles these dermal papillae and the adjacent epidermal ridges produce typical patterns on the fingertips, palms and soles. These are called friction ridges and they increase the gripping ability of hands and feet. These are permanent identification marks of an individual. These patterns are called dermatoglyphics and have genetic basis. Study of these patterns is used in medicolegal investigation, for establishing identity of an individual and in medical genetics (**Figs. 3.8A and B**). It is used as a diagnostic tool in individuals with chromosomal abnormalities (Down's syndrome) and in certain medical conditions (cancers, hypertension, mental illness, and diabetes).
- **Acne vulgaris**: Inflammatory disease of pilosebaceous unit.
- **Albinism**: Congenital disorder. There will be complete or partial absence of melanin in skin, hair and iris. An inborn error in metabolism of tyrosine enzyme results in failure to synthesize melanin pigment by melanocytes.
- **Alopecia areata**: Sudden hair loss especially on scalp with hairless oval patches.
- **Alopecia totalis**: Loss of hair all over the scalp (**Fig. 3.9**).

- **Alopecia universalis**: Loss of hair all over the body.
- **Vitiligo**: An autoimmune disease that results from destruction of melanocytes leading to depigmentation of skin. It presents as glaring white patches **(Fig. 3.10)**.
- **Sun tanning**: When skin is exposed to ultraviolet rays, there will be darkening due to the accumulation of melanin as a protective measure.
- **Skin burns classification**: Depending on the extent of involvement of epidermis and dermis they are classified into:
  - **First degree**: Only epidermis is involved and it heals within one week.
  - **Second degree**: Epidermis and superficial dermis are involved. The wound heals in few weeks.
  - **Third degree**: Both epidermis and dermis are involved. Regeneration is not possible as the hair follicles are destroyed which are the sites of regeneration. Hence it requires skin grafting.
- **Assessment of percentage of surface area of skin involved in burns**: To calculate the percentage rule of nine is followed for taking a decision to start fluid replacement therapy or for transferring to burns unit for special care. The body surface area of an adult with burns is estimated by "rule of 9" using 9% each (head and neck and each upper limb) or multiples of it, i.e., 18% each (front of trunk, back of trunk, each lower limb) and 1% for perineum.
- **Hidradinitis suppurativa**: It is also known as acne inversa. Inflamed, swollen and painful lumps with pus. Commonly seen in axilla and groin **(Fig. 3.11)**.
- **Naevi/moles**: Benign accumulation of melanocytes.
- **Malignant melanoma**: Tumor of melanocytes.
- **Basal cell carcinoma**: Skin cancer arising from cells of stratum basale.
- **Squamous cell carcinoma**: Skin cancer arising from cells in the stratum spinosum.
- **Psoriasis**: A skin disease characterized by erythematous plaques with silvery white scales.
- **Onychmycosis**: Fungal infection of toe or finger nails.
- **Onycholysis**: It is disorder of nail. Onycholysis is separation of nail from its bed **(Fig. 3.12)**.

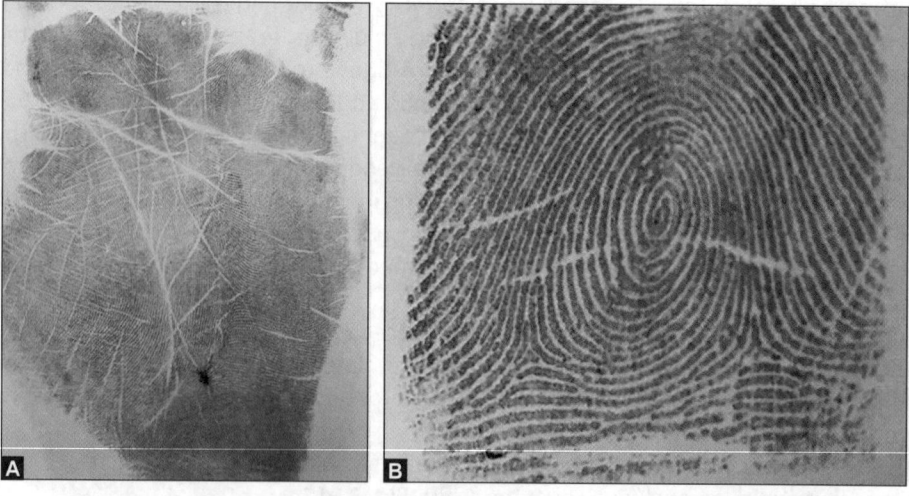

Figs. 3.8A and B: Dermatoglyphic patterns on: (A) Palm of hand; (B) Finger digit.

Chapter 3: Introduction to Skin and Fascia

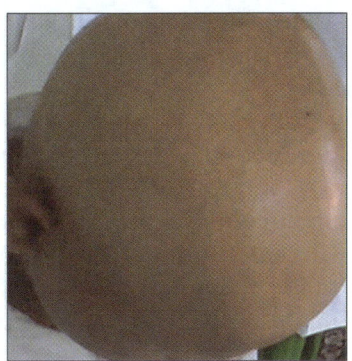

Fig. 3.9: Alopecia totalis.
Source: Dr T Ram Sharan, Dermatologist, SVIMS, Tirupati.

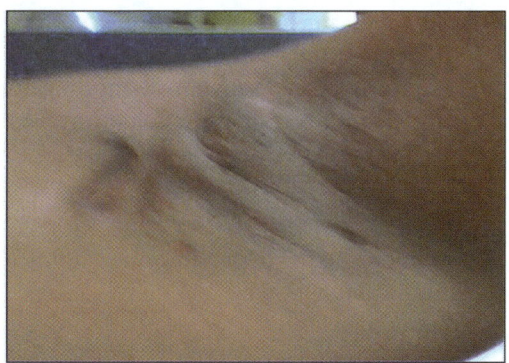

Fig. 3.11: Hidradenitis suppurativa in axilla.
Source: Dr T Ram Sharan, Dermatologist, SVIMS, Tirupati.

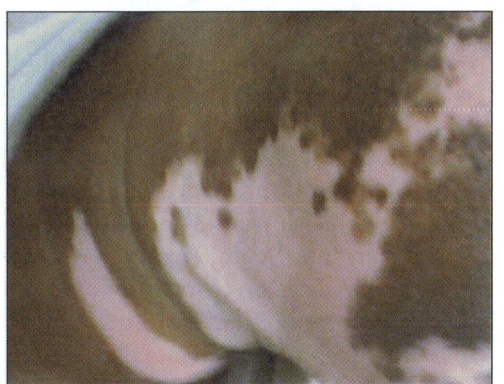

Fig. 3.10: Vitiligo.
Source: Dr T Ram Sharan, Dermatologist, SVIMS, Tirupati.

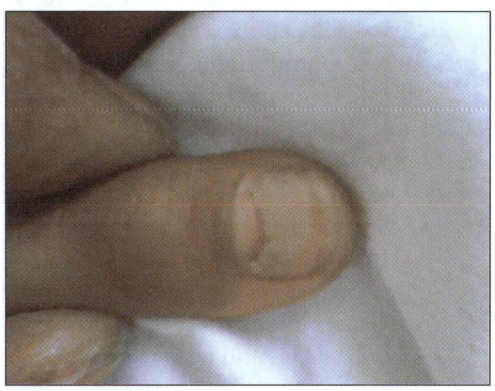

Fig. 3.12: Onycholysis.
Source: Dr T Ram Sharan, Dermatologist, SVIMS, Tirupati.

The structure of skin and its appendages and their regional variations are represented in Table 3.1.

FASCIA

> **AN 4.3:** Describe superficial fascia along with fat distribution in body.
> **AN 4.4:** Describe modifications of deep fascia with its functions.

The word fascia is derived from Latin = "band". Fascia is singular and fasciae are plural.

Definition

Fibrous tissue network in the form of a sheet or flat band.

Location

Below the surface of the skin, covering and separating muscles, organs and other tissues.

Structure

Dense regular connective tissue. Contains closely packed bundles of collagen fibers. It is oriented in a wavy pattern parallel to the direction of pull.

Functions

- Sliding and gliding surface for muscles to reduce friction.
- Suspends organs in their anatomical location.

- Transmits movement from muscles to the bones to which they are attached.
- Supportive and movable wrapping for nerves and blood vessels as they pass through and between the muscles.

Types

Three different types depending on anatomical location and function.
- Superficial fascia
- Deep fascia
- Subserous fascia

Superficial Fascia (Fig. 3.13)

- *Location:* It is the layer of loose connective tissue and it can expand. It connects the skin to the underlying deep fascia. It is also called *hypodermis* or *subcutaneous tissue*.
- *Composition:* Loose areolar and adipose tissues.
- *Functions:*
  - Determines shape of body
  - Acts as a packing material between delicate structures
  - Storage of fat and water
  - Heat insulation due to the presence of fat
  - Vehicle for neurovascular supply to skin
  - Allowing movement of skin over the underlying structures.
- *Contents:*
  - *Panniculus adiposus:* In some areas the superficial fascia contains more fat that forms a layer known as panniculus adiposus. For example, Gluteal (Buttock) region, front of thigh, mammary gland in female, in the upper part of arm (deltoid region).
  - *Panniculus carnosus (subcutaneous muscles):* Flat sheet of muscles in the panniculus adiposus is known as panniculus carnosus. These muscles are different from other muscles in the body in that they are attached at one end to the skin and at the other end to the deep fascia or bone. *Examples:* face (muscles of facial expression), scalp and auricle (occipitofrontalis muscle, auricular muscles) neck (platysma), palm (palmaris brevis), perianal region (corrugator cutis ani) and scrotum (dartos muscle). Except corrugator cutis ani and dartos all the other muscle are voluntary.
  - Mammary gland in female
  - Deeply situated sweat glands
  - Localized groups of lymph nodes
  - Cutaneous nerves and vessels.
- *Regional differences:*
  - *Distinct*—lower part of the anterior abdominal wall, perineum, and limbs.
  - *Very thin*—dorsum of hands and feet, sides of neck, face and around anus.
  - *Very dense*—scalp, palms, and soles.
  - *Stratification (into two layers):* It presents as two layers in the lower part of anterior abdominal wall, perineum, and uppermost parts of thighs.
  - *Superficial fascia without fat*—in the external ear, eyelid, and some parts of external genital organs (scrotum and penis in male and clitoris in female) the superficial fascia is devoid of fat.

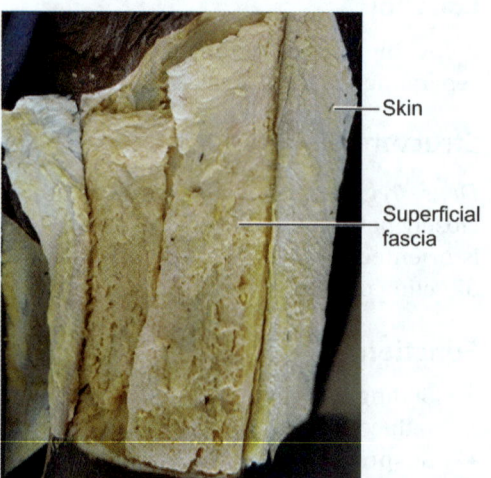

Fig. 3.13: Skin and superficial fascia.

Deep Fascia

- **Peculiarities:**
  - Dense, tough, fibrous and inelastic layer deep to superficial fascia
  - Devoid of fat
  - Covers muscles, nerves, bone, cartilage
  - Avascular
  - Richly innervated with sensory receptors for pain, movement, pressure, vibration, temperature
  - Responds to sensory input by:
    - Contracting and relaxing
    - Changing its composition through the process of fascial remodeling
- **Distribution:**
  - *Best defined* in the limbs and neck
  - *Ill-defined* in:
    - Face—absent to allow facial expressions
    - Trunk—absent in thorax to allow expansion of viscera
  - *Absent* in the anterior abdominal wall to allow expansion
- **Modification of deep fascia:** Extensions or thickenings of deep fascia form the following:
  - *Intermuscular septa:* It sends septa between different functional groups of muscles in the limbs. It also forms septa between various muscles **(Fig. 3.14)**. These septa are especially well developed in the calf muscles of lower limb.
  - *Coverings for muscles*—epimysium, perimysium, endomysium. *Described in Chapter 5.*
  - *Coverings for nerves*—epineurium, perineurium and endoneurium. *Described in Chapter 9.*
  - *Coverings for glands (fibrous capsule):* Deep fascia splits to enclose certain glands (parotid, thyroid, prostate) to form their capsule.
  - *Sheaths around large arteries,* e.g., carotid sheath, axillary sheath.
  - *In relation to joints:* Form the capsule, synovial membrane and bursae in relation to the joints. *Described in Chapter 6.*
  - *Tendon sheaths* wherever tendons cross over a joint. *Described in Chapter 5.*
  - *Fibrous flexor sheath:* Deep fascia on the flexor surface of fingers and toes is thickened **(Fig. 3.15)**. It prevents bow stringing of flexor tendons by retaining them close to the joints.
  - *Aponeuroses:* In the region of palm and sole the deep fascia is thickened

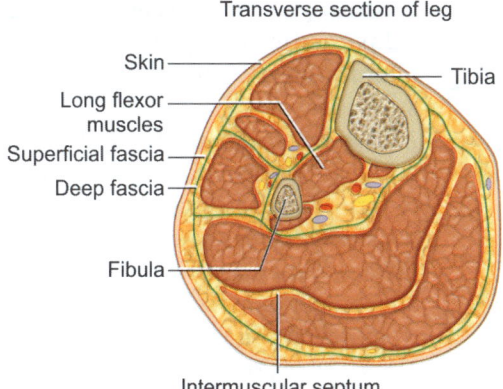

Fig. 3.14: Intermuscular septum.

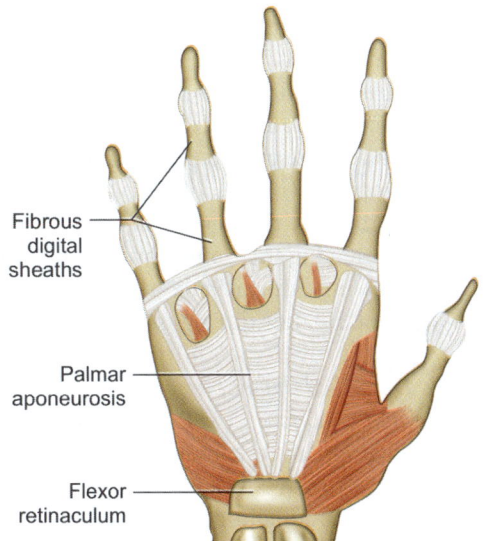

Fig. 3.15: Modifications of deep fascia in hand—fibrous digital flexor sheath, palmar aponeurosis, and flexor retinaculum.

to form aponeuroses (**Fig. 3.15**), e.g., palmar and plantar aponeuroses which afford protection to the underlying-structures.
- *Interosseous membrane:* In the forearm and leg, the deep fascia is modified to form the interosseous membrane, which keeps the two bones at optimum distance, increases surface area for attachment of muscles and transmits weight from one bone to the other. *Described in Chapter 6.*
- *Retinacula:* Near the joints especially at the wrist and ankle, the deep fascia is thickened to form the retinacula that hold the tendons in place preventing their bow stringing (**Fig. 3.11**). Seen where tendons cross the joints. For example, flexor and extensor retinacula are present around the wrist and ankle joint.
- *Ligament*—thickening of deep fascia connecting the bones forming a joint. They hold the articulating bones close to each other during movements and thus provide stability to the joint. *Described in Chapter 6.*
- *Named deep fascia:* Different names are given at different regions.
  - *Neck:* Fascia colli
  - *Back:* Thoracolumbar fascia
  - *Upper limb:* Brachial, antebrachial, palmar fascia
  - *Lower limb:* Fascia lata, crural and plantar fascia
  - *Abdomen and pelvis:* Fascia transversalis and pelvic fascia
  - *Penis:* Buck's fascia.

Subserous Fascia

- Between internal layer of deep fascia and serous membranes lining the body cavities.
- Thin in some areas, e.g., between the pleura and thoracic wall and thick in other areas where it forms a pad of adipose tissue.
- More flexible than deep fascia.
- There is a potential space between subserous and deep fasciae allowing flexibility and movement of internal organs.
- *Examples:* Endothoracic fascia, endo-abdominal fascia and endopelvic fascia.

Clinical Importance of Fascia

Superficial Fascia
Overweight and pregnancy: The superficial fascia stretches in obese people with deposition of fat and in women during pregnancy. Because of the deposition of adipose tissue in the areolar space between the bundles of collagen fibers there will be stretching of the fascia. After weight loss and after delivery it will come back to its normal state.

Deep Fascia
Intermuscular septa: In the limbs the intermuscular septa form fascial compartments that restrict bulging of muscles, loss of energy and infection. Compression of fascia on the muscles causes compression of internal veins and thus facilitates *venous return* to the heart along the unidirectional valves in the veins for example in leg.

CAVITIES OF THE BODY

- A body cavity is a fluid-filled space.
- Anatomical structures are described in terms of the cavity in which they are located. *Example:* Heart in pericardial cavity, brain in cranial cavity.
- These cavities protect the internal organs.
- These cavities are lined by membranes, protected by bones and contain fluid that protects the internal organs.
- Broadly the cavities of the body are divided into dorsal and ventral cavities based on their location in relation to the surfaces of the body (**Fig. 3.16**).
- The dorsal cavities are cranial and vertebral cavities. The cranial cavity contains the

Chapter 3: Introduction to Skin and Fascia

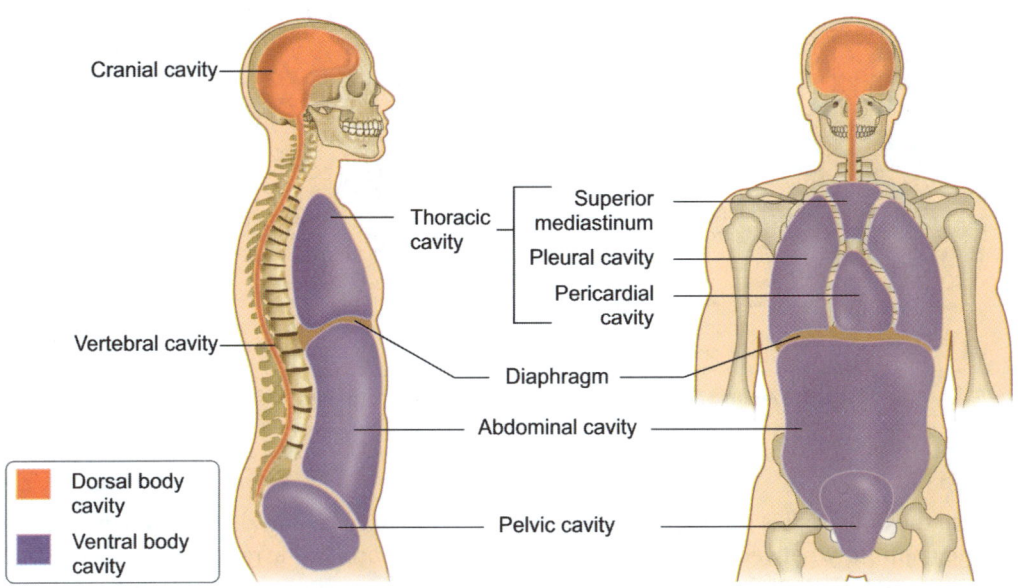

Fig. 3.16: Serous cavities of the body.

brain and the vertebral cavity contains the spinal cord, the continuation of brain. These two are covered with three layers called the meninges that protect them and the cavities within these organs are called ventricles that contain the cerebrospinal fluid that provides nourishment.
- The ventral cavities are broadly divided into thoracic and abdominopelvic cavities.
- The thoracic cavity is protected by musculoskeletal thoracic cage. It contains the lungs and heart each enclosed in a serous cavity the pleural and pericardial respectively.
- The abdominopelvic cavity is partially protected by bones. It houses the organs of digestive, urogenital systems mainly. Most of the viscera are protected by the serous cavity the peritoneal cavity.
- The serous cavities are lined by two layers of serous membranes with fluid in between.

Serous Membranes

- These are thin, delicate connective tissue membranes that line and enclose several body cavities known as serous cavities.
- One surface of this membrane is capable of secreting fluid that acts as the lubricant to reduce friction during the movement.
- Serous membranes surround important organs and structures of the body **(Fig. 3.16)**. They are:
  - Pleura—surrounding the lungs
  - Pericardium—surrounding the heart
  - Peritoneum—surrounding organs of digestive system
  - Tendon sheaths—surrounding the tendons.

Layers of Serous Membrane

- The serous membrane does not surround an organ or a structure like an envelope. But, it folds on itself to form a two layered membranous sac enclosing a cavity that contains thin film of fluid.
- The serous sac can be best described by pushing the fist of your hand into an inflated ball/balloon. The wall of ball or balloon in close contact with your hand is the visceral layer and the one away from your hand is the parietal layer and the air filled space is the cavity **(Fig. 3.17A)**.
- The layer in contact with the structure is called visceral layer and the layer in contact

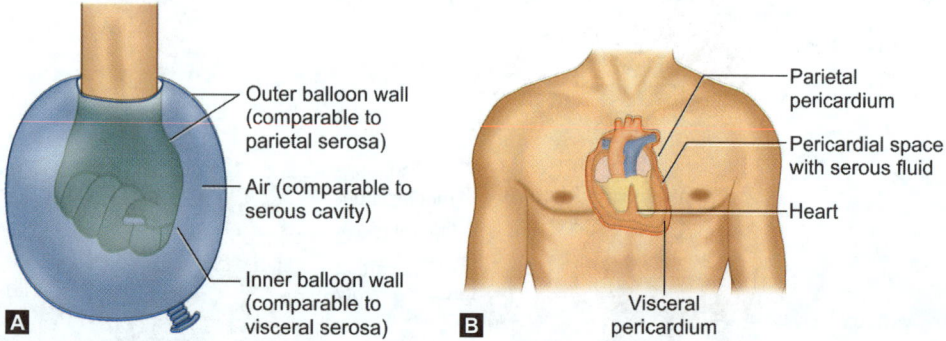

Figs. 3.17A and B: (A) Serous sac—demonstration; (B) Pericardial cavity.

with the body wall is called parietal layer. The continuity between the two layers is maintained. The cavity between the two layers is called serous cavity, the name of which varies depending on the location (pleural, pericardial and peritoneal cavities) (**Fig. 3.17B**).
- The surfaces of visceral and parietal layers facing the cavity are secretory. They secrete the serous fluid that acts as a lubricant and helps in free movement of organs.
- At the point where the parietal and visceral layers are in continuity, a double fold of serous membrane suspends the structures or organs from the body wall and are called *mesenteries* in general. Their specific name differs according to the region as:
  - *Mesogastrium*—in relation to stomach
  - *Mesentery*—in relation to small intestine
  - *Mesocolon*—in relation to large intestine
  - *Mesocardium*—in relation to pericardium
  - Mesotendon—in relation to tendon sheath
- Synovial tendon sheath: In the case of tendons especially the long tendons in the limbs as they pass over the bones and several firm structures are subjected to friction because of frequent movement. To avoid friction and for free movement a lubricating fluid is produced by the wrapping around the tendons, i.e., *synovial tendon sheaths*. Like the two layers in relation to the viscera the tendon sheath has a double layer, i.e., parietal and visceral.

Clinical Importance of Serous Membranes

- *Inflammation of serous membranes:* Pleuritis, pericarditis and peritonitis are inflammation and thickening of pleura, pericardium and peritoneum respectively.
- *Effusion*: It is collection of serous fluid (*ascites*) in the serous cavities due to injury or infection. For example, pleural effusion, pericardial effusion.
- *Tendon sheath inflammation:* Synovial tendon sheaths are present where the tendon passes below the ligament or through osseofibrous tunnel (e.g., *carpal tunnel in hand*) to reduce friction and for easy movement of the tendon. Inflammation of these sheaths is called *tenosynovitis*.

Chapter 3: Introduction to Skin and Fascia

Anatomical Basis for Clinical Condition

Case Scenario

Problem: A marathon runner of 50 years age complained to his orthopedic surgeon about pain at the bottom of heel and stiffness in the right foot which was worse in the morning once he gets up from the bed and gradually decreases as the day passes.

Questions:
1. What could be the cause for the pain?
2. Explain the anatomical basis.
3. What advice to be given to the patient?

Anatomical explanation:

1. The cause for the pain is the inflamed *plantar aponeurosis* or *plantar fascia* called *plantar fasciitis*. This is the most common orthopedic problem.
2. The plantar fascia is a modified deep fascia that connects the heel to the front of the foot. It gives support to the arched foot while walking and acts as a shock absorber in walking, running and jogging.
   Inflammation of plantar fascia is due to the wear and tear of the plantar ligament. Too much pressure on this ligament as in the present case of a marathon runner results in inflammation of the fascia, stiffness, heel pain and it can even tear the fascia.
3. Nonsurgical line of management is giving rest to the feet, avoiding running on hard surfaces, wearing shoes with good shock absorption and pain relief medication. In 95% cases the person gets relief with these methods. Surgical management is required in about 5% of cases by cutting a small bit of plantar fascia to relieve inflammation and to release tension on the ligament.

☞ Key Concept

Take Home Message—Skin, Fasciae, Serous Membranes

- *Langer's lines:* Knowledge of direction of Langer's lines is important for giving surgical incisions on skin for cosmetic reason. Incisions parallel to the Langer's lines generally heal better and produce less scarring than those at right angles to it.
- *Dermatome:* Pain or rash along the distribution of a dermatome indicates disease of the related nerve root. Most common cause is viral infection (*Varicella zoster* that causes *chicken pox* and *Herpes Zoster* that causes *Shingles*).
- *Referred pain:* It is conscious perception of visceral sensations in specific regions of the body **(Fig. 3.18)** as certain sensations from the viscera are felt locally where as others are perceived at distant areas from the affected organ. For example, pain in the teeth or jaws in a case of heart attack. Only deep pain is referred not the superficial. Knowledge of areas where the visceral pain of vital organs like heart are referred helps in early medical attention.
- *Serous cavities:* Knowledge of serous cavities facilitates understanding of clinical conditions resulting from inflammation of serous membranes and collection of fluid in serous cavities and for undertaking procedures to drain the fluid for investigation or for treatment, i.e., *pleural/pericardial tap*. Excess accumulation of pericardial fluid can result in a serious condition called *cardiac tamponade* which is a medical emergency.

Contd...

Contd...

❑ *Tendon sheaths:* Knowledge of tendon sheath is important for understanding and treating inflammations of tendon sheath that is more common. Local inflammation of tendon sheath of a finger can pull the affected finger inward towards the palm (flexion) and this condition is called *trigger finger*. Treatment is by giving rest for the finger for six weeks by applying a splint and anti-inflammatory medicines.

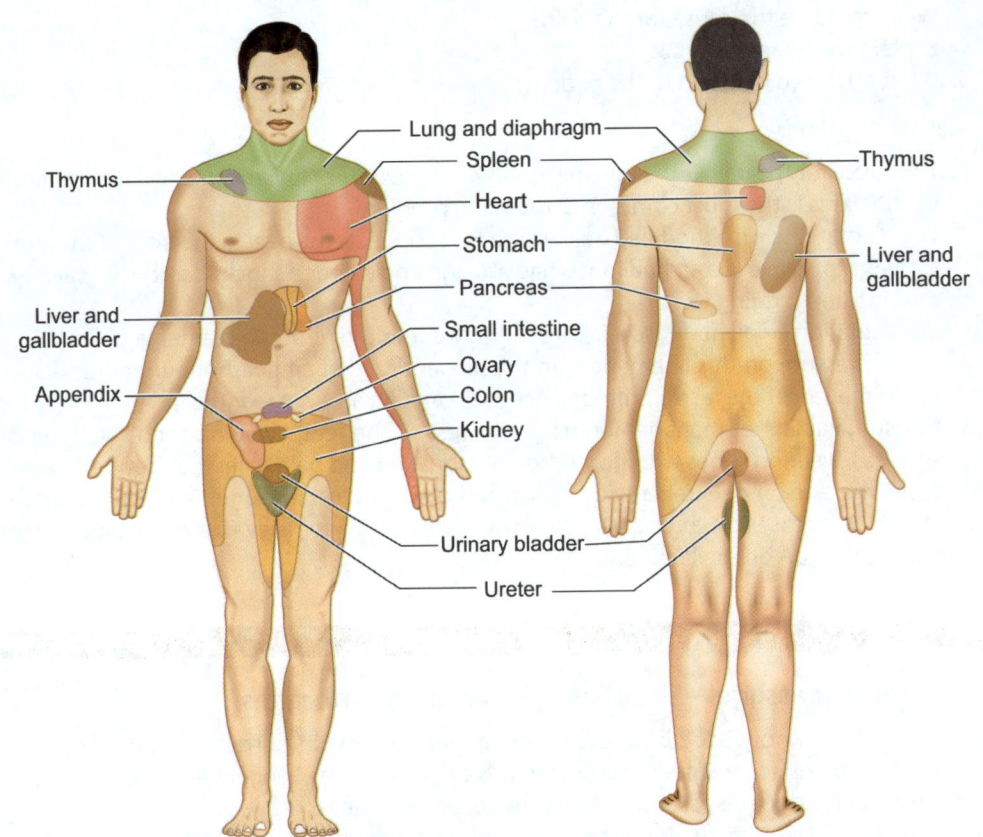

Fig. 3.18: Referred pain areas of various viscera.

QUESTIONS

1. Describe the appendages of skin.
2. Superficial fascia and its contents.
3. Functions of superficial fascia.
4. Deep fascia and its modifications.
5. Describe serous membranes.
6. Langer's lines.
7. Arrectores pilorum
8. Pilosebaceous unit

MULTIPLE CHOICE QUESTIONS

1. Which one of the following is no avascular?
   A. Epidermis

B. Dermis
C. Nail
D. Hair follicle

2. All the following are modified apocrine sweat glands, *except:*
   A. Meibomian glands
   B. Mammary glands
   C. Ceruminous glands
   D. Glands of Moll

3. All the following are subcutaneous muscles, *except:*
   A. Dartos
   B. Palmaris brevis
   C. Levator palpebrae superioris
   D. Platysma

4. Deep fascia is absent in all the following areas, *except:*
   A. Face
   B. Thorax
   C. Anterior abdominal wall
   D. Front of thigh

5. All are modifications of deep fascia, *except:*
   A. Retinacula
   B. Aponeuroses
   C. Fibrous flexor sheaths
   D. Mesocolon

6. All the following muscles of panniculus carnosus are skeletal muscles, *except:*
   A. Platysma   B. Occipitalis
   C. Palmaris brevis   D. Dartos

ANSWERS

1. B   2. A   3. C   4. D   5. D   6. D

CHAPTER

4

Skeletal System

LEARNING OBJECTIVES

- ❖ Structure of different types of cartilage
- ❖ Classification of bones
- ❖ Different parts of a long bone
- ❖ Blood supply of a long bone
- ❖ Structure and composition of bone
- ❖ Clinical case with anatomical explanation

INTRODUCTION

Locomotor system is an organ system that gives the ability to move using muscular and skeletal systems. It is made up of bones, muscle, cartilage, tendons, ligaments, and joints. Its main function is to support the body (standing), protect the vital organs (brain, heart, stomach, liver, kidneys, etc.), and facilitate movements (walking, holding objects with hands, etc.). Cartilage prevents friction at the bone ends that are coming in contact with one another. Ligaments attach one bone to other bone. Tendons attach muscle to bone. The three major subdivisions of locomotor system are:
1. Skeletal system
2. Muscular system
3. Joints.

For convenience these three systems will be discussed as separate chapters.

SKELETAL SYSTEM

- The word skeleton is derived from Greek skeletos = "dried body"; "mummy".
- *Osteology* is the study of all the bones in the body with their associated cartilages and membranes. *Osteon* means bone.
- Skeleton is the bony and cartilaginous framework of the body.
- Bones and cartilage are specialized connective tissues.
- Skeleton is made up of 206 bones and is divided into *axial skeleton* and *appendicular skeleton*.

Number of Bones in Newborn versus Adult

The number of bones in a newborn are 300 whereas in the adult the number is 206. The reduction in number is due to the fusion of certain bones. The non-fusion is more in the axial skeleton than appendicular skeleton. The bones of skull are unfused in the fetus to facilitate the passage of the fetal head through the narrow female pelvis at the time of delivery. The unfused areas between skull bones are called fontanelle. The five vertebrae of sacral region fuse to form the single sacrum. Similarly the four pieces of coccygeal vertebrae fuse to form single coccyx. In the appendicular skeleton also there are unfused parts that fuse at different times during the growth of the child.

Axial Skeleton (Fig. 4.1)

- It is in the center (axis) of the body. It is responsible for upright or erect position of the body.

Chapter 4: Skeletal System

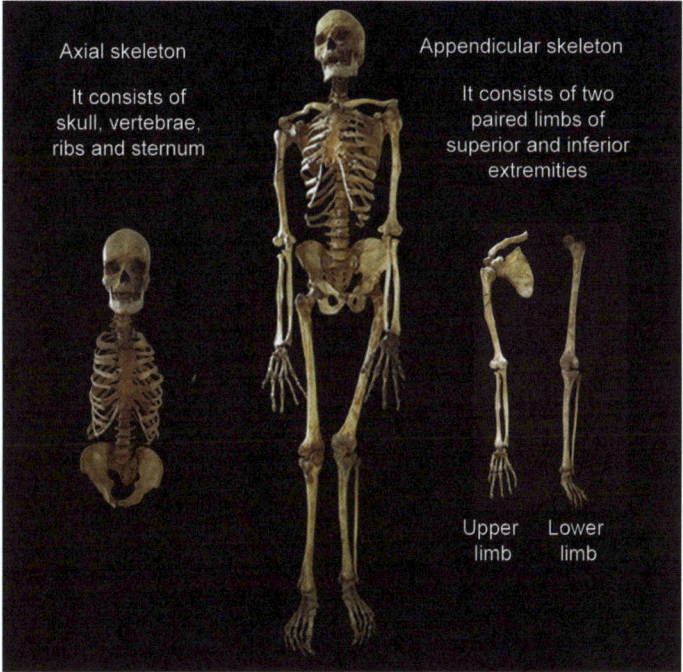

Fig. 4.1: Skeleton: Axial and appendicular skeleton.

- It is formed by 80 bones. It consists of *skull, vertebrae, ribs, mandible, hyoid and sternum*.
- Skull is the cranial expanded end of axis and protects the brain located in it.
- The vertebral column is in the central axis of the body. It consists of vertebrae and the intervening intervertebral discs. It protects the spinal cord and transmits weight from upper limbs to lower limbs.
- Ribs and sternum form the thoracic cage along with vertebrae and facilitate respiratory movements.
- The hyoid bone is located below the mandible and above the larynx. It is the only bone in the body that is not articulating with another bone.

Appendicular Skeleton (Fig. 4.1)

- It is formed by two paired limbs of superior and inferior extremities which are divided into joints for locomotion, grasping, etc.
- It consists of 126 bones.

Functions of Bone

It provides:
- Shape to the body
- *Support to body:* Lower limb bones
- Surface for muscle and tendon attachment
- *Protection for important organs:* Skull (brain), vertebrae (spinal cord), ribs, and sternum (lungs and heart)
- *Storage of mineral:* Calcium, phosphate, and inorganic component
- *Movement:* Walking, grasping objects
- *Blood cells production:* Red blood cells (RBCs), white blood cells (WBCs), and platelets in red bone marrow by the process of hemopoiesis
- *Storage of fat:* Yellow marrow.

CARTILAGE

AN 2.4: Describe various types of cartilage with its structure and distribution in body.

- Cartilage is a *specialized* form of connective tissue.

- *Location:* It is present in areas where rigidity and elasticity are required.
- *Composition:* It contains cells and extracellular fibers embedded in intercellular substance (matrix).
  - The cells of cartilage are called *chondrocytes*. The cells are located in lacunae or little spaces in intercellular matrix. They are either singly placed or in groups of two or more cells. Collection of number of cells in a single lacuna is known as *cell nests*. The young cells are capable of multiplication. The older cells cannot multiply and produce alkaline phosphatase enzyme, which is responsible for ossification of cartilage in advanced age.
  - It contains both collagen and elastic fibers.
  - The intercellular substance gives firmness to the cartilage. Presence of large amount of hyaluronic acid in cartilage makes it capable of weight bearing especially at the freely movable synovial joints. Other constituents of ground substance in cartilage are chondroitin sulfate and proteoglycans.
- *Peculiarities*:
  - Cartilage has no nerves hence *insensitive to pain*.
  - It has no blood vessels (*avascular*) of its own. It has poor regenerative capacity after its injury due to its avascularity.
- *Perichondrium:* The cartilage is enclosed in a dense fibrous connective tissue membrane called the *perichondrium* which is rich in blood vessels. The cartilage cells receive nutrition from these blood vessels by diffusion through ground substance. Perichondrium is absent in articular cartilages covering articulating surfaces of the bones. The perichondrium consists of two layers: (1) An outer fibrous and (2) Inner chondrogenic layers. The chondrogenic layer contains chondroblasts. The outer fibrous layer contains collagen fibers and is vascular.
- *Growth of cartilage:* It is by two processes. They are:
  1. *Interstitial* (internal/inside growth by chondrocytes). Chondrocytes increase in number by mitosis from the center of cartilaginous model. This causes increase in length.
  2. *Oppositional* (external/outside growth by cells of perichondrium). Layers of cartilage cells develop underneath the perichondrium. This causes increase in width of cartilage model.
- *Functions:* Provides support to the soft tissues and a sliding surface for the joints and for growth of a long bone.
- *Clinical importance:* Because of their location in cell nests and lower antigenicity of the cartilage matrix, homogeneous cartilage transplantation can be done without tissue rejection.
- *Types of cartilage:* There are three types of cartilage based on histological appearance and the extracellular matrix (**Figs. 4.2, 4.3** and **Table 4.1**). They are:
  1. Hyaline cartilage
  2. Elastic cartilage
  3. White fibrocartilage.

Clinical Applications of Cartilage

Chondrodystrophies: These are a group of diseases where there will be disturbance of growth and subsequent ossification of cartilage.

Traumatic rupture or detachment of cartilage: It is more common in knee where the white fibrocartilage in menisci is affected and is treated by partial replacement.

Costochondritis: Inflammation of cartilage in the ribs that can cause chest pain.

Herniation of intervertebral disc: This is due to compression of intervertebral disc causing herniation of its contents that often compress the adjacent nerves and causes back pain.

Tumors of cartilage: These can be benign or malignant. Benign tumors are called chondromas and the malignant are called chondrosarcomas.

Chapter 4: Skeletal System

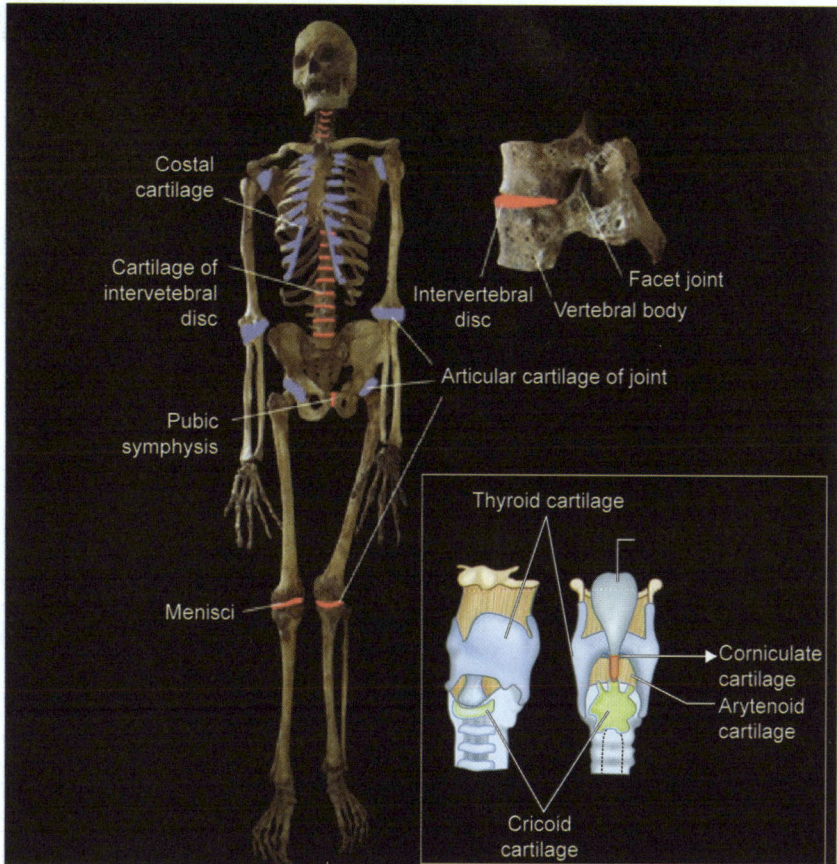

Fig. 4.2: Location of different cartilages.

Cartilage transplantation: Matrix of cartilage acts as an immunological barrier preventing entry of lymphocytes or immunoglobulins. Because of this property cartilage from one individual can be transplanted without tissue rejection to another.

BONE

To understand the structure and classification of bones parts of a long bone and its blood supply are to be studied.

Parts of a Long Bone

AN 2.1 : Describe parts, blood and nerve supply of a long bone.

A young long bone presents **(Figs. 4.4 and 4.5)**:
- Shaft (*diaphysis*)
- Ends (*epiphyses*)
- Epiphyseal cartilage
- Epiphyseal end of shaft (*metaphysis*)
- Outer *periosteum*
- Inner *endosteum*
- Marrow cavity in diaphysis.
- *Shaft/diaphysis (Greek dia = in between, physis = growth):*
  - It is the part between the two ends (epiphyses) in a developing long bone.
  - It corresponds to the shaft of a long bone.
  - It is that part where primary ossification starts and forms major part (shaft) of a long bone.

Table 4.1: Different types of cartilage—description.

Cartilage and features	Structure (Figs. 4.3A to C)
Hyaline cartilage: □ *Cells*: The chondrocytes reside in little spaces in the intercellular substance called *lacunae or capsules*. Chondrocytes have a round or oval nucleus □ *Intercellular substance*: It contains type II collagenous microfibrils and fibers. It is a firm gel and appears bluish, homogeneous, amorphous, and semitransparent (glossy appearance). The matrix is of two types, i.e., (1) *Territorial* and (2) *Interterritorial* according to location and intensity of staining. The territorial matrix is more basophilic and surrounds the lacunae. In between the lacunae is the less basophilic interterritorial matrix □ *Perichondrium*: It is the connective tissue surrounding the cartilage □ With age it undergoes *calcification and ossification* □ *Examples*: It is the most common cartilage. Trachea, larynx, bronchi, and costal cartilages on the articular surface of the bones. Developing bone is a hyaline cartilage	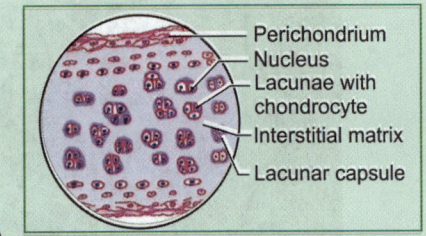 A
Elastic cartilage: □ *Cells*: These are round, surrounded by lacunae or capsules, and scattered singly or in isogenous groups of two or three cells □ *Intercellular substance*: It is permeated by large number of elastic fibers and the ground substance is reduced □ With age it does not undergo calcification and ossification □ *Perichondrium*: It presents perichondrium □ *Examples*: External ear, external auditory canal, Eustachian tubes, and epiglottis (**All E's**)	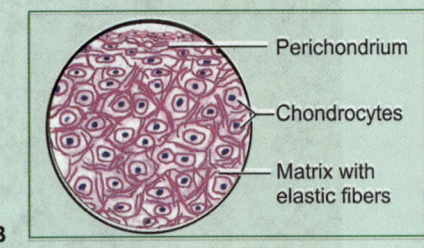 B
Fibrocartilage: □ *Cells*: The encapsulated cartilage cells lie singly or in pairs □ *Intercellular substance*: Bundles of collagen fibers with little ground substance □ *Perichondrium*: It has no perichondrium □ *Examples*: Secondary cartilaginous joints (symphysis pubis, manubriosternal, and intervertebral), menisci of knee joints, articular disc of temporomandibular joint, glenoidal labrum, and acetabular labrum	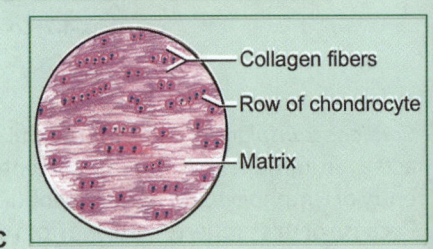 C

- The primary center of ossification is formed before birth.
- The wall of the shaft is composed of *compact bone*.
- The hollow within the diaphysis is called *medullary cavity or marrow cavity*. It contains adipose tissue and forms the yellow marrow.
- End/epiphysis (Greek epi = upon, physis = growth):
  - A typical long bone presents epiphysis at each end. It is that part that is *ossified from secondary center*, i.e. after birth.
  - At birth both ends of a long bone are cartilaginous and are known as *cartilaginous epiphyses*. After birth these ends undergo ossification resulting in *bony epiphyses*. The epiphyses develop by *endochondral ossification*.
  - The epiphyseal ends of a long bone fuse with diaphysis.
  - The epiphyseal union does not take place simultaneously at both ends. On

epiphysis fuses with diaphysis earlier than the other one. The epiphysis which unites last with the diaphysis grows for a longer period before union

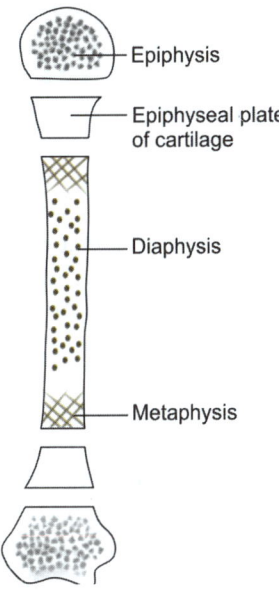

Fig. 4.4: Parts of a long bone.

and is known as the *growing end of a bone*.
- The epiphysis is filled with *spongy/cancellous* bone. The spaces in the spongy bone are filled with red marrow where RBCs are formed (hemopoiesis).
- There are some bones where there is *epiphysis at one end only*. They are the metacarpals, metatarsals, phalanges, and ribs.
- *Types of epiphyses:* There are four types of epiphyses (**Figs. 4.5 and 4.6**). They are:
  1. *Pressure epiphysis:* It develops at the articulating ends of long bones that take part in the formation of a joint complex. It facilitates weight transmission. It is seen in the parts of the bone that is under pressure during movement, e.g., head (**Figs. 4.5 and 4.6**) and condyles of femur; head, capitulum, and trochlea of humerus; and condyles of tibia.

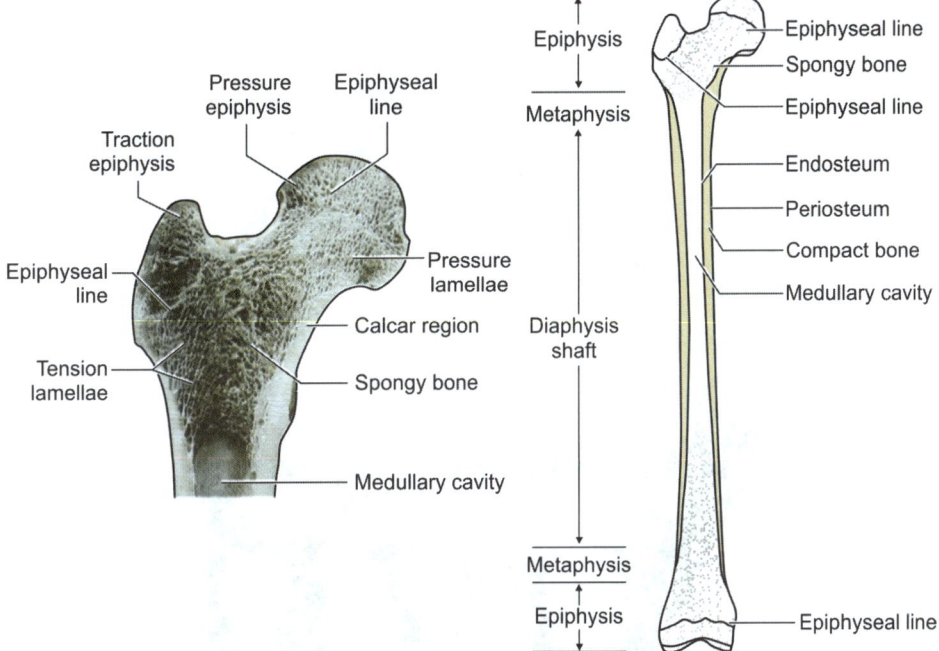

Fig. 4.5: Sagittal section of an adult femur.

2. *Traction epiphysis:* It develops along the line of muscle pull in the nonarticular parts (that do not take part in the formation of a joint) of a long bone that is not involved in weight transmission **(Figs. 4.5 and 4.6)**. This type of epiphyses is nearer to pressure epiphyses. These epiphyses ossify after the pressure epiphyses. Supporting tendons and ligaments are attached to these regions, e.g., trochanters (greater and lesser) of femur, tubercles (greater and lesser), mastoid process and epicondyles (medial and lateral) of humerus.
3. *Atavastic epiphysis:* It is seen as a separate bone in lower animals. But in human skeleton it fuses with other bones, e.g., coracoid process of scapula **(Fig. 4.6)** and posterior tubercle of talus.
4. *Aberrant epiphysis:* It is a deviation from the normal and is not always present, e.g., epiphysis at the head of 1st metacarpal and base of other metacarpals **(Fig. 4.6)**.

♦ *Epiphyseal cartilage* **(Fig. 4.7)**:
  – This is the plate of hyaline cartilage intervening between epiphysis and diaphysis of a growing long bone. It is also called *growth plate*.

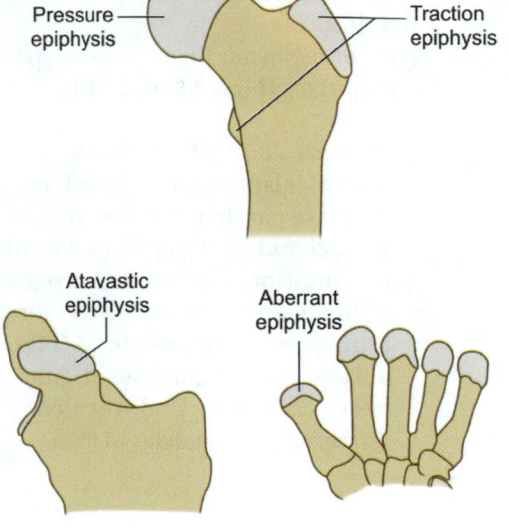

Fig. 4.6: Types of epiphyses.

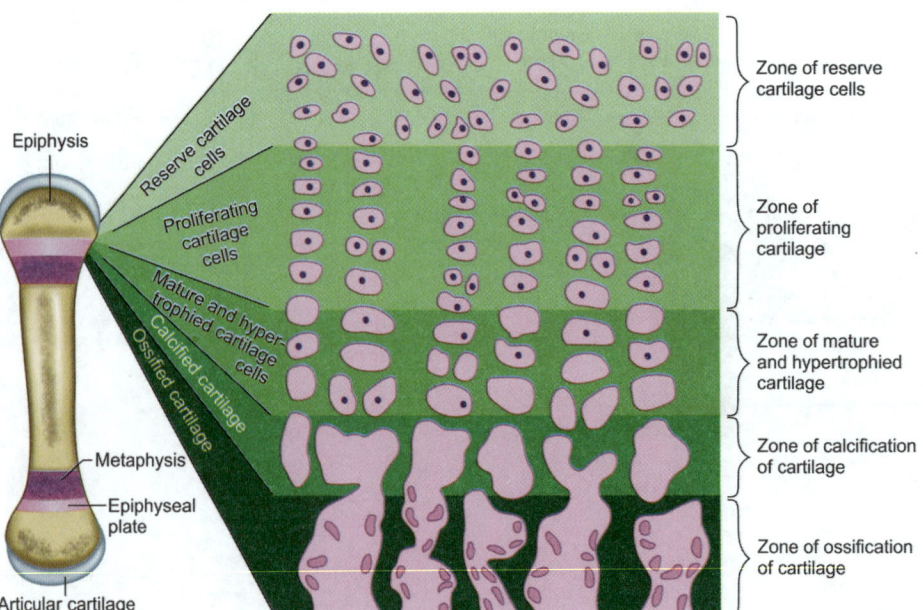

Fig. 4.7: Various zones in epiphyseal plate.

- It persists as long as the bone grows in length. When full length of a bone is reached around puberty (18–21 years) the epiphyseal cartilage is replaced by bone and the epiphyseal plate becomes *epiphyseal line (see **Fig. 4.5**)*.
- This epiphyseal growth plate shows five zones (**Fig. 4.7**):
  1. *Zone of reserve cartilage:* Contains small groups of chondrocytes.
  2. *Zone of proliferating cartilage:* There is rapid mitosis of chondrocytes. The chondrocytes are stacked one above the other in the form of columns, parallel to the long axis of future bone.
  3. *Zone of mature and hypertrophied cartilage:* The mitotic activity of chondrocytes stops. There is enlargement of chondrocytes and their lacunae.
  4. *Zone of calcification of cartilage:* This is a narrow zone where calcification of matrix and resorption of dead cartilage cells are observed.
  5. *Zone of ossification of cartilage:* Osteoblasts accumulate. The osteoid is formed by the osteoblasts and is mineralized.
- *Clinical importance:* Epiphyseal cartilage is temporary. This is the place where growth in length takes place. Disorders of growth plate takes place in children of growing age. Injury to growth plate causes shortening of the limb. In inflammation of the growth plate excess growth in length of a limb occurs due to increased vascularity.

♦ Metaphysis:
- It is the epiphyseal end of diaphysis of long bone facing epiphyseal cartilage. This is the growing region of diaphysis where a bone grows in length.
- Metaphysis is the site from where advancement of ossification occurs. It is the most actively growing area of long bone.
- It gives attachment to muscles, ligaments, and capsules of joints. Hence, it is subjected to stress and strain and is likely to be damaged.
- *Clinical importance:* This region is very vascular and is supplied by nutrient, periosteal, and juxtaepiphyseal arteries. Here, the nutrient arteries form hairpin-like capillary loops (bends). Infected emboli or bacteria circulating in blood will be lodged here. So, infection of a long bone starts from this region of metaphysis (**Fig. 4.8**). In children this region of bone is at high-risk of hematogenous spread of infection as in osteomyelitis. Metaphysis is also affected by different types of bone tumors like chondrosarcoma, osteosarcoma, etc. In rickets, a condition resulting from defective demineralization of bone results in cupping of the metaphysis.

♦ *Periosteum (peri = around or surrounding):*
- It is the thin membrane covering the outer surface of the diaphysis and the epiphyses, where articular cartilage is absent.
- It contains *osteoblasts* (bone-forming cells), *osteoclasts* (bone-destroying cells), nerve fibers, blood vessels, and lymphatic vessels.
- Ligaments and tendons attach to the periosteum.
- It is protective and serves as a channel through which passes the blood vessels and nerves for blood supply and nutrients for bone tissue.
- Because of sensory innervation it is sensitive to pain.

♦ *Endosteum (end = inside):*
- It is the membrane lining the marrow cavity.
- Bone growth, repair, and remodeling occur here.

♦ *Marrow cavity:*

> **AN 1.2 :** Describe composition of bone and bone marrow.

- It is also known as medullary cavity.
- It is the central cavity in the shaft of a long bone.
- It contains red bone marrow and/or yellow bone marrow.
- The red marrow contains hematopoietic cells that produce RBC's. In children red marrow is found in the shafts of long bones. As the child ages the red marrow is replaced with fatty/adipose/yellow marrow. In infants the entire marrow cavity including the bones of digits contains red marrow.
- In adults the red marrow is seen in the skull, vertebrae, ribs, hip bone, clavicle, sternum, and ends of long bones.

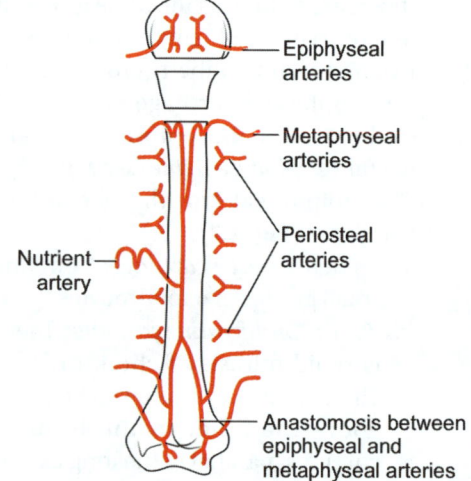

Fig. 4.8: Blood supply of a long bone.

Clinical Importance

- Bone marrow aspiration is the clinical procedure to remove a small amount of bone marrow cells and fluid through a needle inserted into the bone. The collected fluid and cells are observed for blood disorders (of RBC, WBC, or platelets) as in thrombocytopenia, leukemia, anemia, etc.
- Bone marrow biopsy is done to diagnose the spread of cancer cells to the bones that facilitates treatment of cancers.
- Bone marrow transplant is the treatment to replace unhealthy marrow with healthy one through an intravenous injection. The healthy blood forming cells reach the bone marrow for forming the new cells.

Blood Supply of a Long Bone (Fig. 4.8)

AN 2.1: Describe parts, blood and nerve supply of a long bone.

Arteries

Typical long bone is supplied by four arteries. They are nutrient, metaphyseal, periosteal, and epiphyseal arteries. These arteries anastomoses with one another at the metaphysis. Hence, the highly vascular part of a long bone is the metaphysis.

- *Nutrient artery*:
  - This is the main source of blood supply to the long bone.
  - It supplies bone marrow and inner two-thirds of compact bone.
  - It enters through the periosteum at nutrient foramen and travels through nutrient canal to enter the medullary cavity.
  - It presents tortuous course to reduce blood pressure and to allow movement within bone.
  - In the medullary cavity it divides into ascending and descending branches that travel toward the ends of the diaphysis.
  - The ascending and descending branches are close to the endosteum and supply the inner two-thirds of the compact bone of the shaft.
  - It presents hairpin bends at places of anastomosis with epiphyseal, metaphyseal and periosteal arteries. In a growing bone, at the metaphysis the nutrient artery anastomoses with metaphyseal arteries.
  - Number of nutrient foramina may vary, e. g., several in femur and single in tibia.

Chapter 4: Skeletal System

- *Metaphyseal arteries:* These are branches of neighboring systemic arteries (arterial anastomoses) and enter the vascular foramina located beyond the articular capsule and supply epiphysis and diaphysis. Metaphysis is the most vascular part of a long bone.
- *Epiphyseal arteries:*
  - At the epiphysis the bone contains epiphyseal arteries (branches of arterial anastomosis).
  - Epiphyseal arteries reach via capsular ligament to supply articular capsule and end in intertrabecular sinuses.
  - If articular cartilage is continuous with epiphyseal cartilage, e.g., head of femur the arteries pierce the epiphyseal cartilage and is prone for avascular necrosis of epiphysis in injury.
  - If articular cartilage is not continuous with epiphyseal cartilage the arteries enter directly. Hence, avascular necrosis is not possible.
- *Periosteal arteries:*
  - These are branches of muscular arteries and supply outer one-third of compact bone.
  - Articulating surface of a bone is avascular and gets nutrition from synovial fluid and capillary network in the synovial membrane.

Clinical Importance of Blood Supply of a Long Bone
- The blood supply of bone enables rapid growth and remodelling of bone.
- Periosteal stripping in treatment of fractures—causes ischemia and necrosis of outer 1/3rd of cortex followed by periosteal new bone formation.
- Intramedullary nailing (surgery to repair fractured bone)—reaming (making a whole to enlarge medullary canal in a bone) de-vascularizes 50–80% of cortex. Unreaming preserves endosteal blood supply.

Veins
Venous drainage of a bone is by veins (e.g. basivertebral veins) running through red marrow and Volkmann's canals (accompanying arteries) in compact bone. Lymphatics follow the same route.

Nerves
Nerves are mostly present at the articular ends of long bones and vertebrae. They are present freely in the layers of periosteum. The branches enter through nutrient foramen and supply blood vessels. Few sensory branches are distributed to the articular ends and periosteum. Most of the nerves are autonomous (sympathetic and parasympathetic).

Structure and Composition of Bone

AN 1.2: Describe composition of bone and bone marrow.

- Bone is the main component of the skeleton.
- It is a specialized form of dense connective tissue.
- Bone gives skeleton the necessary rigidity to function as attachment and lever for muscles and supports the body against gravity.
- All bones are composed of an outer dense (hard) layer called *compact bone* that is protective in function and an inner less dense part called *spongy bone* that contains network of spicules (trabeculae) with spaces in between. The spaces are filled with red and yellow marrow (*see* **Fig. 4.5**).
- *Composition of bone:* It contains cells and extracellular matrix. The extracellular matrix cis 1/3rd organic and 2/3rds inorganic. *Refer* **Flowchart 4.1** for details.

Microscopic Structure of Bone
- Bone is a sclerous (hard) connective tissue **(Flowchart 4.1)**.
- It is made up of cells and intercellular substance (extracellular matrix).

Chapter 4: Skeletal System

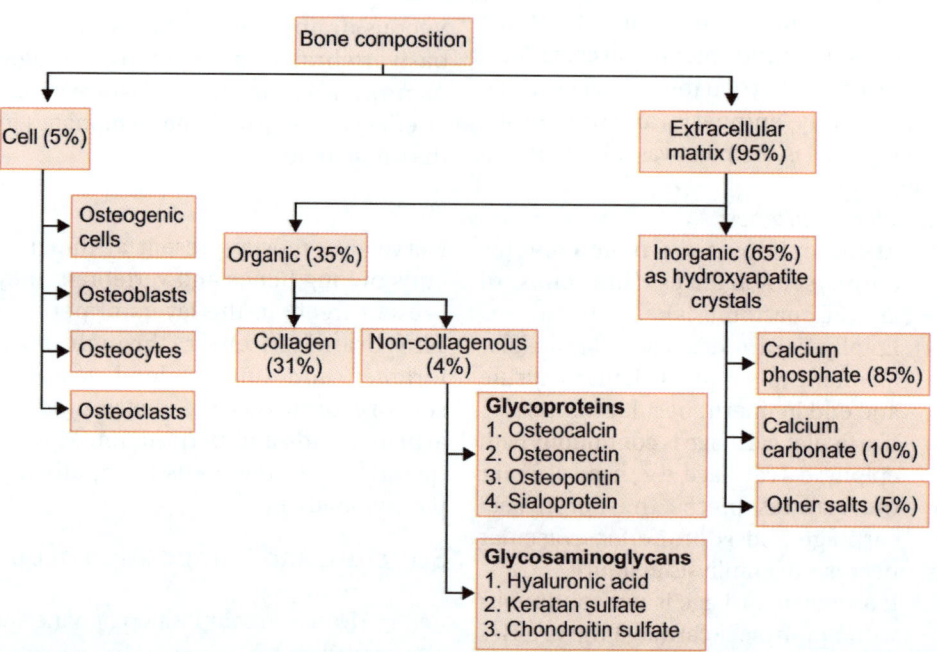

Flowchart 4.1: Composition of bone.

Table 4.2: Cells of bone—structure and function.

Cells	Location	Structure and function
Osteogenic	❑ Periosteum ❑ Endosteum ❑ Haversian canals	❑ Less differentiated cells ❑ Act as stem cells and form osteoblasts
Osteoblasts	❑ Lie along bundles of collagen fibers ❑ By means of cytoplasmic processes connected to adjacent cells for transport of nutrition	❑ Round cells with single nucleus and basophilic cytoplasm ❑ Form matrix-osteoid (collagen fibers and ground substance) ❑ Secrete alkaline phosphatase for mineralization of osteoid ❑ Help in calcification
Osteocytes	❑ Main cells of bone tissue ❑ Trapped in mineralized matrix ❑ Seen in lacunae within matrix ❑ Send their cytoplasmic processes into canaliculi for joining the processes of adjacent osteocytes	❑ Along with bundles of collagen fibers in between them form the lamellar bone
Osteoclasts	❑ Large, multinucleated cells containing nearly 50 nuclei ❑ Surface of the osteoclast in contact with the bone shows ruffled border ❑ They are located in shallow depressions called Howship's lacunae	❑ Involved in bone resorption ❑ The origin and function of osteoclasts is similar to macrophages

- The extracellular matrix contains collagen fibers (protein), ground substance, and inorganic salts (calcium phosphate, calcium carbonate that form hydroxyapatite crystals) making it hard for providing strength and rigidity. The calcium and fibers give strength and flexibility.

Various cells of bone and their structure, their location and function are presented in **Table 4.2** and **Figures 4.9A and B**.

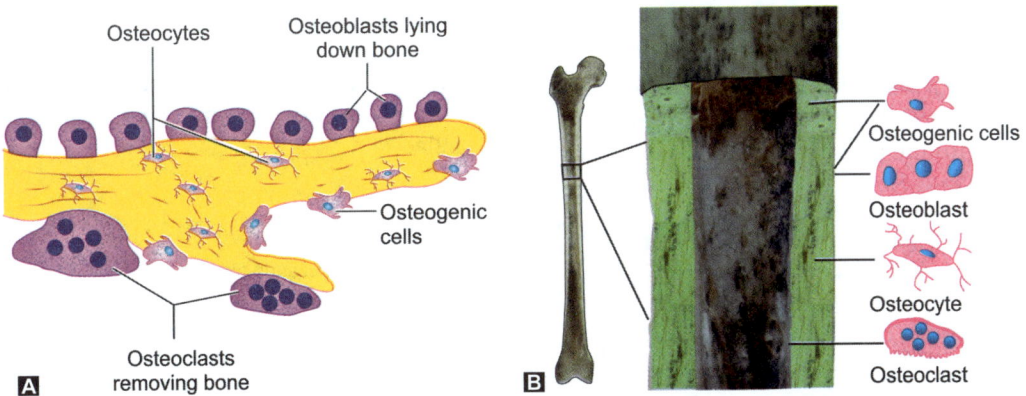

Figs. 4.9A and B: (A) Bone cells in relation to a spicule of bone; (B) Bone cells in compact bone at diaphysis of long bone.

Microscopic Structure of Compact Bone
- *Formation of bone lamellae* **(Fig. 4.10)**:
  - Compact bone contains more of extracellular matrix which is seen in the form of thin sheets called lamellae. In a lamella the collagen fibers are arranged parallel to each other.
  - The thickness of bone depends on the number of lamellae of collagen fibers stacked one above the other.
  - Osteoblasts form the extracellular matrix. While depositing the matrix, the osteoblasts get trapped in the small spaces within the matrix called lacunae. Now they are called osteocytes.
  - The thin cytoplasmic processes of osteocytes that are extending from the lacunae travel through small channels within the matrix called canaliculi through which they communicate with adjacent osteocytes and with blood vessels for nutritive exchange.
- *Structure of compact bone:* This can be observed in a transverse or a longitudinal section of a small piece of compact bone at diaphysis where it is thick and becomes thin at epiphysis **(Figs. 4.11A and B)**. It is covered with periosteum on its outer surface and endosteum on its inner surface. The lamellae of compact bone are arranged in three different patterns:
  - Haversian system of lamellae
  - Interstitial lamellae
  - Circumferential lamellae.

Haversian System of Lamellae
- It is also called *osteon* or Haversian system.
- It is cylindrical in shape.
- 50 μ in size.
- Long axis is parallel to the long axis of the bone.
- The lamellae are arranged concentrically around longitudinal vascular channels called *Haversian canals* within the bone to form cylindrical structure called Haversian system.
- Each osteon is made up of 4–20 lamellae.
- The Haversian canal contains one to two capillaries and nerves.
- The Haversian canals are connected with one another and communicate with the free surface (periosteum) and with marrow cavity via transverse channels called Volkmann's canals.
- The Volkmann's canals are oblique in direction and are not surrounded by concentric lamellae.
- Lacunae and canaliculi connect the Haversian canal with all the lacunae of the osteon. The canaliculi facilitate transport of gases and nutrients to osteocytes from the blood capillaries in Haversian canals.

Interstitial lamellae: These are present between the Haversian systems and are of varying size and irregular shape. These represent disrupted older osteons due to bone remodeling.

Circumferential lamellae: At the external surface of the cortical bone immediately beneath the periosteum and on the internal surface subjacent to the endosteum there are several lamellae that extend uninterrupted around much of the circumference of the shaft. These are the outer and inner circumferential lamellae.

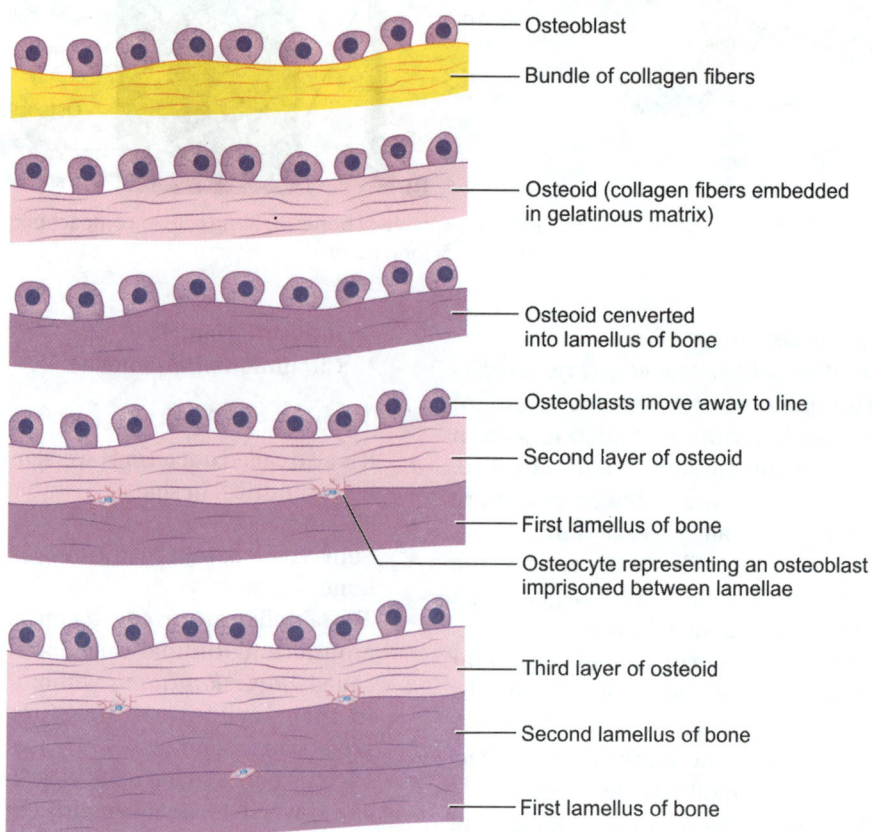

Fig. 4.10: Formation of lamellar bone.

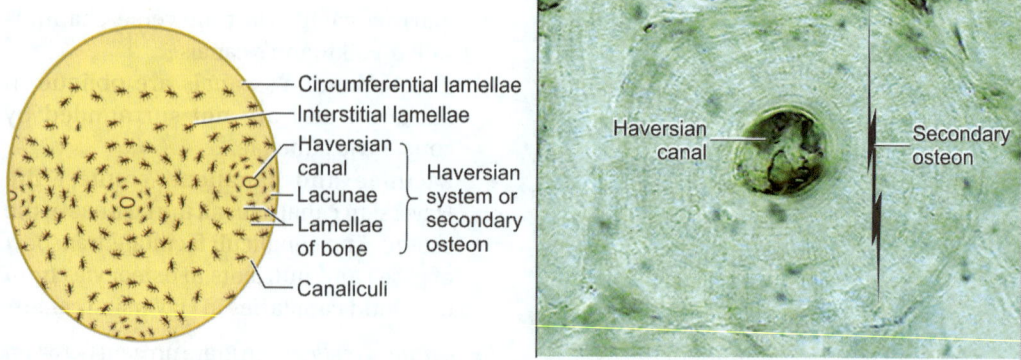

Fig. 4.11A: Transverse section of compact bone.

Chapter 4: Skeletal System

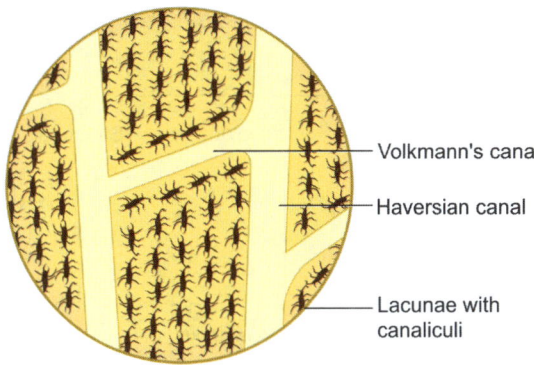
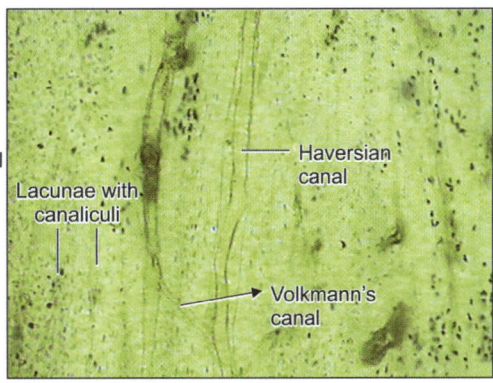

Fig. 4.11B: Longitudinal section of compact bone.

Microscopic Structure of Spongy/Cancellous Bone

- Simple structure of interconnecting trabeculae of lamellar bone forming three-dimensional lattice networks along lines of stress.
- The trabecular surfaces are covered by endosteum.
- It differs from compact bone in not having Haversian system of arrangement.

Diploic (diploe) bones: Flat bones of cranium contain two layers of compact bone with intervening spongy bone. The purpose is to protect the internal organ, the brain in the event of fracture of skull involving the outer compact layer **(Fig. 4.12)**.

Classification of Bones

Bones are classified based on their evolution (phylogenetic), shape (morphological), location in the body (regional), type of development (developmental), and structure (structural) **(Flowchart 4.2)**.

- *Based on evolution (phylogenetic):* It includes:
  - *Exoskeleton:* Remnants are present in human beings as nails, enamel of teeth
  - *Endoskeleton:* It includes all the bones in the body.
- *According to shape (morphological):* They are classified as shown in **Table 4.3** and **Figure 4.13**.

Sesamoid Bones

AN 2.3: Enumerate special features of a sesamoid bone.

- **Definition:** A small independent bone in a tendon where it passes over an angular surface.
- **Origin of the term and meaning:** Derived from Latin word Sesame = sesame seed
- **Location:** Typically seen in
  - Hand—palmar surface
  - Knee—both anterior and posterior surfaces
  - Feet—plantar surface
- Often form in response to strains – Rider's bone
- Present as cartilaginous nodules in the fetus, and in greater numbers than in the adult
- **Best example:** Patella or knee cap is the largest sesamoid bone (Refer Table 4.3 for other examples)
- **Special features:**
  - No periosteum

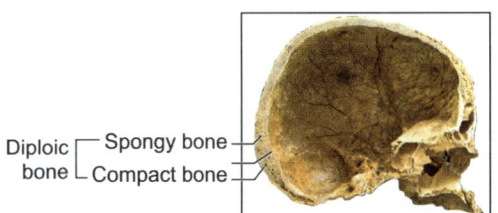

Fig. 4.12: Sagittal section of skull showing diploic bone.

Chapter 4: Skeletal System

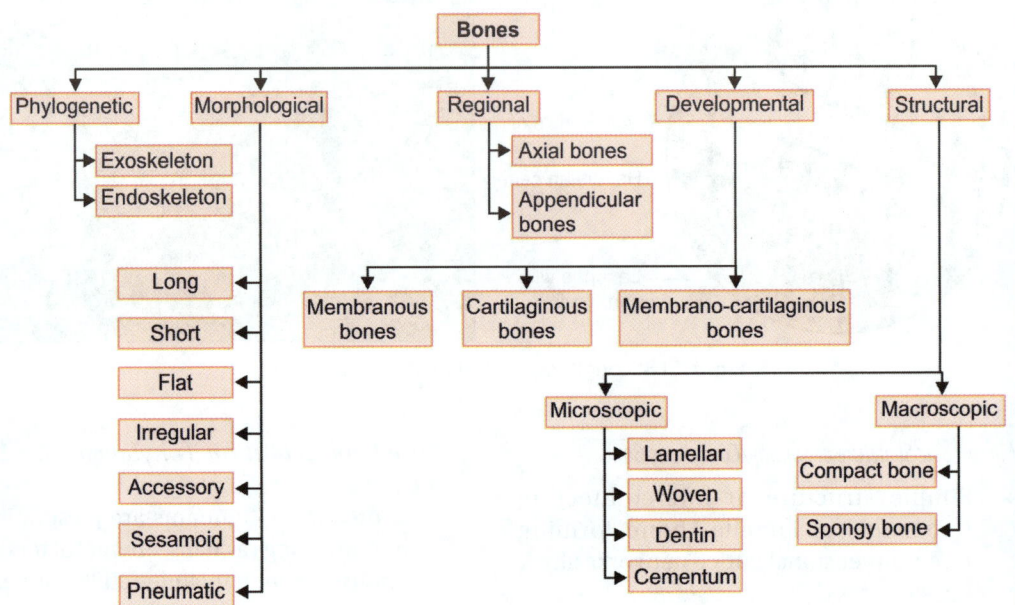

Flowchart 4.2: Classification of bones.

Table 4.3: Morphological classification of bones.			
Bone shape	Features	Examples	Functions
Long bones	Length is more than their breadth and thickness	❑ *Long bones*: Femur, tibia, fibula, humerus, radius, and ulna ❑ *Miniature long bones*: Metatarsals, metacarpals, and phalanges	Levers for muscles
Short bones	❑ Cuboidal in shape ❑ Length, width, and thickness are equal.	Carpals and tarsals	❑ Stability ❑ Support ❑ Slight movement.
Flat bones	Thin, curved	❑ *Bones of vault of skull*: Frontal, parietal, and occipital ❑ *Bones of thoracic cage*: Ribs, sternum, and scapula	❑ Provide attachment for muscles ❑ Protect internal organs
Irregular bones	Atypical shape	❑ Vertebrae ❑ *Bones of base of skull*: Temporal, sphenoid ❑ *Face*: Maxilla, mandible ❑ Hip bone	Protect internal organs
Sesamoid bones	Small, rounded bones in tendons	Patella in quadriceps tendon; Fabella in lateral head of gastrocnemius; Pisiform bone of wrist; At 1st metatarsophalangeal joint	Protection of tendons from compression
Pneumatic bones	Bones with air-filled spaces	*Bones around nose*: Maxilla, frontal, ethmoid, and sphenoid	❑ Lighten the skull ❑ Add resonance to the voice

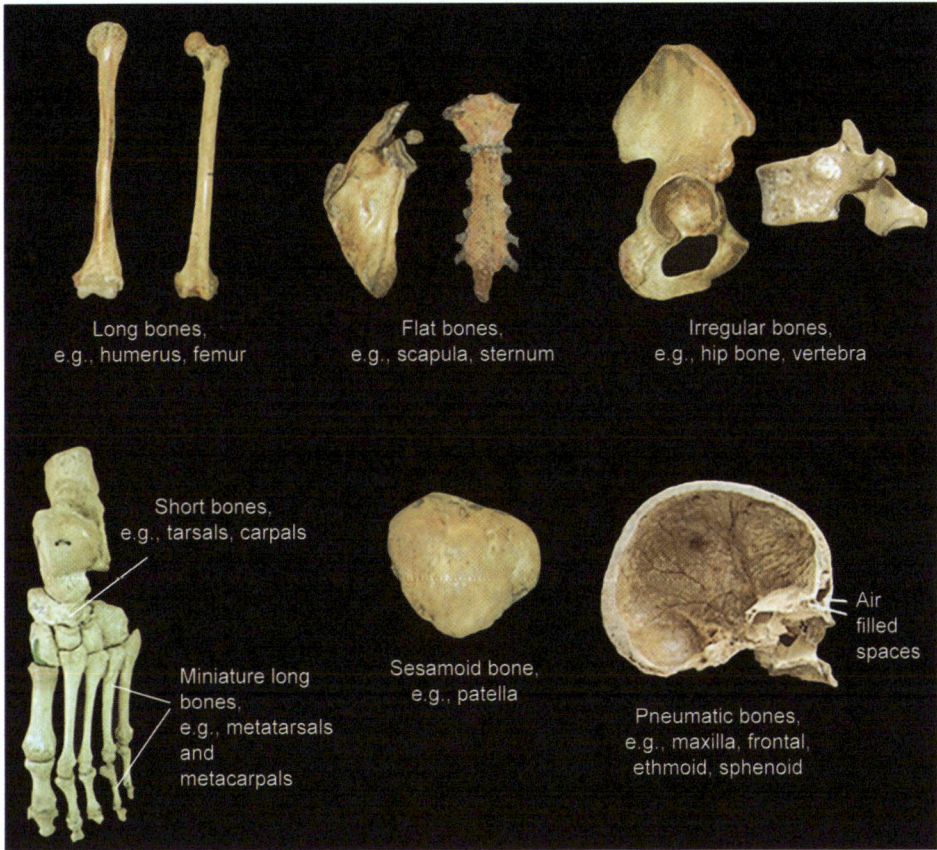

Fig. 4.13: Morphological classification of bones.

- No haversian system
- No primary center of ossification
- Appear after birth
- No separate arterial supply
- Rubbing surface covered with articular (hyaline) cartilage

♦ *According to location with reference to anatomical position (regional):*
  - *Axial bones:* Located along the central axis of the body. They are a total of 80 bones (**Table 4.4**).
  - *Appendicular bones:* Limb bones that are attached to axial skeleton as appendages. They are bones of upper limb (64 no's) and lower limb (62 no's). In each limb they are further divided into girdle (*pectoral and pelvic*) bones and free bones (**Tables 4.5 and 4.6**).

♦ *According to process of bone formation (developmental):* The process of formation of bone is called *ossification*. There are two types of ossification or formation of bone. They are *intramembranous* and *intracartilaginous (endochondral)*. Based on the method of formation of bone the bones are classified as follows:

Table 4.4: Bones of axial skeleton.

Bones	Number
Skull	22
Vertebrae	26
Ribs	24
Sternum	1
Hyoid	1
Auditory ossicles	6
Total	80

Table 4.5: Appendicular skeleton—bones of upper limb.

Bones	Number
Pectoral girdle bones	
Clavicle	2
Scapula	2
Free bones	
Humerus	2
Radius	2
Ulna	2
Carpals	16
Metacarpals	10
Phalanges	28
Total	64

Table 4.6: Appendicular skeleton—bones of lower limb.

Bones	Number
Pelvic girdle bones	
Hip bone	2
Free bones	
Femur	2
Patella	2
Tibia	2
Fibula	2
Tarsals	14
Metatarsals	10
Phalanges	28
Total	62

- *Membranous bones:* Bones are laid down first as thick connective tissue (mesodermal) condensations. These mesodermal models are converted directly into bone. As these bones are developing in membrane the development is called *intramembranous ossification* or bone formation. The bones that are formed by this method are called membranous or dermal bones, e.g., bones of vault of skull (parietal bone), face, mandible, and clavicle. Direct mineralization of highly vascular connective tissue takes place in this method.
- *Cartilaginous bones:* In some bones the mesodermal condensation/model is converted to cartilaginous model. Later calcification of the cartilaginous model and its conversion into bone takes place. This method of formation of bone is known as *intracartilaginous* or *endochondral ossification* and such bones are called cartilaginous bones. Majority of the bones are formed by this method, e.g., vertebra that forms vertebral column, bones of limbs, and bones of thoracic cage.
- *Membranocartilaginous:* Some bones develop partly in membrane and partly in cartilage, e.g., occipital, mandible, temporal, and sphenoid bones.

♦ *According to structure (structural):*
  - *Macroscopically:* There are two types of bone:
    1. *Compact/dense bone:* Outer covering of bone that is ivory like and extremely porous. It is more *radiopaque* and appears white in radiographs. The fundamental functional unit of compact bone is *osteon* or *Haversian system*. Shaft of long bones contain thick outer covering of compact bone surrounding the central marrow or medullary cavity.
    2. *Spongy or trabecular or cancellous bone:* It fills the inner part of bone except:
       - Shaft of a long bone where it is replaced by marrow cavity.
       - In maxilla, sphenoid, ethmoid, and frontal bones that lie around nasal cavity that are filled with air forming large spaces called *paranasal air sinuses*.
       - Spongy bone consists of network of bars of bone called *trabeculae* that are arranged along the lines of stresses and are adapted to withstand stress and strain to which bone is subjected. It is more *radiolucent* and appears darker in radiographs.

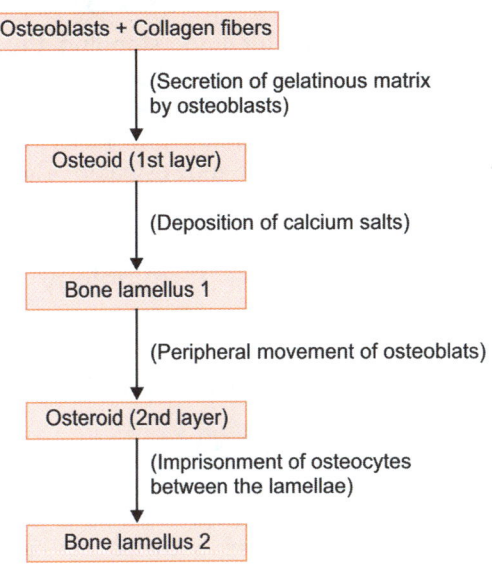

Flowchart 4.3: Formation of bone lamellus.

- Microscopically: They are classified into:
  - Lamellar bone: It presents a regular, parallel alignment of collagen fibers in the form of sheets (lamellae). It is mechanically strong (refer **Fig. 4.10 and Flowchart 4.3**).
  - Fibrous (woven) bone: It presents a haphazard organization of collagen fibers. It is mechanically weak.
  - Dentin: It is one of the four major components of the teeth (enamel, cementum, dentin, and pulp). It surrounds the pulp.
  - Cementum: It is a specialized calcified substance covering root of tooth.

Calcification

It is simply deposition of calcium salts without the presence of osteoclasts, e.g., calcified cartilage.

Ossification

AN 2.2 : Enumerate laws of ossification.

It includes proliferation of collagen and ground substance with subsequent deposition of calcium salts.

A *primary ossification center* is the first area to start ossification.

Laws of Ossification

- *Type:* The ossification may be intramembranous/intracartilaginous/membranocartilaginous.
- *Extension of ossification centers:* These centers extend radially from the site of ossification.
- *Centers of ossification:* There are two centers of ossification. They are primary and secondary. Ossification begins around 8th week of fetal life and is completed by around 25 years. The cartilage cells die and are replaced by osteoblasts that are grouped in the *ossification center*.
- *Primary centers:* These are the first to appear. They appear before birth usually during 6–8th weeks of intrauterine life with *exceptions—cuneiform, navicular*. Diaphysis (shaft) of a long bone is formed from the primary center. If multiple they appear simultaneously.
- *Secondary centers:* These appear after birth (late appearance) with few *exceptions—lower end of femur, upper end of tibia*. Epiphyses (ends) of a long bone are formed from secondary centers. They are multiple and do not appear simultaneously. Fusion of ends (epiphyses) with shaft (diaphysis) starts around puberty and is completed by 25th year. After completion of fusion of epiphyses with diaphysis there is no further increase in growth. The growing end of a long bone is the one that is the last to fuse with the diaphysis.
- *Growing end of a bone:* When there are two ends, at one end secondary center of ossification begins first, grows for a longer period, and fuses with the shaft later. This end which grows for a longer time is known as growing end. In the upper limb the upper end of humerus and lower ends of radius and ulna are the growing ends. In the lower limb lower end of femur and upper ends of tibia and fibula are the growing ends.

- *Law of union of ossification:* The epiphyseal center which appears first unites last with the diaphysis and the one that appears last fuses first. *Exception—fibula where distal epiphysis appears first and unites first.*
- *Direction of nutrient foramen and artery:* The nutrient foramen is situated near the middle of the shaft of a long bone through which the nutrient artery enters. The direction of nutrient foramen and artery are away from the growing end in a long bone. In the case of upper limb bones it is directed towards the elbow in humerus, radius, and ulna. In the case of lower limb bones it is directed away from the knee in femur, tibia, and fibula. *To the elbow I go and from the knee I flee is the dictum* **(Fig. 4.14)**. In the upper limb shoulder and wrist ends are the growing ends. In the lower limb knee ends of the femur, tibia, and fibula are the growing ends.
- *Union of various epiphyses:* Different secondary centers of ossification of an epiphysis first unite with one another and then join with diaphysis with an *exception—upper end of femur where lesser trochanter, greater trochanter, and head join shaft at different times.*
- *Sex differences:* Ossification begins earlier in females than in males. Fusion of epiphysis with diaphysis is completed 2 or 3 years earlier in females than in males.

Clinical Application of Ossification

It is important for understanding the maturity of the individual and for age estimation in medicolegal practice. The time of appearance and fusion of epiphyses in both pre and postnatal life are represented in **Tables 4.7** and **4.8**.

Markings on Bone—Terminology

- *Elevations:* Markings which are raised up from the surface.
  - *Spine:* A sharp elevation, e.g., spine of scapula
  - *Line/ridge/crest:* Linear elevations, e.g., iliac crest, linea aspera of femur, supracondylar ridge
  - *Tuberosity/tubercle/trochanter/malleolus:* Rounded elevation, e.g., gluteal tuberosity.
- *Depressions:* Markings which run lower to the surface.
  - *Pit/fovea:* A very small depression, e.g., fovea on head of femur

Table 4.7: Chronology of prenatal ossification centers.

Age	Time of appearance of ossification centers
5th–6th week	Skull bones and clavicle
7th–8th week	Long bones
5th month	Calcaneum, ischium and pubis
7th month	Talus
9th month	Lower end of femur, cuboid

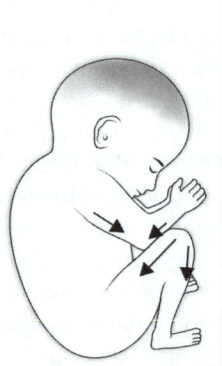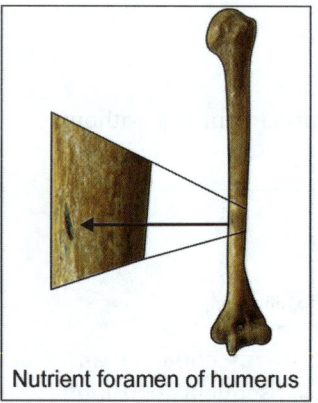

Nutrient foramen of humerus

Fig. 4.14: Direction of nutrient foramen in a long bone.

Chapter 4: Skeletal System

Table 4.8: Chronology of postnatal development of bone.

Age (in years)	Appearance and fusion of centers of ossification or sutures or parts of bones
1st	Appearance of head of femur, humerus, tibia
2nd	Lower end of tibia and radius
3rd	Appearance of patella
4th	Appearance of upper end of fibula, greater trochanter of femur
5th	Appearance of lower end of fibula
6th	Appearance of head of radius, lower end of ulna
7th	Appearance of scaphoid, union of ischial and pubic rami
8th	Appearance of medial epicondyle of humerus, olecranon process of ulna
10th	Appearance of lesser trochanter of femur
11th	Appearance of trochlea of humerus
12th	Acetabular y-shaped cartilage, pisiform
13th	Appearance of lateral epicondyle of humerus and its union with trochlea and capitulum
14th	Union of coracoid process with scapula
16th	Union of olecranon process with ulna
18th	Union of head of femur and radius with shafts
20th	Union of lower ends of radius, ulna and femur with shafts. Union of iliac crest with the body
21st–25th	Appearance of secondary epiphyseal center at the medial end of clavicle and its fusion with articular facets of 1st ribs
25th–50th	Closure of skull sutures in sequence—sagittal (<35 years), coronal (<40 years), lambdoid <50 years), parietomastoid and squamous sutures (<60 years), sphenoparietal suture (<70 years)
	Union of xiphisternum with body (40 years) and greater cornu with body of hyoid (60 years)
	Early degenerative changes occur in articular surfaces of the long bones
50–70 years	Calcification of laryngeal and costal cartilages
	Pathological changes in the skeleton

Clinical Application

- *Growing end*: Injury or infection of the growing end in young age makes the bone stunted in growth.
- *Periosteum*: Contains cells called osteoblasts that help in bone growth and in healing of fracture. It is supplied by sensory nerves. Hence, sensitive to pain. Drilling of periosteum without giving anesthesia should not be done.
- *Osteoarthritis*: Degeneration of articular cartilage that lacks perichondrium. It can affect any joint. Most common joints affected are knee, hip, lower back, and small joints of fingers. It causes painful movements of the joints **(Figs. 4.15A to D)**.
- *Osteoporosis*: Disease of bone where bones become brittle and fracture easily. Usual in elderly and in postmenopausal women.
- *Osteomyelitis*: Bacterial infection of bone.
- *Fibrous dysplasia*: Excessive growth or swelling of bone.
- *Achondroplasia*: It is a genetic disorder that results in abnormally short stature, e.g., circus dwarfs. Achondroplasia means without cartilage formation. The long bones will be shortened. Growth plate at the junction of diaphysis and epiphysis is defective **(Fig. 4.16)**.
- *Acromegaly*: Overgrowth of bones. It is caused by excess production of growth hormone.
- *Rickets*: Weak and brittle bones that fracture easily. It is seen in children. It results from deficiency of vitamin D.
- *Osteomalacia*: It is similar to rickets but is seen in adults.
- *Sesamoiditis*: Inflammation of sesamoid bones.
- *Avascular necrosis of sesamoid bone*: More prone for bone death.

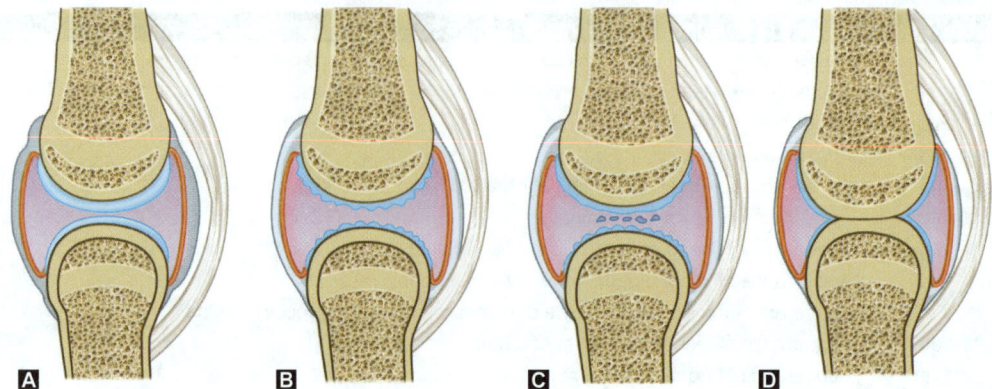

Figs. 4.15A to D: Osteoarthritis of knee joint. (A) Normal joint; (B) Thinning of cartilage; (C) Remnants of cartilage; (D) Decrease of joint space.

Anatomical Basis for Clinical Condition

Case Scenario

Problem: A primigravida delivered a baby that died immediately after birth. The picture of the dead fetus is presented in **Figure 4.16**. By looking at the photograph what abnormality could be diagnosed? Where lies the defect? What is the cause for the abnormality?

Questions:
1. What is the name given to this condition?
2. Describe your observations.
3. What is the cause for this condition?
4. How this condition can be detected prenatally?
5. Explain the anatomical basis.

Anatomical explanation:
1. It is a case of dwarfism or achondroplasia.
2. There is disproportionate head, trunk, and limbs. Large head with prominent forehead (frontal bossing), depressed nasal bridge.
3. It is caused by a mutation in fibroblast growth factor receptor 3 (FGFR3) gene. A person with this gene can transmit it to 50% of his children who can become dwarf. If both the parents are having the defective gene then the results are fatal.
4. This condition can be detected by prenatal ultrasound examination.
5. In this condition, there is insufficient, or disorderly, formation of bone in the region of the epiphyseal plate of cartilage/growth plate. This interferes with growth of long bones. The individual does not grow in height and becomes a dwarf **(Fig. 4.16)**.

- *Fossa:* Cup-like depression, e.g., iliac fossa
- *Groove or sulcus:* Linear depression, e.g., bicipital groove
- *Notch:* A depression in a border and this notch may be bridged by a ligament, e.g., suprascapular notch of scapula.

Chapter 4: Skeletal System

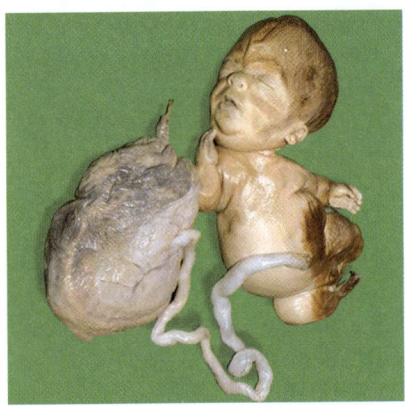

Fig. 4.16: Achondroplasia.

- *Foramen:* A hole or opening, e.g., foramen magnum in base of skull.
- *Canal or meatus:* A tubular tunnel-like structure. The canal will have at both its ends, an opening called the *orifice* or *ostium*, e.g., external acoustic meatus.
- *Head or capitulum:* A large and prominent rounded area, e.g., in the humerus.
- *Condyles:* Smaller rounded areas, e.g., in humerus.
- *Epicondyle:* A smaller eminence superior or adjacent to a condyle, e.g., in femur.
- *Trochlea*: A pulley-shaped part, e.g., in humerus.

☞ Key Concept

Take Home Message—Skeletal System

Cartilage
- Cartilage is aneural (insensitive to pain) and avascular. Nutrition is provided to chondrocytes by diffusion.
- Perichondrium is absent in articular cartilage.
- Cartilage transplantation can be done without tissue rejection.

Bone
- There are two types of bone—compact and spongy.
- The eight important components of a developing long bone are:
  1. Shaft (diaphysis)
  2. Upper end (upper epiphysis)
  3. Lower ends (lower epiphysis)
  4. Epiphyseal cartilage
  5. Epiphyseal end of shaft (metaphysis)
  6. Periosteum
  7. Endosteum
  8. Marrow cavity.
- Epiphyseal cartilage is the place where growth in length of a long bone takes place. This plate is temporary. Knowledge of this epiphyseal plate is important for understanding growth disorders in children and for shortening of a limb after injury and lengthening of the limb after inflammation of the growth plate.
- Knowledge of metaphysis and the blood vessels in this region are important especially in children for understanding the hematogenous spread of infection in long bones.
- Knowledge of structure of bone and bone marrow is important for understanding the importance of bone marrow aspiration, biopsy and transplantation.
- Knowledge of time of appearance of ossification and their fusion is required for age estimation and in medicolegal practice for ruling out a case of juvenile delinquency.

QUESTIONS

1. Describe the different types of cartilage giving examples for each.
2. Describe the parts of a long bone.
3. Describe the blood supply of a long bone.
4. Classify bones giving examples for each.
5. Mention the various laws of ossification.
6. Different types of epiphyses with examples for each.
7. Name the different types of epiphyses of humerus.
8. Metaphysis.
9. Laws of ossification.
10. Sesamoid bone.

MULTIPLE CHOICE QUESTIONS

1. **All the following are true about Volkmann's canals, except:**
   A. Connect the osteons with one another
   B. Connect the osteons with periosteum
   C. Connect the osteons with endosteum
   D. Surrounded by concentric lamellae

2. **Find the wrong statement in the following for examples of epiphyses.**
   A. Pressure epiphysis—capitulum of humerus
   B. Traction epiphysis—greater tubercle of humerus
   C. Atavastic epiphysis—coracoid process of scapula
   D. Aberrant epiphysis—epiphysis at the base of 1st metacarpal

3. **Perichondrium is absent in all of the following, except:**
   A. Articular cartilage
   B. Glenoidal labrum
   C. Intervertebral disc
   D. Epiglottis

4. **Growth in length of a long bone is affected in fracture at which of the following region?**
   A. Epiphyseal end of diaphysis
   B. Metaphysis
   C. Epiphysis
   D. Epiphyseal cartilage

5. **Blood cells are formed in ---- part of bone.**
   A. Bone marrow
   B. Periosteum
   C. Epiphysis
   D. None of the above

6. **Spongy bone is present in all the following bones, except:**
   A. Maxilla
   B. Sphenoid
   C. Ethmoid
   D. Shaft of femur

7. **Which one among the following is an example for traction epiphysis?**
   A. Tibial condyles
   B. Trochanters of femur
   C. Coracoid process of scapula
   D. Head of femur

8. **Perichondrium is absent in all the following, except:**
   A. White fibrocartilage
   B. Articular cartilage
   C. Elastic cartilage
   D. Costal cartilage

9. **All the following are examples of white fibrocartilage, except:**
   A. Acetabular labrum
   B. Menisci of knee joints
   C. Costal cartilage
   D. Intervertebral discs

10. **The direction of nutrient artery is:**
    A. Towards metaphysis
    B. Away from metaphysis
    C. Away from epiphysis
    D. None

11. **Untrue about articular cartilage is:**
    A. Covers the articular surfaces of all synovial joints

Chapter 4: Skeletal System

B. Is of hyaline variety in all synovial joints
C. No ossification with age
D. Is generally devoid of nerves, vessels and perichondrium

12. **Importance of metaphysis is because of all of the following reasons, *except*:**
    A. High vascularity
    B. Hair pin bends of nutrient vessels
    C. Cupping of metaphysis in osteomyelitis
    D. Infection of long bone starts here

13. **All secondary centers of ossification appear after birth, *except*:**
    A. Upper end of femur
    B. Lower end of tibia
    C. Lower end of femur
    D. Upper end of humerus

14. **All the following are examples for membranous bones, *except*:**
    A. Parietal
    B. Mandible
    C. Clavicle
    D. Scapula

15. **All the following are sesamoid bones, *except*:**
    A. Patella
    B. Calcaneus
    C. Pisiform
    D. Part of cuboid

ANSWERS					
1. D	2. D	3. D	4. D	5. A	6. D
7. B	8. A	9. C	10. A	11. B	12. C
13. C	14. D	15. B			

Chapter 5

Introduction to Muscular System

LEARNING OBJECTIVES

- General features of muscular tissue
- Classification and types of muscles
- Structure of skeletal muscle
- Structural components of skeletal muscle
- Blood supply and innervation of skeletal muscle and its significance
- Classification of skeletal muscles
- Naming of muscles
- Clinical case with anatomical explanation

INTRODUCTION

- The bones are the supportive connective tissue and joints are meant for locomotion. Muscular system brings out movements of these components by pulling the bones through the mechanism of nerve impulse.
- In the human body muscles form the major bulk of limbs and some other parts of the body.
- Muscular tissue is a contractile tissue and is primarily designed for various movements which the individual can perform. Thus, the muscles are also part of the locomotor apparatus.
- Study of muscles is called *myology*.
- The word muscle is derived from *Latin musculus = little mouse* because of the resemblance of many muscles to the shape of a mouse. Most of the skeletal muscles have a bulkier, fleshy part, the body or the belly and a thinned out fibrous part, the tendon; thus they appear to have the shape of a mouse, with the tendon looking like a tail.
- Contractility (to be able to shorten and lengthen itself by contractions and relaxations) is the important property of the muscle.
- Muscle cells (myocytes) are often called muscle fibers as they are elongated (long) when contracted and thin (narrow) when relaxed.

GENERAL FEATURES OF MUSCULAR TISSUE

- The muscular tissue is capable of bringing about different types of movements in the body.
- It is vascular and has limited capacity to regenerate.
- The fundamental protoplasmic property of contractility is highly developed in this tissue.
- The cytoplasmic organelles of muscle fibers are given different names. They are represented in **Table 5.1**.
- The cells are elongated in the direction of contraction and organized as long units of structure called muscle fibers. It is covered by a cell membrane called *sarcolemma*.
- A muscle fiber is made up of actin and myosin proteins that are responsible for contractility.

Chapter 5: Introduction to Muscular System

Table 5.1: Names of cytoplasmic organelle in muscle fiber.

In ordinary cell	Muscle
Plasma membrane	Sarcolemma
Protoplasm	Sarcoplasm
Smooth endoplasmic reticulum	Sarcoplasmic reticulum
Mitochondria	Sarcosomes

Classification

AN3.1: Classify muscles according to structure and function.

It can be classified based on its structure or on its function **(Flowchart 5.1)**.

- *Morphological classification (based on structure)*:
  - Striated
  - Nonstriated or smooth.
- *Functional classification (based on function)*:
  - Voluntary
  - Involuntary.
- *Combination of both (structure and function)*:
  - *Striated voluntary:* Skeletal muscle
  - *Striated involuntary:* Cardiac muscle
  - *Nonstriated involuntary:* Smooth muscle.

TYPES OF MUSCLE

There are three types of muscles:
1. *Skeletal, striated, and voluntary muscle*:
   - This is the most common type of muscle. It is attached to skeleton.
   - It is called striated because of the presence of lines or striations when this tissue is seen under the microscope.
   - Supplied by cranial or spinal nerves (motor) and are usually under the control of will hence called voluntary. *Exceptions*—the muscles of pharynx and diaphragm are striated and supplied by motor nerves but are not voluntary.
   - They are also called *skeletal muscles* because of their attachment to skeletal tissue (bone). As the majority are involved in movements of the body (soma) they are called *somatic muscles*.
   - The contraction of skeletal muscle is rapid hence they fatigue easily.
2. *Smooth, nonstriated, and involuntary muscle:*
   - There are no striations in these muscles and they are also called smooth muscles.

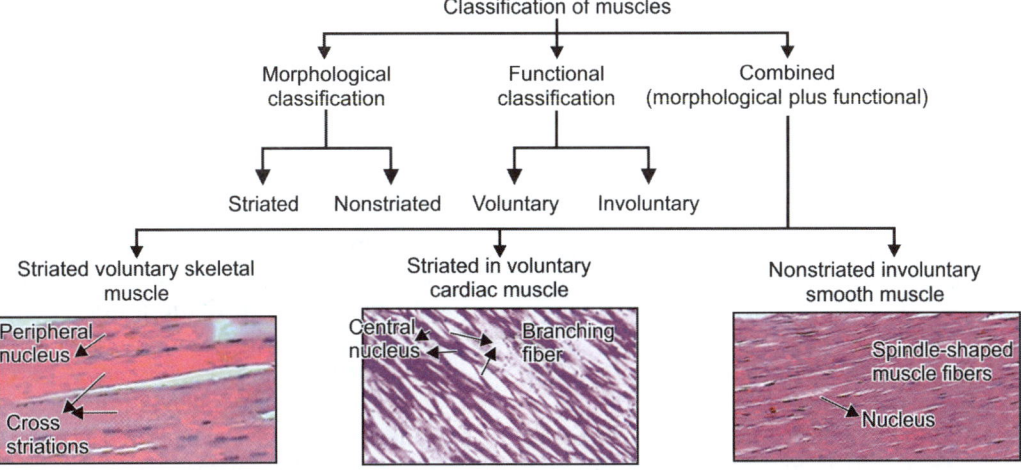

Flowchart 5.1: Classification of muscles.

- They are involuntary as they are innervated by autonomic nerves (both sympathetic and parasympathetic) and their movements are not under the control of will.
- They are concerned with the processes of digestion, secretion, excretion, and circulation. They are also called *visceral muscle* as they are seen in the walls of viscera.

3. *Cardiac, striated, and involuntary muscle:*
   - The musculature of heart is in between striated voluntary and nonstriated involuntary.
   - It shows striations but is involuntary as it acts under the influence of autonomic nerves (both sympathetic and parasympathetic).
   - It is responsible for rhythmic contractions of heart.

The description of various types of muscle fibers and their microscopic structure is presented in **Table 5.2** and **Figures 5.1A to C**.

STRUCTURE OF SKELETAL MUSCLE

AN3.2: Enumerate parts of skeletal muscle and differences between tendons and aponeuroses.

The structural components of a muscle can be divided into those that can be observed (**Fig. 5.2**):
- With naked eye
- Under light microscope
- Under polarized microscope
- Under electron microscope.

Accordingly the structure can be described as follows.

Macroscopic Appearance—Parts of a Skeletal Muscle (Flowchart 5.2 and Fig. 5.3)

- Components: It presents two parts—(1) A fleshy part, and (2) A fibrous part.
  1. *Fleshy part:* Contractile, made up of muscular tissue, and is called the *belly*.
  2. *Fibrous part:* Noncontractile, made up of connective tissue fibers arranged in the form of a cord or rope, i.e., *tendon* or as a flat sheet, i.e., *aponeurosis*.
- It presents two ends—(1) Origin, and (2) Insertion.
  1. *Origin:* More fixed part—proximal (limbs) in location. It is relatively fixed during contraction.
  2. *Insertion:* Movable—distal (limbs) in location. It moves during contraction. Depending on the types of insertion, the muscles are classified into those inserted:
     - Near the *proximal end of bone* close to the joint. In this type of insertion the range of movement is more than the power of contraction, e.g., *biceps brachii, psoas major*.
     - Near the *distal end of bone* away from the joint where the power of contraction is more than the range of movement, e.g., *brachioradialis*.
     - At the *middle of shaft* of bone, e.g., *coracobrachialis, pronator teres*.

Tendon

- Fibrous cord-like end of a muscle.
- Noncontractile.
- Composed of bundles of collagen fibers. It is an example for *dense regular connective tissue*. It is surrounded by *epitendineum*.
- Less vascular because of which whenever injured it heals slowly.
- In areas where it is subjected to friction a *synovial sheath* or a *bursa* interposes.
- At the junction of muscle and tendon (myotendinous junction) the muscle fibers are not continuous with the fibers of tendon. Instead they are contiguous with one another giving a *dove-tailed appearance* (**Fig. 5.4**).
- *Functions:*
  - Concentrate the pull of a muscle on a narrow area, i.e., at insertion.
  - Can bear the weight.

Chapter 5: Introduction to Muscular System

Table 5.2: Different types of muscular tissue—microscopic structure.

Types of muscle	Structure (Figs. 5.1A to C)
Skeletal muscle: ☐ *Location*: Seen throughout the body ☐ Attached to bones ☐ Appears in bundles called fascicles that are visible to the naked eye ☐ The unit of muscle is called *muscle* fiber or *cell* ☐ These are extremely long, cylindrical, and unbranched ☐ The muscle fiber is multinucleated. The nuclei are peripherally located in the muscle fiber ☐ Skeletal muscle presents longitudinal and transverse striations because of alternating pattern of light and darks bands in ultrastructure A	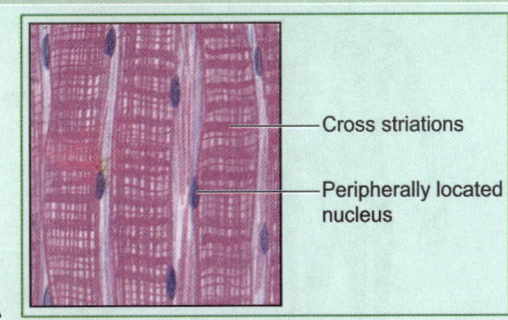
Cardiac muscle: ☐ *Location*: In heart ☐ Muscle fibers are striated and the striations are less prominent than in skeletal muscle ☐ The fibers branch and join with adjacent fibers to form a complex network ☐ The nucleus is single, elongated, and centrally placed ☐ The muscle cells are joined by specialized structures called *intercalated discs* that run transversely B	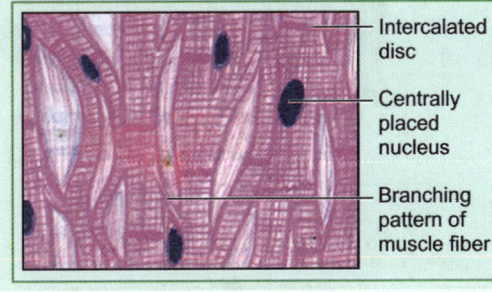
Smooth muscle: ☐ *Location*: In the walls of hollow organs like gastrointestinal tract, respiratory tract, and blood vessels ☐ Muscle fibers are long, spindle-shaped cells arranged in bundles or sheets ☐ Striations are lighter in appearance when compared to skeletal muscle ☐ The fibers branch or bifurcate and join with adjacent fiber to form a complex network ☐ The nucleus is single, elongated, and is seen in the thickest part of the cell C	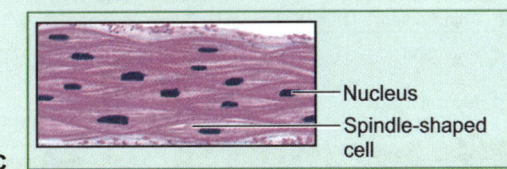

- Can alter the direction of muscle pull by using bony projections as pulleys.
- Keeps the main bulk of muscle at a distance from insertion.

Functional Importance of Fleshy Belly and Fibrous Tendon

- *Cross-sectional area of a tendon:* It is much less than that of the fleshy belly. This factor is important in the functioning of a muscle. The pull of a muscle is exerted at the tendon.
- *Extent of muscle:* Many of the striated muscles of the body run from one bone to another across a joint. When the muscle contracts, the two bones are approximated and movement occurs at the joint.

- *Force and movement:*
  - When the muscle is attached to the bone through a tendon, the tendon converges to a smaller area of attachment; the force of muscle pull is concentrated and focused. This will make the movement smoother, faster, and more powerful.
  - When the muscle is attached to the bone directly by means of fleshy fibers, the force is low and widespread. In many muscles, such a fleshy attachment can be seen at the origin.
  - If the origin remains fixed and the insertion (the tendinous portion of the muscle) moves, cumulative addition

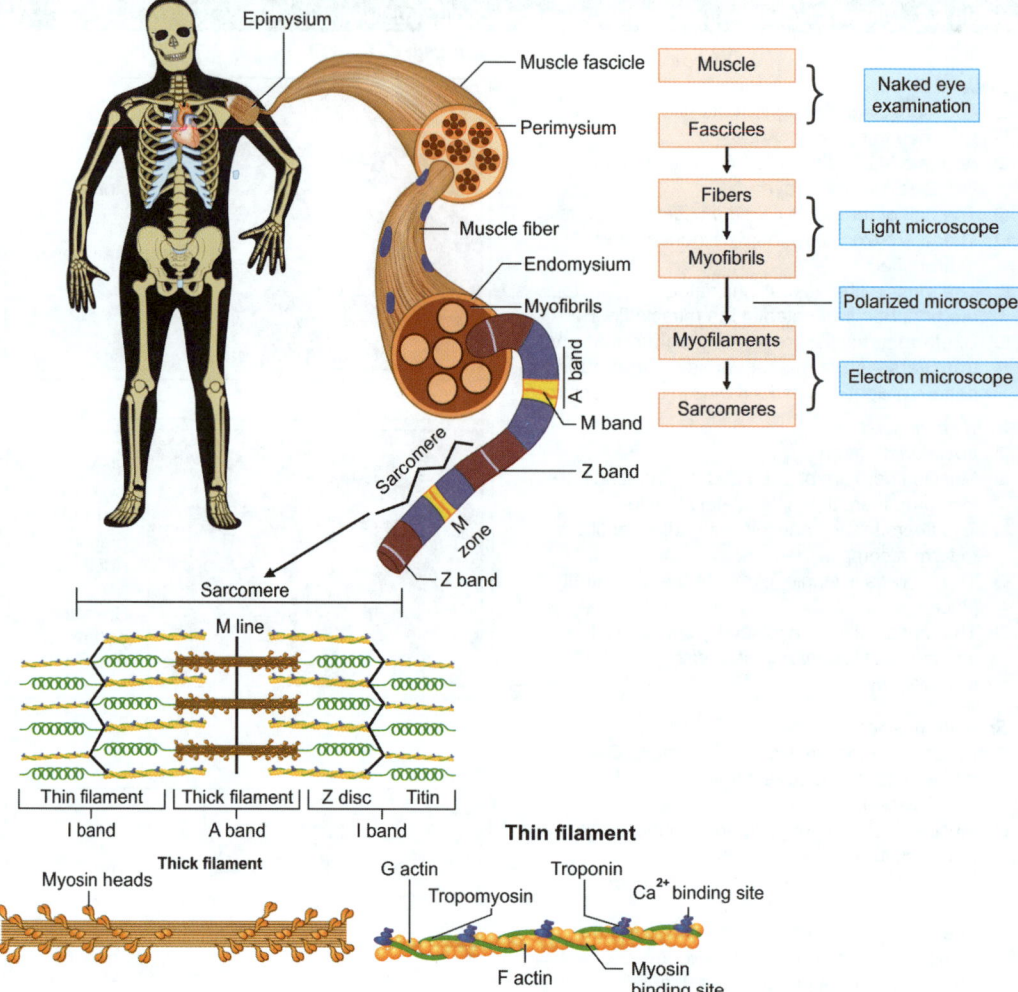

Fig. 5.2: Structural components of skeletal muscle and their observation.

of force occurs from the origin to insertion as the muscle contracts and all the force is focused on the tendinous insertion to give an effective pull.
- *Bony prominences produced by muscle attachments:*
  - Points of fleshy attachments do not produce bony ridges or tubercles but points of tendinous attachments have bony prominences like ridges, tubercles, facets (*please refer to Chapter 4 for the bony prominences mentioned*).
  - This is due to the fact that force is concentrated at the tendinous attachments and is responsible for producing marks on the bone.

Clinical Importance
- Rupture of tendon makes the muscle ineffective.
- Traction of a tendon at the insertion causes bone fracture without rupture of tendon.
- Site of insertion and movement of the muscle are important in assessing the integrity of tendon.

Chapter 5: Introduction to Muscular System

- Most common tendons that can be injured are biceps, Achilles, quadriceps, and rotator cuff.
- Healing is prolonged in cases of tendon injury due to poor blood supply.

Aponeurosis

- Aponeurosis is the attachment of a muscle by thin, broad sheet.
- It is composed of parallel bundles of collagen fibers.
- Act as shock absorbers to bear extra pressure and tension.
- Very poor blood supply and nerve supply.
- Examples:
  - Anterior abdominal wall—external oblique and internal oblique aponeuroses
  - Limbs—palmar and plantar aponeuroses, bicipital aponeurosis **(Fig. 5.3)**
  - Scalp—epicranial aponeurosis
  - Soft palate—palatine aponeurosis

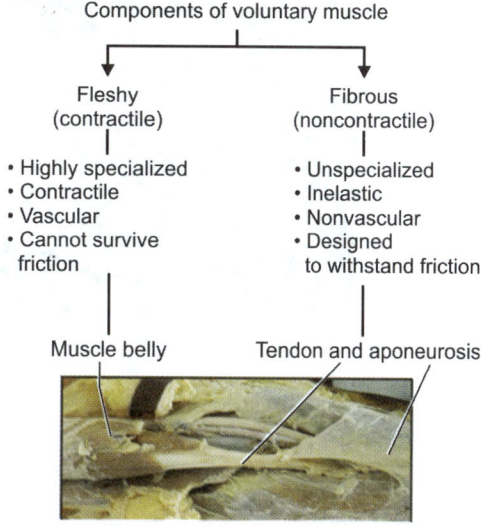

Flowchart 5.2: Components of voluntary muscle.

Raphe

Interdigitation of tendinous ends of a flat muscle is called raphe.
Example: Mylohyoid raphe.

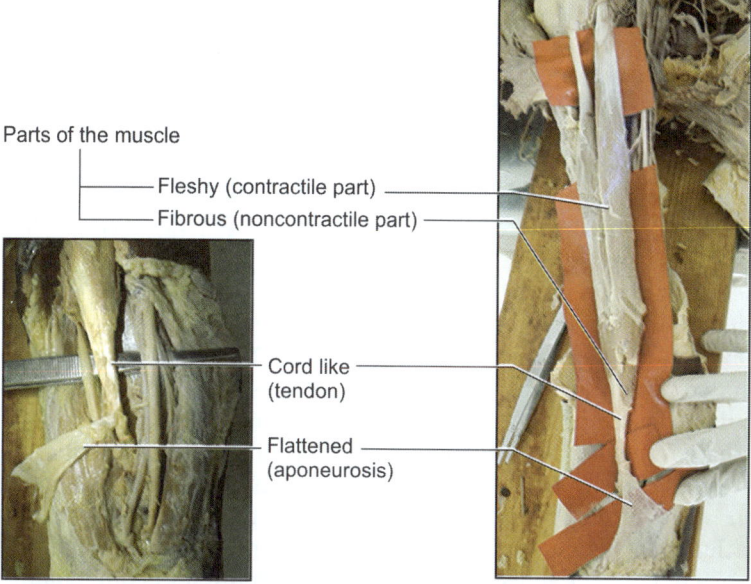

Fig. 5.3: Parts of muscle (biceps).

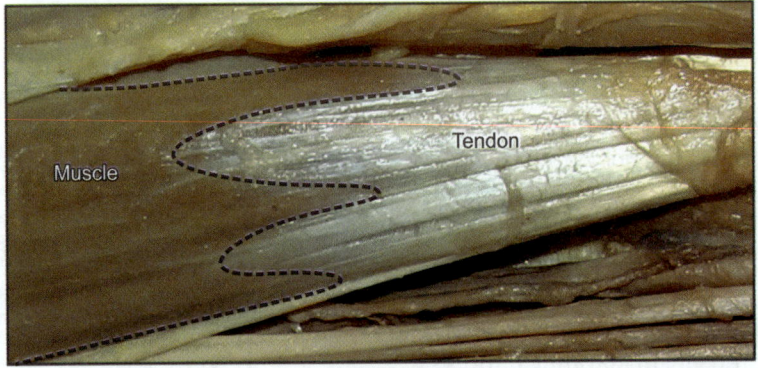

Fig. 5.4: Myotendinous junction showing "dove-tail" appearance.

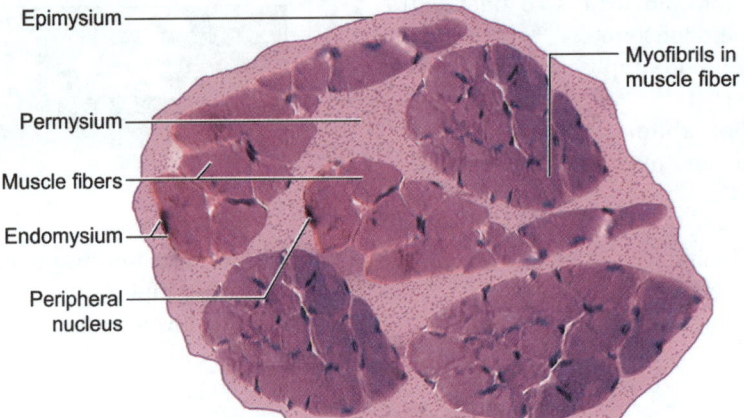

Fig. 5.5: Connective tissue present in relation to skeletal muscle.

Connective Tissue Coverings of Muscle (Fig. 5.5)

- Each muscle fiber is surrounded by a delicate (loose) connective tissue covering called the *endomysium*.
- Around a bunch of fibers called fascicles, there is another sheath of connective tissue called the *perimysium*.
- Many fascicles join up to form a muscle. Around the entire muscle is yet another sheath called the *epimysium*. The epimysium sometimes blends with the layers of deep fascia present near the muscle. The connective tissue contains collagen and elastic fibers and is continuous with tendon and bone at the site of attachment of the muscle.
- The presence of connective tissue in the form of endo, peri, and epimysia permits gliding and swelling of the individual fiber or bunch of fibers enclosed.

STRUCTURAL COMPONENTS OF A SKELETAL MUSCLE

Muscle Fascicles (Fig. 5.6)

- Bundles of muscle fibers that can be seen with unaided eye.
- The individual muscle fascicles and in turn the muscle fibers are arranged either parallel or at an angle to the long axis of the muscle.
- Based on the arrangement of fascicles, i.e., longitudinal, circular, spiral, etc., the muscles can be classified (*vide infra*).
- The range of movement of a muscle depends on the arrangement of fascicles e.g., parallel arrangement with greater range of movement.

Chapter 5: Introduction to Muscular System

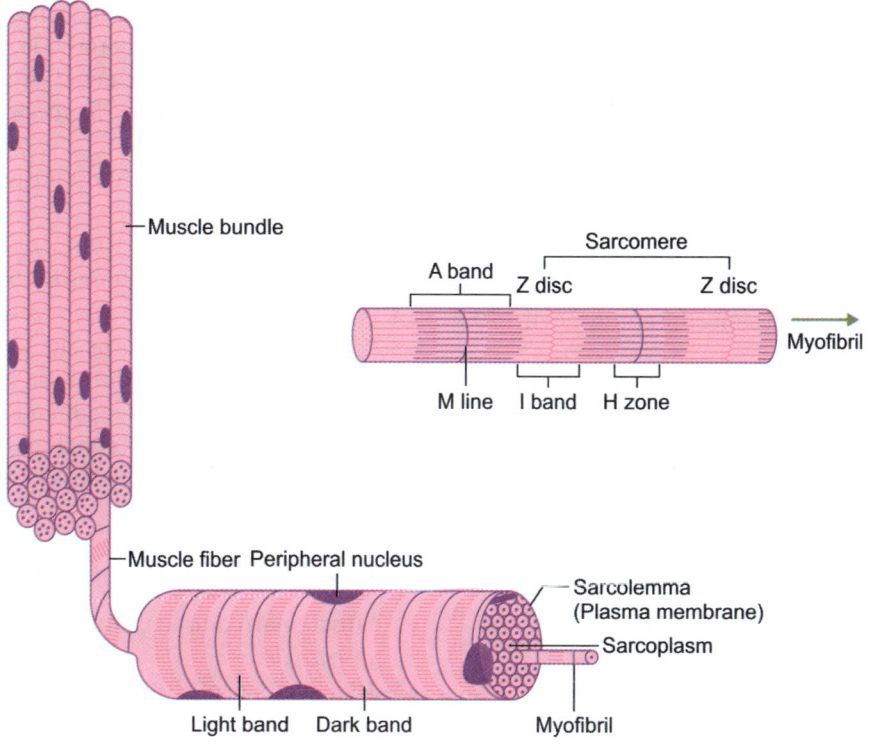

Fig. 5.6: Structure of skeletal muscles: Muscle bundle, muscle fiber, myofibril, and sarcomere.

- The number of fascicles also influences their movement, e.g., muscles that take part in highly controlled fine movements (e.g. extraocular muscles of eyeball) contain less number of fasciculi than those concerned with gross movements (e.g. gluteal muscles).

MICROSCOPIC APPEARANCE OF SKELETAL MUSCLE (FIGS. 5.2, 5.5 TO 5.8)

Muscle Fibers

- These can be observed under the light microscope **(Table 5.2 and Fig. 5.1A)**.
- These are extremely long, cylindrical, unbranched, cross striated, and multinucleated.
- The nuclei are peripherally located in the muscle fiber underneath the sarcolemma.
- Each muscle fiber, actually, is a muscle cell called the *myocyte*. However, each muscle fiber is a fusion of several embryonic muscle cells and therefore, has several nuclei. The muscle cells are elongated in the direction of contraction and organized in long units of muscle fibers.
- It has a *sarcolemma* [cell membrane of the myocyte; (Greek sarx = flesh; lemma = husk/skin)] which encloses the *sarcoplasm* (cytoplasm of the myocyte). Within the sarcoplasm, several nuclei can be seen arranged at the periphery beneath the sarcolemma **(Fig. 5.6)**.
- The diameter of skeletal muscle fibers in different parts of the body ranges from $10\,\mu$ to $100\,\mu$. This is about ten times larger than the average body cell. Similarly, the length of the fiber is many centimeters.
- The muscle fibers present cross striations. The striations observed under light microscope are due to the presence of myofibrils.

Myofibrils (Fig. 5.6)

- These can be observed under the electron microscope.
- These are seen inside each fiber and are responsible for the contraction mechanism.
- Each muscle fiber is made up of longitudinally arranged cylindrical sub-units called myofibrils that are arranged parallel to the long axis of muscle fiber.
- These extend along the entire length of the muscle fiber.
- These myofibrils give striped appearance to the muscle fiber.
- Each myofibrils presents repeating cross striations due to the orderly arrangement of *myofilaments*, i.e., contractile proteins (actin and myosin).
- The bundle of myofilaments in a myofibril is surrounded by sarcoplasmic reticulum (smooth endoplasmic reticulum of muscle).
- Cross striations of parallel myofibrils are in register and are responsible for the striated appearance observed under light microscope.

Myofilaments (Figs. 5.6 and 5.7)

- These are the ultramicroscopic structures and require the use of polarized microscope and electron microscope.
- Under the polarized microscope they present dark and light bands and show the property of *birefringence* (doubly refractive).
- The dark bands are called *A (anisotropic) bands* and are birefringent (doubly refractile) as they alter the polarized light in two planes.
- The light bands are called *I (isotropic) bands* and are mono-refringent as they do not alter the plane of polarized light.
- Both dark and light bands are bisected by two lines.
- The dark A band is bisected by a less dense region called *H [Heller = light—(German)] band* which is further bisected by a narrow dense line called *M [Mittel scheibe = middle—(German)] band* which is best seen under electron microscope.
- The light I band is bisected by a dense Z *[Zwischen scheibe = between discs—(German)] line*.
- *Types of myofilaments:* There are two types of myofilaments:
  1. *Thick filaments*: Contain protein *myosin*. 1.5 µ in length. 15 nm in diameter. They are seen only in the center of sarcomere, i.e., in A band.
  2. *Thin filaments*: Contains protein *actin*. It is 1.0 µ in length and 6 nm in diameter. They are attached to the Z line and extend into the A band up to the edge of H band.

Sarcomere (Figs. 5.6 and 5.7)

- Functional/contractile unit of myofibril is the *sarcomere*.
- It is a segment of myofibril between Z lines.
- Each sarcomere is 2–3 µ in relaxed state and more than 4 µ when stretched and about 1 µ in contracted state.
- The entire muscle fiber presents cross striations as the sarcomeres of adjacent myofibrils are in register (i.e. one below the other).
- The cross striations are due to the orderly arrangement of myofilaments (contractile proteins) within myofibril.
- *Arrangement of contractile proteins in various bands of sarcomere* are:
  - *Light I band:* It is parts of two sarcomeres on either side of Z line. This is the portion that contains only thin filaments (actin only).
  - *Dark A band:* Contains thick myosin filaments and overlapping thin filaments (myosin and actin).
  - *H band:* It is the area of A band containing only thick myosin filaments without overlapping thin actin filaments (myosin only).
  - *M line:* It is the point where the thick filaments join.

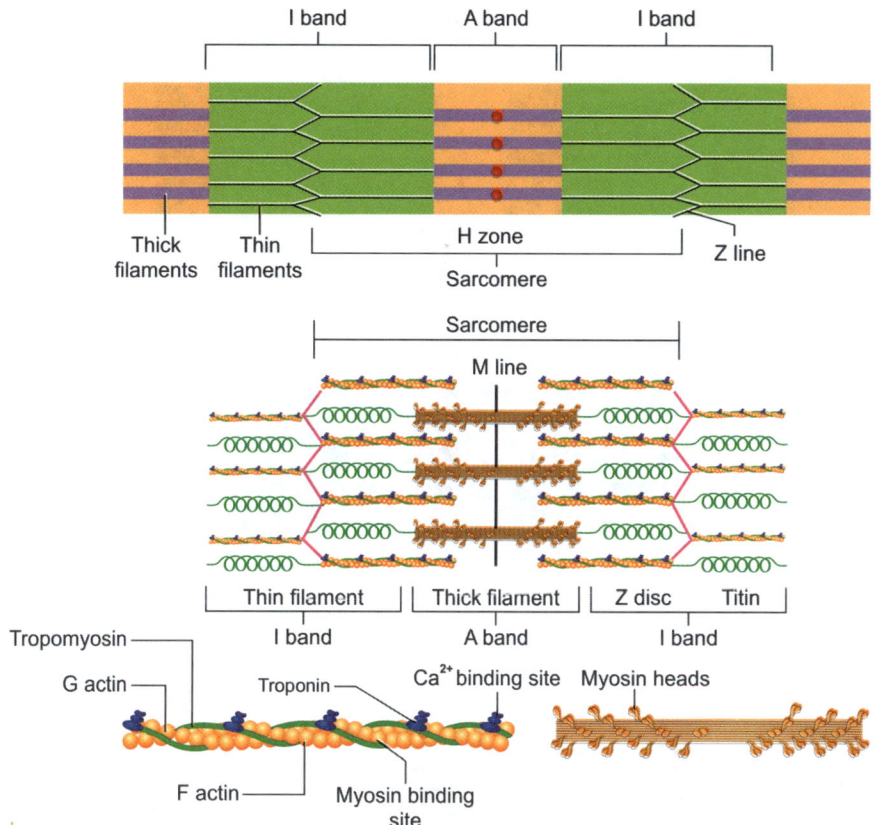

Fig. 5.7: Myofilaments and sarcomere.

- *Z line:* One end of thin actin filament runs parallel with thick myosin filament in A band for some distance. Other end is attached to the Z line in I band.

- Apart from *actin* and *myosin* a number of accessory contractile proteins, i.e., *tropomyosin* and *troponin* play an important role in the contraction.

Mechanism of Contraction (Fig. 5.8)

- There is no shortening of thick and thin filaments.
- There is only change in the degree of overlap of these filaments under the influence of adenosine triphosphate (ATP) and calcium ions released from sarcoplasmic reticulum.
- A band remains constant and only I and H bands become narrow and the Z lines come closer.
- The basis for these movements is explained by sliding filament theory.

BLOOD SUPPLY OF SKELETAL MUSCLE (FIG. 5.9)

- The muscular tissue is highly vascular because of its high metabolic activity.
- Blood supply is from muscular branches of neighboring arteries.
- Neurovascular hilum is the place where artery, vein, and nerve enter the muscle.
- Small muscles have single artery, two veins. Large muscles have several arteries and veins.
- *Vascular pedicle* of a muscle is one which consists of at least one vein and one

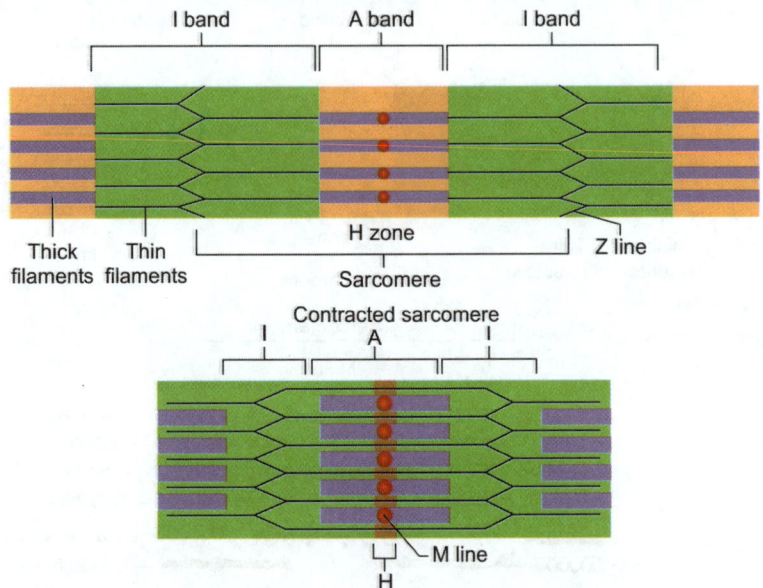

Fig. 5.8: Mechanism of contraction of skeletal muscle.

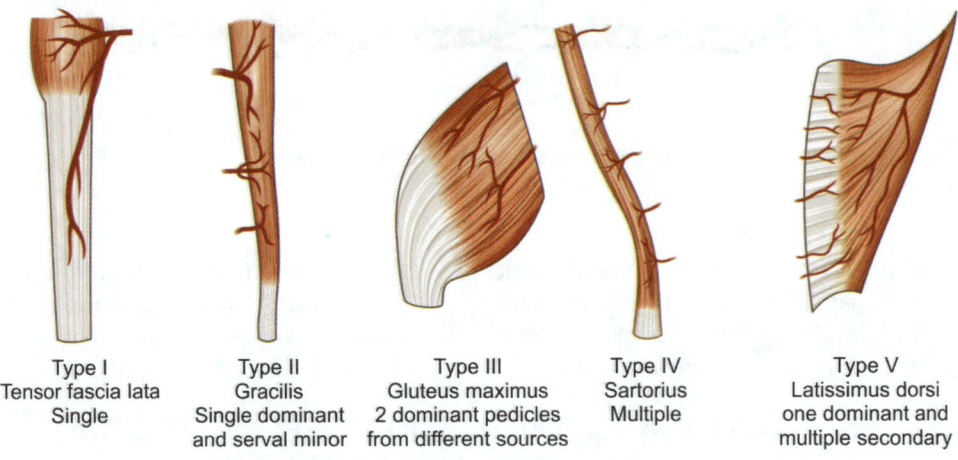

Fig. 5.9: Classification of skeletal muscle: Based on vascular pedicle.

artery. Based on the number of vascular pedicles the muscles are classified into the following types:
- *Type I:* Single vascular pedicle, e.g., tensor fascia lata (ascending branch of lateral circumflex femoral artery).
- *Type II:* Single dominant and several minor pedicles, e.g., gracilis (medial circumflex artery).
- *Type III:* Two dominant pedicles from different sources, e.g., gluteus maximus (superior and inferior gluteal arteries), rectus abdominis (superior and inferior epigastric arteries).
- *Type IV:* Multiple vascular pedicles, e.g., sartorius (5–10 pedicles from superficial circumflex iliac from external iliac, femoral artery and its

branches the profuda femoris, lateral circumflex femoral, and descending genicular); tibialis anterior.
- *Type V:* One dominant and multiple secondary pedicles, e.g., latissimus dorsi [thoracodorsal artery (dominant pedicle) and perforating branches from lower six posterior intercostal arteries and lumbar arteries as secondary pedicles].

Clinical Importance
- There will be stiffness of muscle after strenuous exercise. Due to strain on muscles there will be accumulation of lactic acid. In a physically fit individual it is removed by venous flow.
- The vascular pedicle is important in muscle graft and in determining which muscle will survive when used as graft in plastic and reconstructive surgery.

INNERVATION OF SKELETAL MUSCLE

AN7.5: Describe principle of sensory and motor innervation of muscles.
AN7.6: Describe concept of loss of innervation of a

The nerve to skeletal muscle contains motor (60%) and sensory (40%) fibers.

Motor Point

- It is the site/sites where motor nerve enters the muscle.
- Electrical stimulation of nerve at the motor point is more effective in initiating nerve impulse or action potential.

Motor Unit (Fig. 5.10)

- Motor unit is the number of muscle fibers in a skeletal muscle that are supplied by a single alpha motor neuron.
- The motor unit is large if it is supplying 100–200 muscle fibers. Large motor units are seen in muscles that are bulky and concerned with gross movements, e.g., muscles of gluteal region and thigh.
- Small motor units are those where a single motor neuron supplies 5–10 muscle fibers and such muscles are concerned with finer movements, e.g., extraocular muscles of eyeball, muscles of thumb.

Neuromuscular Junction (Fig. 5.11)

- It is also called myoneural junction. It is a chemical synapse between motor nerve fiber and muscle fiber where the neurotransmitter acetylcholine is released.
- The axon of a motor nerve, once it enters the muscle divides into number of branches.

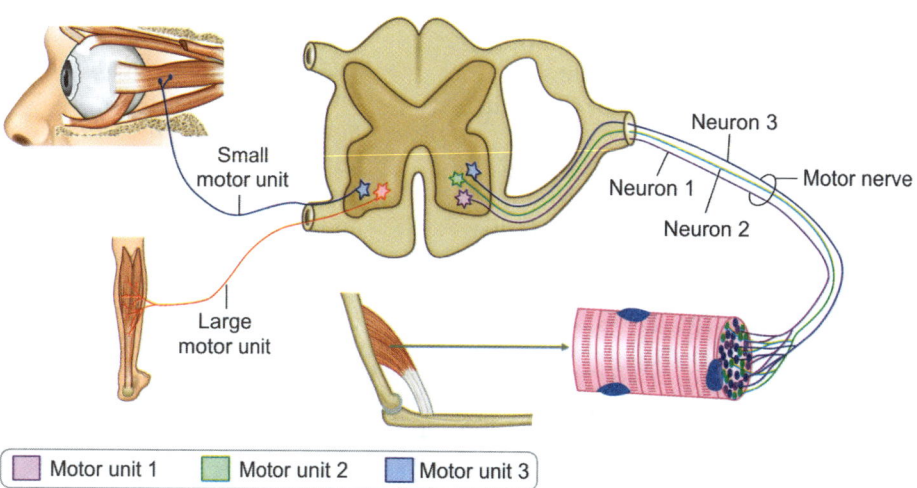

Fig. 5.10: Motor unit.

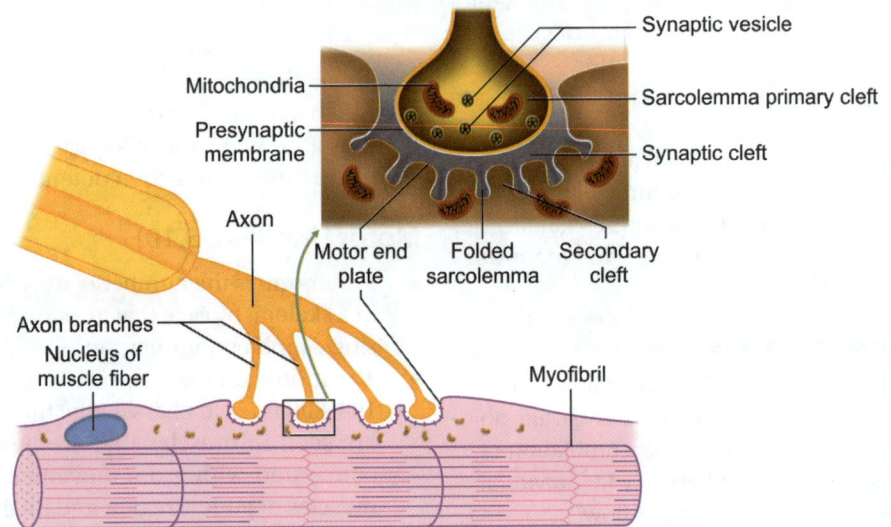

Fig. 5.11: Neuromuscular junction.

- Each of these branches reaches different set of muscle fibers called motor unit.
- Near the midpoint of muscle fiber each nerve fiber forms a synapse with the muscle fiber known as neuromuscular junction for transmission of impulses for precise muscle contraction.
- At neuromuscular junction the nerve fiber again splits forming a cluster of terminal branches.
- There are three parts in the neuromuscular junction. They are:
  1. *Presynaptic motor neuron:* It is presynaptic end bulb containing vesicles filled with acetylcholine.
  2. *Synaptic cleft:* It is the space where the acetylcholine is released.
  3. *Motor end plate:* Invaginated postsynaptic membrane forming the synaptic gutter (primary cleft) that comes in contact with the neurotransmitter and the subneural or secondary clefts of sarcolemma with mitochondria and nicotinic receptors.

Muscles with Dual Innervation

- Certain muscles have double nerve supply by two different motor nerves with different root values.
- They are called *composite* or *hybrid muscles.*
- Usually flexors have dual innervation. They receive from extensors.
- During development, the extensor muscles migrate to flexor compartment for functional reasons. While migrating they bring their original nerve supply with them.
- *Examples:*
  - *Brachialis:* Lateral part is supplied by radial nerve and medial part by musculocutaneous nerve.
  - *Biceps femoris:* Short head is supplied by peroneal part of sciatic nerve and long head by tibial part of sciatic nerve.
  - *Adductor magnus:* Supplied by obturator nerve and tibial part of sciatic nerve.
  - *Flexor digitorum profundus:* Median and ulnar nerves supply this muscle.
  - *Pectoralis major:* Innervated by medial and lateral pectoral nerves.
  - *Subscapularis:* Supplied by upper and lower subscapular nerves.

Sensory Innervation of Muscles

Muscle Fibers (Fig. 5.12)

Functionally the muscle fibers are of two types: (1) Extrafusal, and (2) Intrafusal.
1. Extrafusal fibers make up the bulk of skeletal muscle and are attached to bone. They are

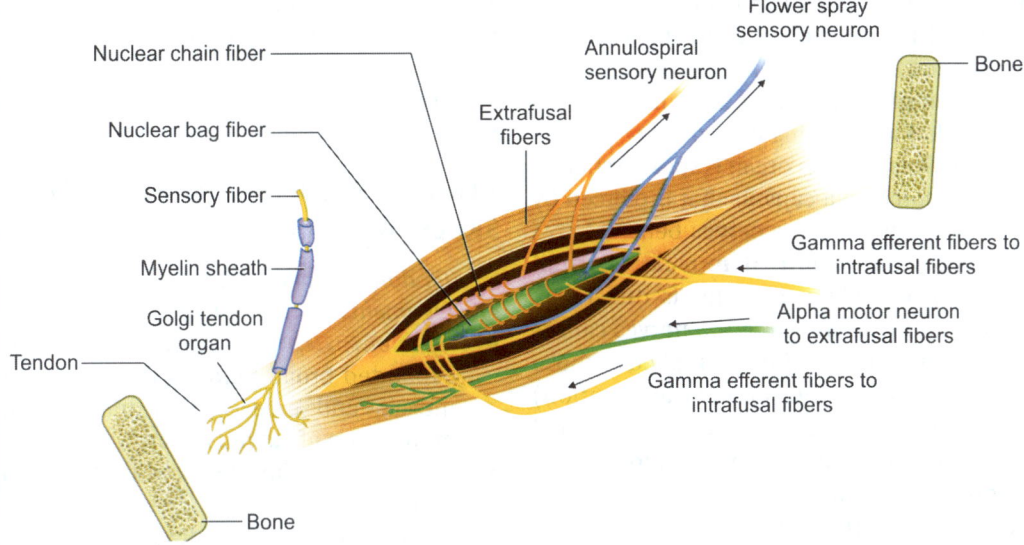

Fig. 5.12: Muscle spindle and Golgi tendon organ.

innervated by alpha motor neurons and are concerned with generating tension by contraction and allowing movement.

2. Intrafusal fibers serve as specialized sensory receptors (proprioceptors) that can detect the change in the length of muscle. They form the *muscle spindle* and are innervated by both sensory and motor neurons.

Muscle Spindle **(Fig. 5.12)**

- The muscle spindle is the peripheral receptor (proprioceptor) located in the muscle belly of skeletal muscles.
- They are parallel to the muscle fibers in orientation.
- Each spindle consists of *intrafusal fibers, sensory nerve endings*, and *gamma motor neuron endings*.
- The intrafusal fibers are of two types, i.e., (1) *Nuclear bag,* and (2) *Nuclear chain.* Nuclear bag fibers are thicker and longer than the nuclear chain fibers.
- The sensory endings in relation to intrafusal fibers are of two types, i.e., (1) *Annulospiral,* and (2) *Flower spray* endings. Annulospiral endings wrap around the center of intrafusal fibers. Flower spray endings are at the ends of intrafusal fibers.
- These respond to changes in the length (stretch) and velocity (speed) when the muscle is stretched (stretch reflex).
- When the muscle is stretched to its maximum the information will be sent to the central nervous system (CNS) to give an alarm not to stretch further and get hurt.
- Gamma motor neurons innervate intrafusal fibers and make them contract. Contraction of intrafusal fibers stimulates the sensory neurons in neuromuscular spindle that stimulates the alpha motor neurons that inturn make the extrafusal fibers to contract.
- The gamma reflex loop consists of gamma motor neuron, neuromuscular spindle, afferent neuron that supplies extrafusal fibers.

Golgi Tendon Organ **(Fig. 5.12)**

- These are peripheral receptors (proprioceptors) located in the tendons that get attached to the bone.

- Here the dendrites of sensory neurons wind round the collagen fibrils in the tendon.
- These sense and limit the tension in the tendon while lifting the weights.
- The Golgi tendon organ is spindle shaped and contains a capsule that is pierced by myelinated sensory nerve fibers.

Loss of innervation of muscle: Normal function of skeletal muscle is due to its nerve supply. Damage to the nerves causes atrophy of the muscle fibers supplied by those nerves. Loss of nerve supply (denervation) of a muscle is due to injury or surgical procedure (sympathectomy, vagotomy) or a disorder (e.g., amyotrophic lateral sclerosis, poliomyelitis). Injury to motor nerve causes paralysis. If the paralysis involves muscles of one limb it is called *monoplegia*. If muscles of one side of body are paralysed it is called *hemiplegia*. If muscles of both lower limbs are paralyzed it is called *paraplegia*. If muscles of all the four limbs are paralyzed it is called *quadriplegia*.

IMPORTANCE OF SKELETAL MUSCLE

- Most common type of muscle tissue in the body. It constitutes 40–50% of body weight.
- There are about 656 muscles in the body.
- Mostly, it is attached to skeleton and closely associated with the bones and joints which it moves.
- Act as levers to move the body.
- It is vascular and has limited capacity to regenerate.
- Commonly paralyzed and can be tested clinically.
- It is subjected to injuries in athletes.
- It is used for giving intramuscular injection.

FUNCTIONS

- *Locomotion:* Performing movement.
- Protection of underlying parts.
- Gives shape to the body parts.
- Storage of glycogen, calcium.
- *Generate heat:* Helps in maintaining body temperature.
- Maintain posture.
- Maintenance of joint stability.

STRUCTURES ASSOCIATED WITH SKELETAL MUSCLE

- *Tendon:* Connects muscle to bone.
- *Ligaments:* Connects bone to bone.
- *Aponeurosis:* Flat fibrous sheet or expanded broad tendons that attach to muscles and serve as the means of origin or insertion of flat muscles.
- *Retinaculum:* Fibrous band that holds a structure in place.
- *Bursae:* Flattened sacs of synovial membrane that contain fluid for facilitating movement by minimizing friction.
- *Synovial tendon sheath:* Tubular sacs filled with synovial fluid that wraps around tendons. Present where tendons pass under ligaments or facilitating movement by reducing friction.
- *Fascia:* Fibrous sheet that envelops the body under the skin and invests the muscles. This may limit the spread of pus.

CLASSIFICATION OF SKELETAL MUSCLES

They are broadly classified according to:
1. Color of muscle fiber.
2. Direction of muscle fibers to the line of pull.
3. Force of action.

- *According to color of muscle fibers*: Depending on the amount of myohemoglobin the muscles are classified into:
  - Red muscle
  - White muscle
  - Intermediate muscle.

  The differences between these three types of muscle fibers are shown in **Table 5.3**.
- *According to direction of muscle fibers to the line of pull:*
  - *Parallel to the line of pull* (**Fig. 5.13**):
    - Direction of muscle fibers are parallel to the line of pull

Chapter 5: Introduction to Muscular System

Table 5.3: Description of muscles classified according to color.

Features	Red muscle	White muscle	Intermediate muscle
Metabolism pathway	Aerobic oxidation of fats and fatty acids	Anaerobic glycolysis	Intermediate between slow oxidative and fast glycolytic fibers
Myoglobin (muscle hemoglobin providing a source of oxygen) content	Large	Less	Moderate
Mitochondria	More number	Less number	More number
Adenosine triphosphatase (ATPase) activity	More	Less	-do-
Cytochrome complexes that are essential for oxidative phosphorylation	Large number	Few	-do-
Oxidative enzyme levels	High	Low	High
Blood supply	Rich	Poor	Rich
Contraction (motor units)	Slow, sustained continuous (slow twitch motor units)	Rapid, less sustained, and short time (fast twitch motor units)	Fast twitch
Force and period of contraction	Small force for prolonged period	Strong force for short period	Moderate
Structure	Less cross striations, more sarcoplasm	More cross striations, less sarcoplasm	Moderate striations and sarcoplasm
Number of neuromuscular junctions	Less	More	Moderate
Fatigue	Not easily fatigued (resistance to fatigue)	Fatigued easily	-do-
Diameter	Smaller	Larger	Larger
Location	In deep muscles	In superficial muscles	Both
Function	Maintenance of posture	Rapid and precise movement	On training they act rapidly
Examples	❑ Antigravity muscles of trunk ❑ *Limbs*: One joint muscles ➢ Soleus and brachialis	❑ Extraocular muscles of eyeball ❑ *Limbs*: Two joint muscles: ➢ Biceps brachii ➢ Gastrocnemius ➢ Hamstring ➢ Muscles for finer movements of digits	Most of the body muscles

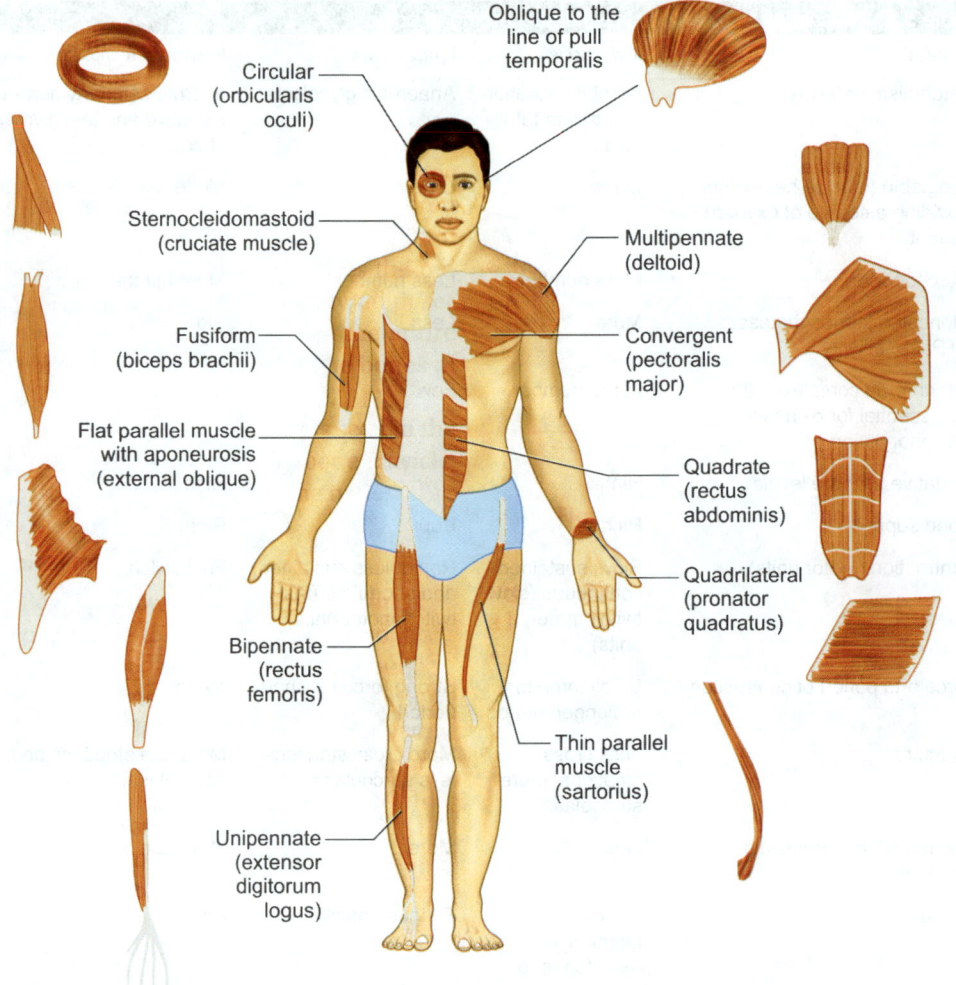

Fig. 5.13: Classification of muscles according to direction of muscle fibers.

- The fibers are long and few in numbers
- Maximum range of movement because of long fibers
- Less force of contraction because of small numbers
- Good endurance/tolerance.
- *Subtypes with examples*:
  » Strap like: Sartorius, rectus abdominis, and infrahyoid muscles
  » Fusiform: Biceps, digastric
  » Quadrilateral: Thyrohyoid, pronator quadratus, and quadratus lumborum.
- *Oblique to the line of pull* (**Fig. 5.13**):
  - Fibers converge at insertion
  - Maximization of contraction
  - Muscles are made powerful
  - Range of movement less.
  - *Shapes with example:*
    » Triangular: Adductor longus
    » Fan shaped: Temporalis.
- The arrangement of the fibers and the fascicles determines the power and range of movement of the muscle. When a muscle contracts, it shortens by one-half or one-third of its resting length; so, a muscle

whose fibers are parallel to the long axis and thereby the line of pull, will bring about greater movement than the one whose fibers are oblique.
- *Spiral/twisted arrangement* **(Fig. 5.13)**:
  - Some muscles are twisted at the insertion.
  - The twisting provides flexibility.
  - *Examples:*
    » Trapezius
    » Pectoralis major
    » Latissimus dorsi
    » Supinator.
- *Cruciate arrangement* **(Fig. 5.13)**:
  - The muscle fibers are arranged in superficial and deep planes and cross like letter X.
  - *Examples*:
    » Sternocleidomastoid
    » Masseter
    » Adductor magnus.
- *Sphincteric* **(Fig. 5.13)**:
  - Fibers surrounding an orifice
  - Closure of aperture.
  - *Examples:*
    » Orbicularis oculi
    » Orbicularis oris.
- *Pennate (feather like):*
  - Pennate fasciculi
  - Fleshy fibers-like bars of feather and are oblique to the line of pull
  - Fibers are short hence the range of movement is decreased
  - Force of contraction is greater as the number of fibers is more
  - All inserted by tendon
  - Strong muscles.
  - *Types with examples* **(Fig. 5.13)**:
    » Unipennate: Fleshy fibers slope to one side of the tendon. The tendon is formed along one margin of the muscle, e.g., extensor digitorum longus, flexor pollicis longus, and peroneus tertius.
    » Bipennate: Tendon is formed in the central axis and muscle fibers slope on to two sides of the tendon like a feather, e.g., rectus femoris, dorsal interossei of hand and foot.
    » Multipennate: Series of bipennate fibers lying side by side form this type, e.g., deltoid, subscapularis.
    » Circumpennate: The muscle is cylindrical with a central tendon. Oblique muscle fibers converge into the central tendon from all directions, e.g., tibialis anterior.

The power of a muscle depends on the total number of fibers it contains and the power is more if the contraction is oblique to the long axis. Hence, pennate and convergent (oblique) muscles are more powerful.

AN3.3: Explain shunt and spurt muscles.

- *According to force of action:*
Two types of muscles are present. They are spurt and shunt muscles.
  1. *Spurt muscles*
  2. *Shunt muscles.*

In a simple joint one bone is more mobile than the other. A muscle acting on a mobile bone exerts force that can be described as two components acting at right angles to each other. The two components are: (1) *Swing/spurt* (transaxial) component, and (2) *Shunt* (paraxial) component. The swing component produces angular or rotational movement of the joint. The shunt component draws the bone along the shaft toward the joint, compresses the articular surface, and thus stabilizes the joint. Accordingly, the muscles are classified into spurt and shunt muscles that are described in **Table 5.4** and **Figure 5.14**.

ACTIONS OF SKELETAL MUSCLES

Movements occur by coordinated action of several muscles rather than by a single muscle. Flexion or bending of the elbow involves shortening of muscles on the front of arm with associated lengthening of muscles of the back of arm. It is essential that various muscles should act in harmony to produce

Table 5.4: Differences between spurt and shunt muscles.

Features	Spurt muscle	Shunt muscle
Swing component/shunt component	Swing component is more powerful	Shunt component is powerful
Origin	At a distance from the joint on which it acts	Near the joint on which it acts
Insertion	Near the joint on which it acts	Away from the joint on which it acts
Direction of force	Across the bone	Along the bone
Stabilizing function	Less	Greater
Rotation function	Greater	Less
Action	Prime movers	Synergists
Examples	Biceps brachii, brachialis, triceps brachii	Brachioradialis, brachialis

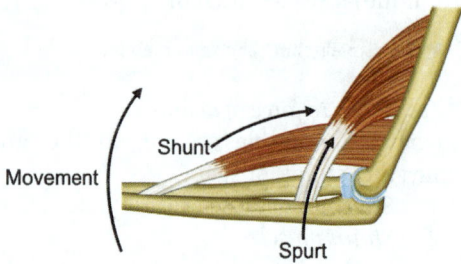

Fig. 5.14: Classification of muscles according to force of contraction.

different kinds of movements. The muscles are classified into the following four groups according to their contribution for producing a particular movement.

1. *Agonists (prime movers):* These are the chief muscle responsible for a particular movement. Active in initiation and maintenance of a particular movement. Examples:
   - Quadriceps femoris is a prime mover for extension of knee.
   - Biceps brachii is a prime mover for flexion of elbow.
2. *Antagonists:* These oppose the action of the prime mover (for that particular movement). Examples:
   - Biceps femoris is an antagonist for extension of knee.
   - Triceps is antagonist for flexion of elbow.
3. *Fixators:* These muscles stabilize (fix) the origin of the prime mover so that the latter can act efficiently. Examples:
   - The muscles of the shoulder girdle (rhomboideus major and rhomboideus minor) that attach it to the vertebral column fix the scapula so that the deltoid muscle can act efficiently on the shoulder joint.
   - In weight training exercises that are targeted at contraction of biceps brachii (biceps curl) the rotator cuff muscles act as fixators and are called the guardians of the shoulder joint.
4. *Synergists:* A prime mover sometimes crosses more than one joint before reaching its main point of action, because of which unnecessary movements can occur in the intermediate joint. To avoid this kind of a movement, another muscle contracts and fixes the intermediate joint. Such muscle is called synergist. These help the prime mover to act efficiently. Example:
   - When flexor digitorum profundus crosses the wrist joint before reaching the fingers, it can cause flexion of the wrist. But its efficiency and power will be reduced. Flexor carpi ulnaris and flexor carpi radialis contract and fix the wrist so that flexor digitorum profundus can act efficiently.

Note: The same muscle can act in different capacities during different movements.

NAMING OF MUSCLES

Each muscle has a name. A muscle is named after considering its:
- Action
- Size
- Shape
- Region in which it lies.

Any of these factors can be associated with the name and the name usually consists of two or more words based on these characteristics. However, from the name of a given muscle, it is easy to understand its location and to some extent its action **(Table 5.5)**.

Table 5.5: Naming of muscles based on certain features.

Features	Examples
Location	☐ Anterior aspect of tibia: Tibialis anterior ☐ In relation to spine of scapula: Supraspinatus (superior to spine), infraspinatus (inferior to spine) ☐ In between bones: Interossei
Location and size	☐ Pectoral = front of chest: Pectoralis major (major = significant); pectoralis minor ☐ Palm of hand: Palmaris longus, palmaris brevis ☐ Lateral aspect of leg: Peroneus longus, peroneus brevis, and peroneus tertius ☐ Buttock = gluteal region: Gluteus maximus, gluteus medius, and gluteus minimus
Location and action	☐ Flexor aspect, superficial/deep stratum, and acting on digits: Flexor digitorum superficialis, flexor digitorum profundus ☐ Depressing the lower lip: Depressor labii inferioris
Location and significance	☐ Head: Longus (linear) capitis, longissimus (longest) capitis ☐ Trunk: Latissimus (broadest) dorsi
Shape	☐ Trapezoid: Trapezius—quadrilateral muscle ☐ Deltoid: The fourth letter of Greek alphabet delta ☐ Broad sheet: Platysma ☐ Worm like: Lumbricals
Shape and location	☐ Quadrate shape and in relation to femur: Quadratus femoris ☐ Quadrate shape and in lumbar region: Quadratus lumborum ☐ Serrated and anterior location: Serratus anterior ☐ Straight and in abdominal wall: Rectus abdominis ☐ Straight and in relation to femur: Rectus femoris
Shape and significance	☐ Rhomboid: Rhomboideus major and rhomboideus minor ☐ Round: Teres major and teres minor
Attachments	Sternocleidomastoid (sternum, clavicle, and mastoid)
Action	☐ Supinator ☐ Sartorius (sartor = tailor)
Action and shape	Pronator quadratus
Number of bellies and location	☐ Biceps brachii (two heads and in relation to arm or brachium) ☐ Biceps femoris (two heads and in relation to femur) ☐ Triceps brachii (three heads) and in relation to arm or brachium ☐ Quadriceps femoris (muscle with four heads and in relation to femur) ☐ Digastric (di = two; gaster = bellies)
Action and significance	☐ Flexor digiti minimi ☐ Extensor pollicis longus
Size and action	Adductor longus (linear), adductor magnus (large), and adductor brevis (small)
Orientation of muscle fibers and location	☐ Rectus abdominis ☐ Superior oblique ☐ Transversus abdominis
Action and part on which it acts	☐ Abductor pollicis ☐ Abductor hallucis ☐ Abductor digiti minimi ☐ Adductor pollicis ☐ Opponens pollicis

Clinical Applications of Skeletal Muscle

- *Paralysis:* Muscle is unable to contract. It is due to damage to motor pathway that consists of upper motor neuron and lower motor neuron.
  - Upper motor neurons originate in the motor region of cerebral cortex or brainstem. Damage to upper motor neuron causes spastic paralysis with exaggerated tendon reflexes.
  - Lower motor neurons originate in the motor neurons located in the anterior gray column of spinal cord (spinal lower motor neurons) or in the cranial nerve nuclei of the brainstem (cranial nerve lower motor neurons). Damage to lower motor neuron causes flaccid paralysis with loss of tendon reflexes.
- *Muscular spasm*: It is due to spontaneous or involuntary contraction of a muscle. It may be localized (caused by muscle pull) or generalized (seen in tetanus and epilepsy).
- *Hypertrophy*: Excessive use of a particular muscle results in its hypertrophy. It is usually seen in athletes and body builders.
- *Atrophy*: If muscle is not used for a long time it becomes thin and weak. There will be reduction in size of muscle (muscle wasting). It is seen in paralysis and in generalized debility.
- *Regeneration:* Muscle is capable of limited regeneration. If large regions are damaged regeneration does not occur. The damaged muscle is replaced by connective tissue.
- *Muscular dystrophy:* It is progressive weakness and degeneration of muscles that control movement. These are a group of about 30 genetic disorders. There will be inherent defect in cell membrane of muscle and there is rupture of muscle fibers, e.g., Duchenne muscular dystrophy, Baker's muscular dystrophy. Duchenne muscular dystrophy is an X-linked recessive disorder. In this there is mutation in the gene for muscle protein dystrophin attached to cell membrane. This results in ineffective contraction of muscle leading to progressive damage and death of muscle cells.
- *Myasthenia gravis:* My = muscle, asthen = weakness, gravi = heavy. It is an autoimmune disease. There will be reduction in acetylcholine (ACh) receptors at neuromuscular junction as autoimmune antibodies attack the ACh receptors. It is characterized by progressive muscular weakness. Muscles of head and neck are affected first.
- *Intramuscular injections:* The muscles commonly used for intramuscular injection are deltoid (shoulder region), gluteus maximus (gluteal region), and vastus lateralis (thigh region) **(Fig. 5.15)**.
- *Muscle biopsy:* This is done for the diagnosis of certain muscle diseases by inserting a needle into a muscle under local anesthesia and collecting a small bit of muscle tissue. By this procedure diseases of connective tissue and blood vessel (*polyarteritis nodosa*) and inflammatory (*polymyositis*) and infectious (*toxoplasmosis*) diseases of muscle can be diagnosed.
- *Electromyography:* It is a diagnostic procedure performed to assess the health of the muscles and the motor neurons that control their movements.

Chapter 5: Introduction to Muscular System

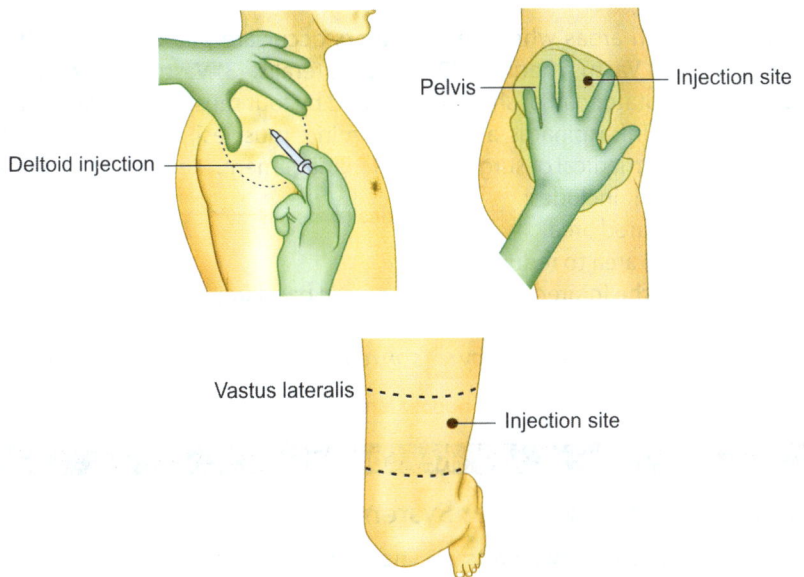

Fig. 5.15: Sites of intramuscular injection.

Anatomical Basis for Clinical Condition

Case Scenario

Problem: A middle aged person complained a snapping sound and sharp pain in the left heel after jumping from a height and landing on his sole and making him unable to walk properly. On examination a swelling above the heel was observed. The patient was unable to bend the left foot downward and unable to stand on the toes of the injured leg. It was diagnosed as rupture of Achilles tendon.

Questions:
1. What is Achilles tendon?
2. What is the site of rupture?
3. What is the cause for rupture of Achilles tendon?
4. What are the conditions in which it can occur?
5. What are the other tendons that rupture commonly?
6. What is the treatment?

Anatomical explanation:
1. Achilles tendon is a fibrous cord that connects the muscles of calf to the calcaneus.
2. Rupture of Achilles tendon occurs about 6 cm above the heel.
3. The tendon can bear forces of more than five times the body weight. Tear of this tendon is due to overstretching of the tendon and the poor blood supply to the tendon.
4. It occurs in recreational sports like jumping, running, etc., The common age at which it can occur is 30–40 years and is five times more common in men. In general rupture of tendon occurs in middle age and old age. In the middle age muscle tissue tears before the tendon will tear. Tendon tears are common in old people and in certain diseases such as gout, hyperthyroidism, and certain drugs like fluoroquinolones, statins, injection of steroids into a tendon, etc.

5. The most common areas where tendon tears occur are patellar tendon [formed by four muscles—(1) Vastus medialis, (2) Vastus lateralis, (3) Vastus intermedius, and (4) Rectus femoris]; rotator cuff of shoulder [formed by four muscles—(1) Subscapularis, (2) Supraspinatus, (3) Infraspinatus, and (4) Teres minor muscles]; and biceps muscle of arm.
6. Treatment is either medical or surgical line of management. Medical line of management is by RICE method. It includes:
   - Rest to the injured area.
   - Ice the injured area to reduce swelling.
   - Compressing the injured area with an elastic bandage.
   - Elevating the injured area.
   - *Surgical line of management is by tendon repair*—Sewing the two ends of the tendon.

☞ Key Concept

Take Home Message—Muscular System
- Skeletal muscle presents two parts: (1) The fleshy contractile part, the belly and (2) The fibrous noncontractile part, the tendon or aponeurosis.
- The various structures associated with the muscles, i.e., tendons; ligaments, aponeuroses, retinacula, etc., facilitate attachment to bone, holding of structures, and facilitate movement, etc.
- Three different connective tissue coverings of the muscle are: (1) Epimysium, (2) Perimysium, and (3) Endomysium.
- Tendon injuries, i.e., rupture, traction, etc., heal slowly because of poor blood supply.
- Muscles with their innervation are important for functioning.
- Sarcomere is the structural and functional unit of muscle.
- The color of the muscles indicates their action.
- The knowledge of blood supply of muscle is important in choosing a muscle for reconstructive surgeries.
- According to their contribution for a particular movement the muscles are classified into agonists, antagonists, fixators, and synergists.
- Naming of muscles facilitates remembering them by their location, action, size, etc.
- Certain muscles are used for intramuscular injection because of their accessibility and their bulky nature.
- Muscle biopsy is the investigation for the diagnosis of certain muscle diseases.

QUESTIONS

1. Microscopic structure of skeletal muscle.
2. Parts of a muscle.
3. Connective tissue coverings of a muscle.
4. Sarcomere.
5. Differences between red and white muscles.
6. Classification of muscles according to the arrangement of muscle fibers.
7. Classification of muscles according to their action.
8. Differences between shunt and spurt muscles.
9. Differences between tendon and aponeurosis.

MULTIPLE CHOICE QUESTIONS

1. **The term myocyte refers to:**
   A. Myofibril

Chapter 5: Introduction to Muscular System

B. Muscle fascicle
C. Muscle fiber
D. Muscle filament

2. **Which of the following statements about sarcomere is incorrect?**
   A. I band is on either side of Z line
   B. I band contains only thin filaments
   C. A band is a light band
   D. M line is the point where thick filaments join

3. **All the following are examples for composite or hybrid muscles, *except*:**
   A. Brachialis
   B. Biceps femoris
   C. Adductor magnus
   D. Supraspinatus

4. **Which pair in the following is wrong?**
   A. Unipennate—flexor pollicis longus
   B. Circumpennate—peroneus tertius
   C. Bipennate—rectus femoris
   D. Multipennate—deltoid

5. **Muscle with parallel fibers are all, *except*:**
   A. Sartorius
   B. Rectus abdominis
   C. Sternohyoid
   D. Tibialis anterior

6. **Which of the following is multipennate muscle?**
   A. Flexor pollicis longus
   B. Extensor pollicis longus
   C. Flexor hallucis longus
   D. Deltoid

7. **Muscles having double nerve supply include all the following, *except*:**
   A. Digastric
   B. Omohyoid
   C. Trapezius
   D. Adductor magnus

8. **A central nucleus and branching fibers are characteristic of:**
   A. Cardiac muscle
   B. Smooth muscle
   C. Skeletal muscle
   D. All the above

9. **Identify the wrong statement about spurt muscles.**
   A. Arises at a distance from site of action
   B. It is a prime mover
   C. Swing component is more powerful
   D. It is inserted away from the joint on which it acts.

ANSWERS

| 1. C | 2. C | 3. D | 4. B | 5. D | 6. D |
| 7. C | 8. A | 9. D | | | |

CHAPTER 6

Introduction to Arthrology/Joints

LEARNING OBJECTIVES

- ❖ Definition of joint
- ❖ Classification of different types of joints with examples
- ❖ General features of a synovial joint
- ❖ Bursa
- ❖ Clinical case with anatomical explanation

DEFINITION

A joint or articulation is a connection or a junction between two or more bones or cartilages to permit movement.

- All the 206 bones of the body with the *exception* of hyoid bone in the neck are connected to at least one other bone.
- Study of joints is called *arthrology* (Greek arthron = joint) or *syndesmology* (Greek syndesmo = fastening or joining).
- A joint can also be called an *articulation* (Latin articulatio = connecting) or an *articulus*.
- Some joints are merely bonds of union between different bones and do not allow movement. Joints of the skull (sutures) belong to this category.
- Some joints allow slight movement (intervertebral discs), while some others (shoulder) allow great freedom of movement.
- The number of joints in a child is more than that of adult. As growth proceeds some of the bones fuse together, e.g., ilium, ischium, and pubis fuse to form hip bone; the two halves of frontal bone

and that of mandible fuse; the five sacral vertebrae fuse to form single sacrum; and the four coccygeal vertebrae fuse to form single coccyx.

Articulating parts in different bones:

- Long bones articulate at their ends
- Flat bones articulate at margins
- Short or irregular bones articulate at their articular surfaces.

CLASSIFICATION OF JOINTS

AN2.5: Describe various joints with subtypes and examples.

Joints are classified based on structure, region, and function **(Flowcharts 6.1 to 6.3)**.

- *Structural:* Depending on the type of material binding articulating bones
- *Regional:* Depending on location
- *Functional:* Depending on the range of movement
- *Combined:* Combination of structure and function.

Subdivision of each with type, its specific identification features with examples was presented in **Table 6.1** and **Figures 6.1A to C**.

Chapter 6: Introduction to Arthrology/Joints

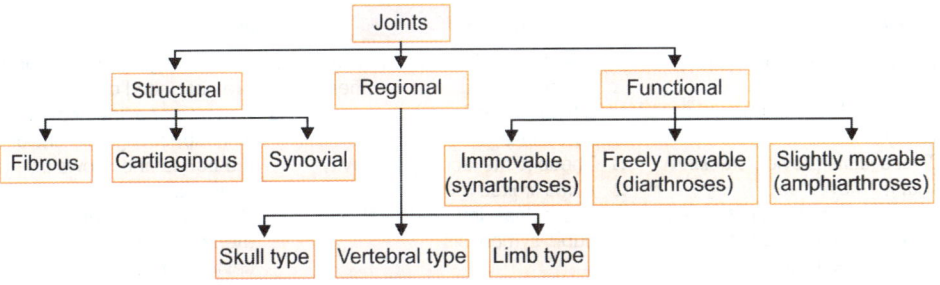

Flowchart 6.1: Broad classification of joints.

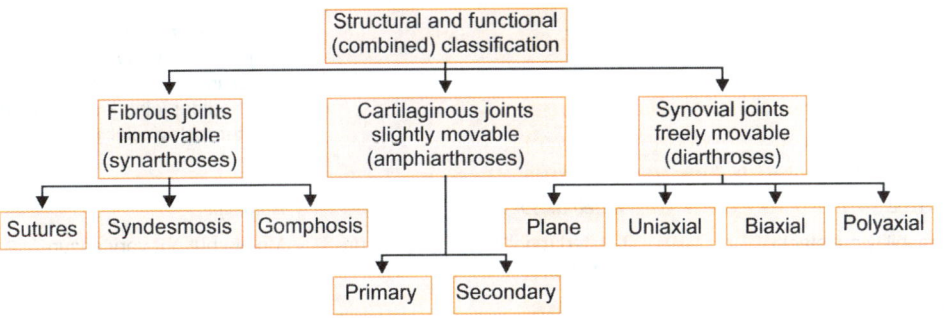

Flowchart 6.2: Combined (structural and functional) classification of joints.

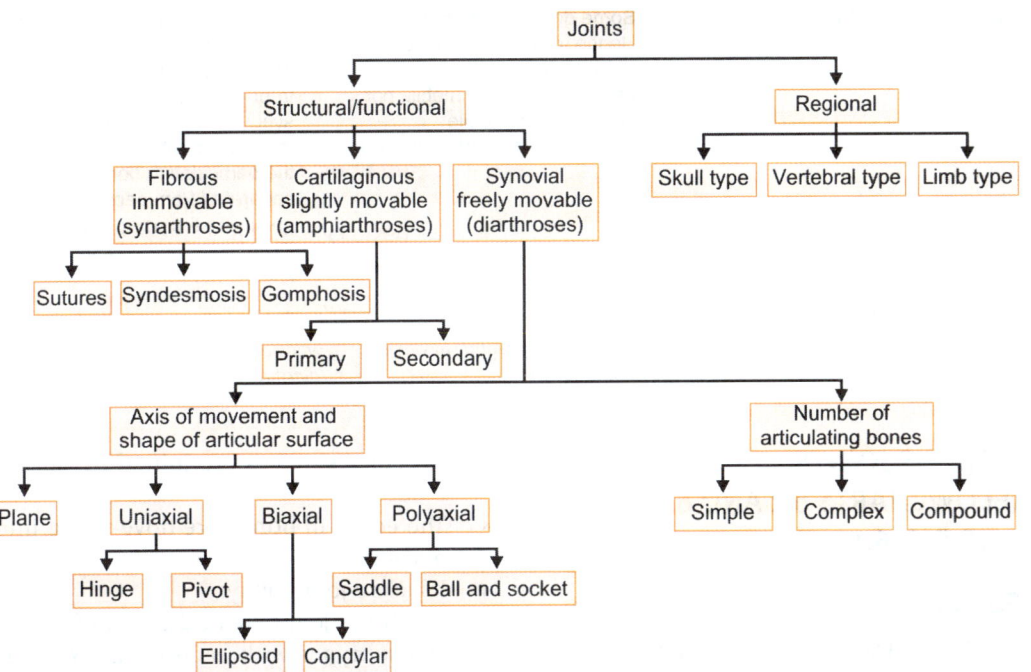

Flowchart 6.3: Combined classification of joints and subtypes.

Table 6.1: Classification of joints.

A. Structural classification

Fibrous joints	Cartilaginous joints	Synovial joints
❑ Fibrous tissue will be binding the articulating ends ❑ It is a solid joint without joint cavity ❑ These joints provide *stability with no movement* ❑ They are protective in function. ❑ Example—joints between bones of skull (sutures)	❑ The intervening tissue between the articulating ends is either a hyaline cartilage or a fibrocartilage ❑ These joints lack a joint cavity ❑ *It has limited mobility* ❑ Examples—intervertebral disc, pubic symphysis	❑ Articulating surfaces of bones are not united directly ❑ A membrane lined cavity filled with lubricating fluid encloses the bones and allows free movement ❑ Cartilage with synovial membrane enclosing a joint cavity is present ❑ These joints allow a wide range of movement ❑ Mobility is greater but stability is less ❑ These are the most common joints of the body ❑ Examples—hip joint, shoulder joint, knee joint, and sternoclavicular joint

B. Regional classification

Skull type	Vertebral type	Limb type
No mobility but stable	Limited mobility but very secure and stable	Mobile but not very secure

C. Functional classification

Synarthroses	Amphiarthroses	Diarthroses
❑ *Immovable joints*: No mobility ❑ Example—sutures of skull	❑ *Slightly movable joints*: Some degree of mobility. Hence, called amphi (two-sided) arthroses because it is neither completely mobile nor completely immobile ❑ Example—intervertebral discs	❑ *Freely movable joints*: Maximum degree (wide range) of mobility ❑ The name "diarthroses" is frequently applied to the synovial type of joint, where the movements are free and the participating bones are separated from each other, qualifying the adjective "two" ❑ Examples—shoulder, hip, and knee joints

D. Combination of structure and function

Fibrous and immovable (synarthroses)	Cartilaginous and slightly movable (amphiathroses)	Synovial and freely movable (diarthroses)

FIBROUS JOINTS (FLOWCHARTS 6.2 AND 6.3 AND FIG. 6.1A)

Features

- These are immovable/fixed joints, i.e., *synarthroses*.
- Articular surfaces are joined by fibrous tissue.
- The edges of bones are dove-tailed into one another.
- It lacks a joint cavity.

The fibrous joints are further classified into various subtypes with each having specific features.

Chapter 6: Introduction to Arthrology/Joints

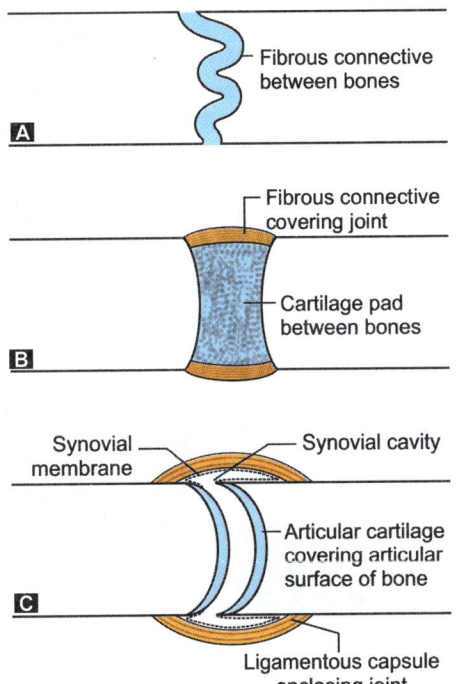

Figs. 6.1A to C: Classification of joints. (A) Synarthrosis—fibrous joint; (B) Amphiarthrosis—cartilaginous joint; (C) Diarthrosis—synovial joint.

Subtypes of Fibrous Joints

- *Sutures (synostosis)* **(Figs. 6.2A to E):**
  - *Latin* Sutura, derived from suo = a sewing or a seam. This type of joint is found only in the skull.
    - *Synostosis:* Obliteration of suture leads to union of the articulating bones by bone tissue itself. This is called synostosis (syn + osteo = joining by bone). When a suture obliterates, *synostosis* occurs first on the deeper aspect of the suture (internal or endocranial aspect) and gradually extends on to the superficial (external or pericranial) aspect. Complete obliteration occurs much later in life.
  - Fibrous tissue connects the bones as *sutural ligament* (thin connective tissue layer).
  - Majority are seen between bones that develop in membrane.
  - These gradually ossify with advancing age.
  - These are immovable.
  - Seen between skull bones, e.g., sagittal and coronal sutures.
  - In a growing child they exhibit little mobility.
  - *Types:* Depending on shape of articulating surfaces and articular margins:
    - *Plane suture:* The articulating margins are plane and united by sutural ligament, e.g., joint between palatine processes of two maxillae **(Fig. 6.2A)**.
    - *Serrate suture:* Saw-toothed appearance of bone edges, e.g., sagittal suture of skull **(Fig. 6.2B)**.
    - *Denticulate suture:* The margins are like teeth, e.g., lambdoid suture **(Fig. 6.2C)**.
    - *Squamous suture:* Edges of bones overlap, e.g., suture between parietal and squamous parts of temporal bone **(Fig. 6.2D)**.
    - *Schindylesis (wedge and groove suture):* Edge of one bone fits into the groove of the other bone, e.g., joint between rostrum of sphenoid and upper margin of vomer **(Fig. 6.2E)**.
- *Syndesmosis* **(Fig. 6.3):**
  - *Greek—Syndesmos* = ligament.
  - Surfaces of bones are united by fibrous connection, most commonly by interosseous ligaments that persist throughout life. It is also represented by slender fibrous cord or aponeurotic membrane.
  - Slight degree of movement is possible depending on the distance between bones and degree of flexibility of uniting fibrous tissue.
  - For example, interosseous membrane between forearm bones and leg bones, inferior tibiofibular joint; ligamenta

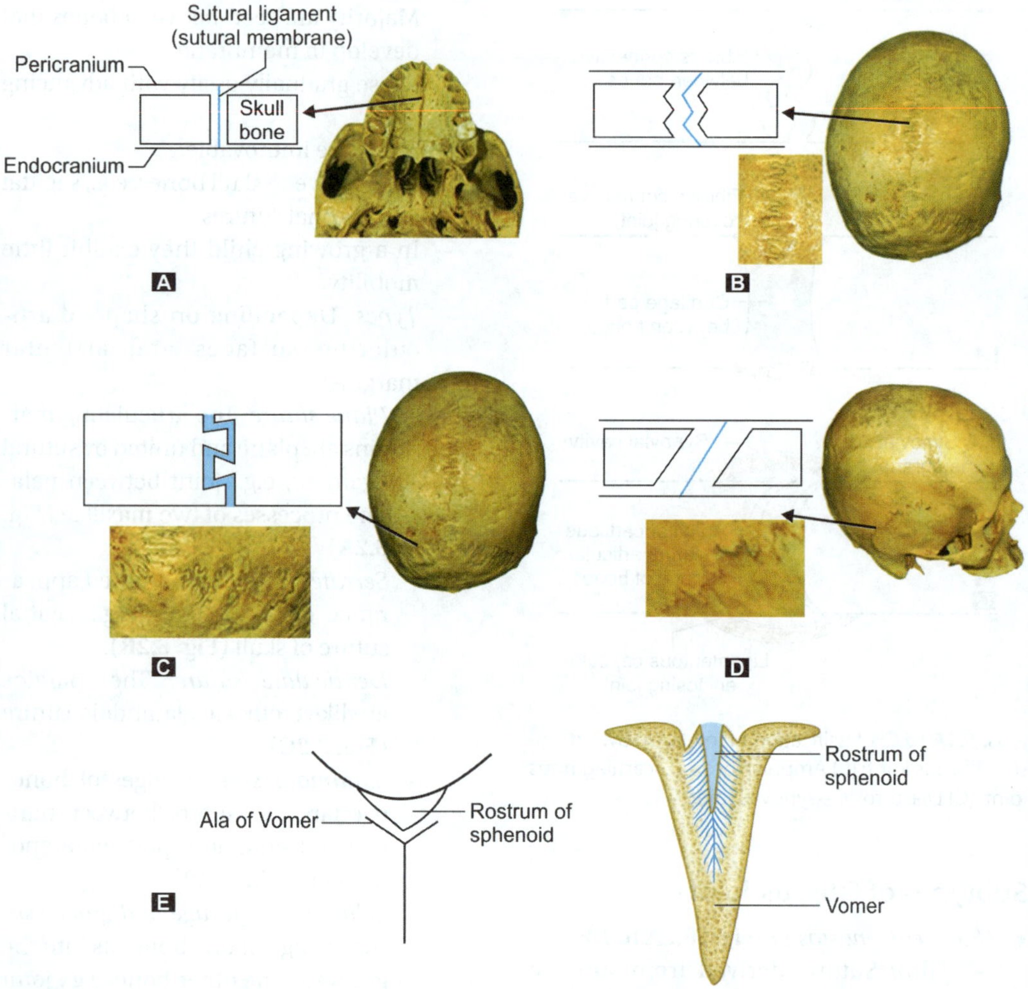

Figs. 6.2A to E: Fibrous joint—sutures: (A) Plane suture (palatine process of two maxilla); (B) Serrate suture (sagittal suture); (C) Denticulate suture (lambdoid suture); (D) Squamous suture (between parietal and squamous part of temporal bone); (E) Schindylesis (wedge and groove suture).

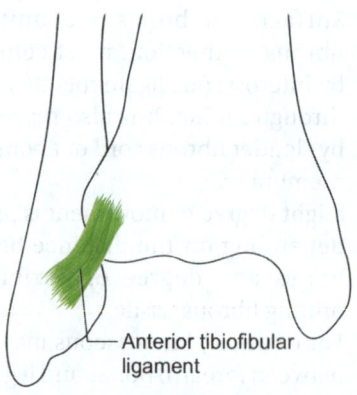

Fig. 6.3: Fibrous joint—syndesmosis.

flava (ligaments between spines of vertebrae).

- *Gomphosis/peg and socket joint* **(Fig. 6.4)**:
  - Gomphos = bolt, Osis = condition.
  - A peg-shaped process gets inserted into a socket and is united by fibrous tissue.
  - For example, articulation of roots of teeth into alveolar sockets anchored by *periodontal ligament*.
  - This type of arrangement does not allow movement of tooth. If movement is allowed it is pathological and results in loosening of tooth.

Chapter 6: Introduction to Arthrology/Joints

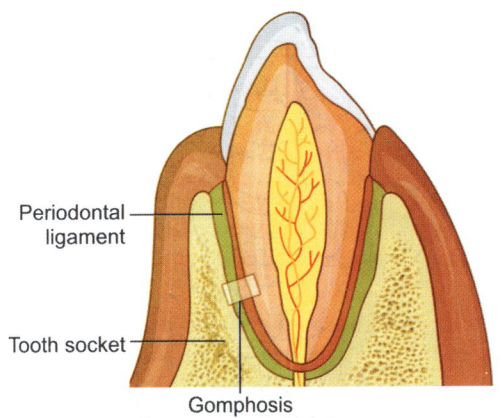

Fig. 6.4: Fibrous joint—gomphosis.

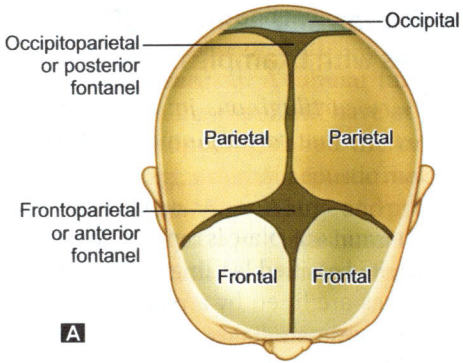

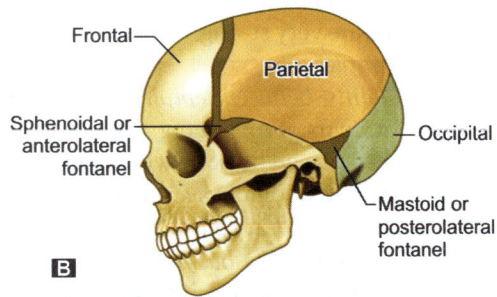

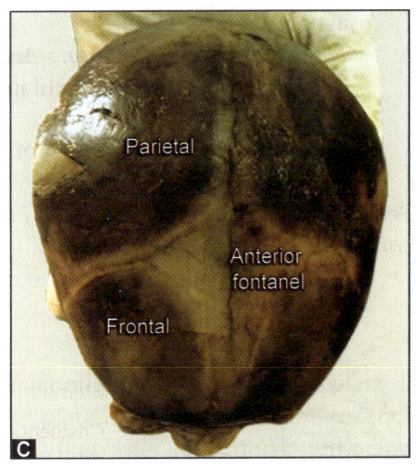

Figs. 6.5A to C: Fontanel.

Fontanel (Figs. 6.5A to C)

- In the newborn and in infants the connective tissue between bones of skull is much wider especially in the skull cap, i.e., between sagittal, coronal, squamous, and lambdoid sutures. These are called fontanels.
- During the time of parturition (delivery of the fetus) the fontanel provides flexibility for the delivery of the fetal head to pass through birth canal by overlapping of bones of vault or skull cap.
- After birth these fontanel allow expansion of skull with enlargement of brain.
- The fontanel decrease in width during 1st year after birth when the skull bones are enlarging and it becomes the suture.
- At some sutures, the connective tissue will ossify and be converted into bone.

CARTILAGINOUS JOINTS (FLOWCHARTS 6.1 TO 6.3 AND FIG. 6.1B)

Features

- These are slightly movable joints, i.e., amphiarthroses.
- Cartilage is present between articulating surfaces.
- Fibrous capsule holds the bones and cartilage in place.
- The cartilage uniting the articulating surfaces is either hyaline cartilage or white fibrocartilage.
- No joint cavity.
- The cartilaginous joints are further classified into various subtypes with each having specific features.

Classification and Features of Subtypes with Examples

- *Primary cartilaginous joints: Synchondroses/hyaline cartilaginous joints* (**Fig. 6.6**).
  - It is temporary. At a certain age cartilaginous plate is replaced by bone, i.e., it is ossified leading to synostosis.
  - Bones are lined by a plate of hyaline cartilage.
  - Primarily designed for bone growth.
  - All primary cartilaginous joints are quite immovable.
  - They are very strong.
  - *Examples:*
    - *Joints between epiphysis and diaphysis of a growing long bones*: It is replaced by bone when growth in length of diaphysis is completed. It is a temporary synchondrosis.
    - *Joint between basiocciput and basisphenoid*: Synchondrosis is converted to synostosis around 25 years of age.
    - *First chondrosternal joint*: Articulation between costal cartilage of 1st rib and manubrium.
    - Anterior ends of 11 pairs of ribs with their costal cartilages.
- *Secondary cartilaginous joints: Fibrocartilaginous/symphyses* (**Fig. 6.7**).

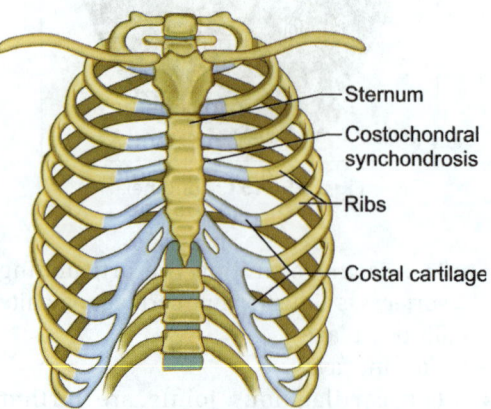

Fig. 6.6: Cartilaginous (primary) joint—synchondroses.

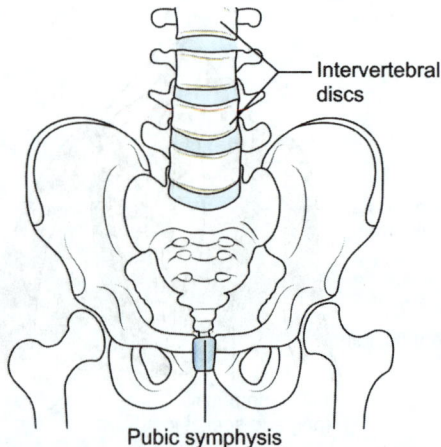

Fig. 6.7: Cartilaginous (secondary) joint—symphysis.

  - These joints are permanent and persist throughout life, *except* symphysis menti which is temporary.
  - Articular surfaces are covered by a thin layer of hyaline cartilage and united by a disc of fibrocartilage/fibrous tissue.
  - Typically they occur in the median plane of the body. Hence, they are also called *midline joints*.
  - These permits limited movements due to compressive fibrocartilage.
  - *Examples:*
    - Intervertebral discs between the bodies of vertebra
    - Manubriosternal joint
    - Symphysis pubis
    - Symphysis menti. This is the only symphysis devoid of fibrocartilage.

SYNOVIAL JOINTS

Features

- These are freely movable joints, i.e., *diarthroses*. Wide range of movement is possible.
- Most of the joints of appendicular skeleton belong to this group.
- Articular surfaces are covered by cartilage.
- Ligaments hold the bones together.
- Joint cavity is present and it contains synovial fluid.

Chapter 6: Introduction to Arthrology/Joints

- Joint cavity is enveloped by articular capsule which consists of an outer fibrous capsule and an inner synovial membrane.
- Sometimes the joint cavity is divided completely or incompletely by articular disc or meniscus of fibrocartilage.
- Movements of joints vary from a simple gliding to a wide range.
- Factors contributing for the stability of the joint are:
  - Bony contour
  - Ligaments
  - Muscles
  - *Atmospheric pressure:* Negligible factor.
- Synovial joints are important in the field of health sciences, i.e., in medicine, nursing, physiotherapy, sports medicine, and massage therapies.

Description of General Structure of Synovial Joint

The basic structure of synovial joint can be described under **Figure 6.8**.

Articulating Bones

- The articulating surfaces are called male and female surfaces.
  - *Male surface:* It is the articulating surface that is larger and always convex in all directions, e.g., head of humerus/femur.
  - *Female surface:* It is the articulating surface which is smaller and concave in all the directions, e.g., glenoid fossa of scapula/acetabulum of hip bone.
- There will be at least two bones forming each joint. For example, hip joint is between head of femur and acetabulum of hip bone.
- Periosteum is the tough collagen fiber sheet covering the outer surface of bones wherever their surface is not covered by articular cartilage.

Articular Cartilage

- Articular surfaces of most joints are covered with hyaline cartilage. *Exception*—those bones that are ossified in membrane

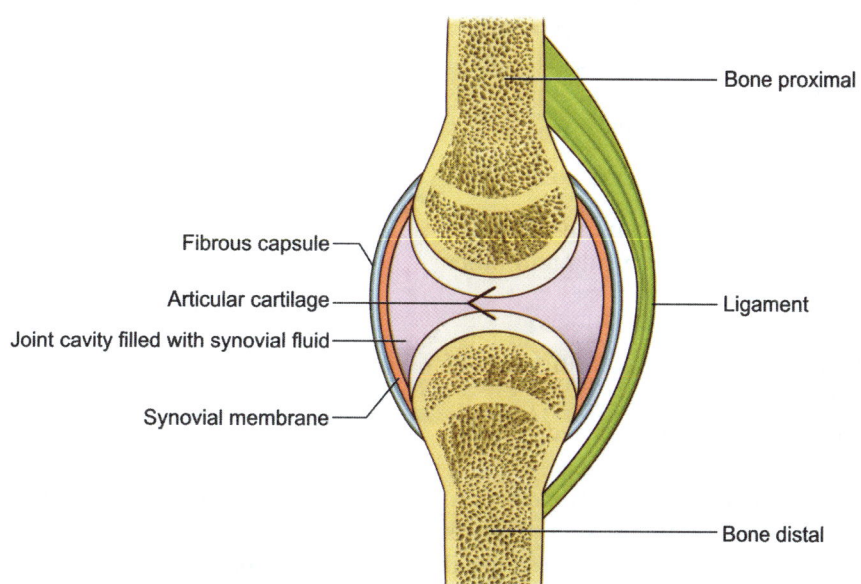

Fig. 6.8: Synovial joint—general structure.

are covered by fibrous cartilage, e.g., sternoclavicular and acromioclavicular joints as the clavicle develops in membrane.
- *Function:* Articular surfaces are lubricated with synovial fluid which provides slippery surface for free movement.
- Articular cartilage is avascular. Nutrition is provided by diffusion through synovial fluid, blood vessels in the medullary cavity, and by vascular network at the periphery of synovial membrane.
- It is non-nervous.
- It has no perichondrium.
- It is not covered by synovial membrane.
- It reduces friction and absorbs shock.
- On the convex (male) articular surface it is thick at the center and thin at the periphery. On the concave (female) articular surface it is thin at the center and thick at the periphery.
- *Age-related changes:* With age degenerative and proliferative changes occur. Degenerative changes occur in the central part and the cartilage is replaced with fibrous tissue. Proliferative changes take place at the periphery where the cartilage cells are replaced with bone cells which are known as *osteophytes*.
- *Clinical importance:* If damaged it cannot be replaced by hyaline cartilage. It is replaced with fibrous tissue.

Articular Capsule

Joint is surrounded by articular capsule which consists of outer fibrous capsule and inner synovial membrane.
- *Fibrous capsule:*
  - It is attached to articulating ends of bones in the form of a cuff.
  - The fibrous capsule is formed by dense irregular connective tissue.
  - It is pierced by blood vessels and nerves.
  - At some places the capsule presents openings through which the synovial membrane comes out as *bursa* near the tendon of a neighboring muscle.
  - The flexibility of fibrous capsule permits movement at the joint and its tensile strength resists dislocation of the joint.
  - The fibrous capsule is reinforced by:
    - *Capsular/true ligaments:* Thickenings of fibrous capsule.
    - *Accessory ligaments:* Intra/extracapsular (distinct from fibrous capsule).
  - *Functions*:
    - Binds the articulating bones.
    - Supports the synovial membrane.
    - *Watchdog action of capsule:* Ramification of nerve ending on the capsule protects it.
- *Synovial membrane*:
  - It is a layer of loose connective tissue formed of elastic fibers and adipose tissue.
  - It lines the whole of the interior of the joint, except for articular surfaces covered by hyaline cartilage.
  - It is highly vascular and cellular.
  - *Functions:*
    - It secretes synovial fluid that provides nutrition to articular cartilage.
    - It is phagocytic and removes particulate matter and worn out cartilage cells.
    - It produces hyaluronic acid that maintains viscosity.

Joint Cavity

- Between articular surfaces there is a joint cavity filled with synovial fluid.
- The cavity may be partially/completely subdivided by an articular disc/meniscus.

Articular Disc or Meniscus

- These are pads of fibrocartilage that facilitate articulating bones of different shapes to fit more snugly together.
- Some of the joints are completely divided by the presence of articular disc of fibrocartilage, e.g., sternoclavicular joint, temporomandibular joint, and inferior radioulnar joint.

Chapter 6: Introduction to Arthrology/Joints

- In some of the joints the disc divides the joint cavity incompletely, e.g., knee joint, acromioclavicular joint.
- *Functions:* Lubrication of the joint to prevent friction, provides surface for increasing the range of movement (gliding movement).

Accessory Ligaments

These are either intracapsular or extracapsular.
- *Intracapsular ligaments*:
  - These are located inside the articular capsule and surrounded by folds of synovial membrane.
  - For example, anterior and posterior cruciate ligaments of the knee joint and ligament of head of femur in hip joint.
- *Extracapsular ligaments*:
  - These are located outside the articular capsule but attached to the articular capsule.
  - For example, tibial and fibular collateral ligaments and ligamentum patella of the knee joint.

Synovial Fluid

- It is a clear viscous fluid.
- It fills the joint cavity.
- It is a dialysate of plasma to which hyaluronic acid is added by the synovial membrane.

Functions of synovial fluid:
- *Lubrication:* Reduction of friction in the joint.
- *Nutritive:* Supplying nutrients to articular cartilage.
- *Removal of metabolic waste products:* As there are no blood vessels in the cartilage.
- *Phagocytic:* Removal of microbes and debris that accumulate due to mechanical damage from use of the joint.

Bursae (Fig. 6.9)

- *Latin:* Bursa = purse; Bursa = singular; Bursae = plural.
- Bursae are small fluid-filled, closed, sac-like structures that are present in some synovial joints.
- They are located between bone and muscle or tendon or ligament. These are seen wherever there is friction between the tendon of a muscle and the bone/cartilage/other tendon. The bursae are common in limbs.

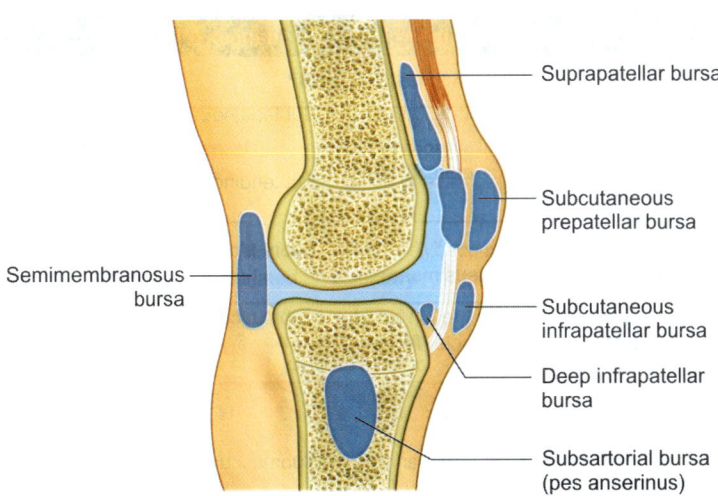

Fig. 6.9: Bursae around knee.

- They are lined by synovial membrane and filled with a capillary layer of viscous fluid called synovial fluid.
- The consistency of synovial fluid is that of raw egg white.
- The function of bursae within synovial joints is to reduce the mechanical friction between bone and the other structure (tendon/muscle) by acting as a cushion. They allow free movement.
- The bursae are present in almost all major joints of the body.
- There are four types of bursa:
  1. **Synovial bursa:** Majority of the bursae are synovial, e.g., knee joint, and shoulder joint.
  2. **Adventitious bursa:** This bursa develops if any surface of the body is subjected to repeated stress. They are called accidental bursa, e.g., bunion.
     - *Bunion* is a deformity of great toe. The bursa at the metatarsophalangeal joint of big toe is swollen and the head of first metatarsal tilts to a side and a large bump is seen.
  3. **Subcutaneous bursa:** It is located between the skin and the bony prominence near the joint. For example, Olecranon bursa (students elbow), prepatellar bursa (housemaids bursa), superficial infrapatellar bursa, and Achilles bursa.
     - *Students elbow* (olecranon bursa)—located between the loose skin of the elbow and the ulna. When inflamed there will be pain, swelling, and redness of elbow with restriction of movement. If infected, the bursa will open and the pus gets drained.
     - *Prepatellar bursa* (housemaids bursa)
  4. **Subtendinous bursa:** It is present between the tendon and bone or between adjacent tendons or between tendon and ligament. They are seen in the limbs, e.g., retrocalcaneal bursa. It is present from birth.
  5. **Submuscular bursa:** It is seen between muscles, e.g., greater trochanteric bursa, iliopsoas bursa, medial and lateral gastrocnemius bursae, and subpopliteal bursae.

Different types of bursae in the body, their location, and type are presented in **Table 6.2**.

Table 6.2: Location of various bursae and their clinical importance.

Name of bursa	Location	Type	Clinical importance
Ulnar bursa	Begins at wrist and ends at the middle of palm	Subtendinous	Horse shoe abscess results from infection of radial or ulnar bursa
Radial bursa	Extends from wrist crease to distal phalanx of thumb	Subtendinous	
Subpopliteal bursa	Between the lateral condyle of the femur and the popliteus muscle	Submuscular	
Iliopsoas bursa	Between the front of the hip joint and the iliopsoas muscle (flexor of hip)	Submuscular	Largest bursa in the body Iliopsoas bursitis—pain at the front of the hip radiating down to the knee or even into the buttocks
Greater trochanteric bursa	Superficial to greater trochanter of femur	Submuscular	Inflammation of this bursa is the common cause of hip pain

Contd…

Contd…

Name of bursa	Location	Type	Clinical importance
Medial gastrocnemius	Between the medial head of the gastrocnemius and the capsule of knee joint	Subtendinous	
Lateral gastrocnemius	Between lateral head of the gastrocnemius and the capsule of knee joint	Subtendinous	
Anserine bursa	Between the medial (tibial) collateral ligament and the tendons of the sartorius, gracilis, and semitendinosus (i.e. the pes anserinus)	Submuscular	Inflammation of the bursa due to constant friction because of certain positions, constant movement, certain diseases
Bunion	At the metatarsophalangeal joint of big toe	Adventitious bursa	Inflammation pushes the big toe against next toe. The surface skin is red.
Acromial bursa	Between the acromion process and the skin	Subcutaneous	
Subacromial bursa	Between the acromion process and supraspinatus muscle	Submuscular	
Subcoracoid bursa	Between the tendon of coracobrachialis and subscapularis muscles	Submuscular	
Subtendinous bursa of subscapularis	Between the neck of scapula and subscapularis muscle	Subtendinous	
Intertubercular bursa	Between the tendon of biceps brachii and the intertubercular sulcus of the humerus	Submuscular	
Retrocalcaneal bursa	Between Achilles tendon and calcaneus	Subtendinous	
Achilles bursa	Between Achilles tendon and the skin in the lower part of the ankle toward the heel	Subcutaneous	
Suprapatellar bursa	Between the anterior surface of the lower part of the femur and the quadriceps femoris	Synovial	It allows for movement of the quadriceps tendon over the distal end of the femur
Superficial infrapatellar bursa	Between the patellar ligament and skin	Subcutaneous	
Deep infrapatellar bursa	Between the upper part of the tibia and the patellar ligament	Synovial	Allows movement of the patellar ligament over the tibia
Prepatellar bursa	Between patella and skin	Subcutaneous	Allows movement of the skin over the underlying patella. When inflamed it is known as housemaids knee
Olecranon bursa	Between loose skin of the elbow and ulna	Subcutaneous	

Classification of synovial joints **(Flowchart 6.3)**:

A. **Based on number of articulating bones:** Presented in **Table 6.3**.

Table 6.3: Classification of synovial joints based on number of articulating bones.

Simple	Compound	Complex
Only two bones enter in the articulation. E.g. Hip joint, talotibial (ankle) interphalangeal joints	More than two articular bones are involved sharing a common articular capsule. E.g. radiocarpal joints (4 bones articulate)	A joint is divided into two compartments by an articular disc or meniscus. E.g. Knee joint, sternoclavicular joint

B. **Based on axis of movement and shape of articular surfaces:**

1. *Plane joint* **(Fig. 6.10A)**:
   – No axis
   – Articular surfaces are more or less flat (plane)
   – They permit gliding movement (translation) in various directions
   – Examples:
     – Acromioclavicular joint
     – Intercarpal joints
     – Intertarsal joints
     – Intermetacarpal and intermetatarsal joints
     – Joints between articular processes of vertebrae.

2. *Uniaxial joint:*
   – Axis of movement: Moves in one axis
   – Degrees of freedom: It has only one degree freedom of movement
   – Subtypes: There are two subtypes. They are hinge and pivot joints.
     – *Hinge (ginglymus)* **(Fig. 6.10B)**:
       - Movement along transverse axis
       - One articular surface is convex and the other is reciprocally curved
       - Bones united by strong collateral ligaments, e.g., interphalangeal joints, humeroulnar (elbow) joint, and ankle joint.
     – *Pivot (trochoid)* **(Fig. 6.10C)**:
       - Axis of movement: Movement along vertical axis
       - One bone acts like a pivot and surrounded by an osseoligamentous ring
       - Examples:
         * Atlantoaxial joint (pivot is the dens of axis which is fixed and the ring is the anterior arch of atlas and transverse ligament of atlas)
         * Radioulnar joint (pivot is the head of radius that rotates with in the ring formed by annular ligament of ulna that is fixed)

3. *Biaxial joint:*
   – Movement occurs in two axes
   – It has two degrees freedom of movement
   – Presents two varieties: (1) Ellipsoid and (2) condylar
     – *Condylar joint* **(Fig. 6.10D)**:
       - It is a modified hinge joint
       - Articular surfaces are known as condyles. Each bone has two distinct articular surfaces called condyles
       - The pair of articular condyles will be enclosed in the same articular capsule or separate articular capsules
       - Permit movement mainly in one axis—(flexion/extension in transverse axis and partly rotation in vertical axis)
       - Examples:
         * Knee joint
         * Temporomandibular joint
     – *Ellipsoid joint* **(Fig. 6.10E)**:
       - Articular surfaces are reciprocally curved. One articular surface is convex and elliptical. Other is concave and reciprocally curved.
       - Movement occurs in transverse and anteroposterior axes. Flexion and extension along transverse

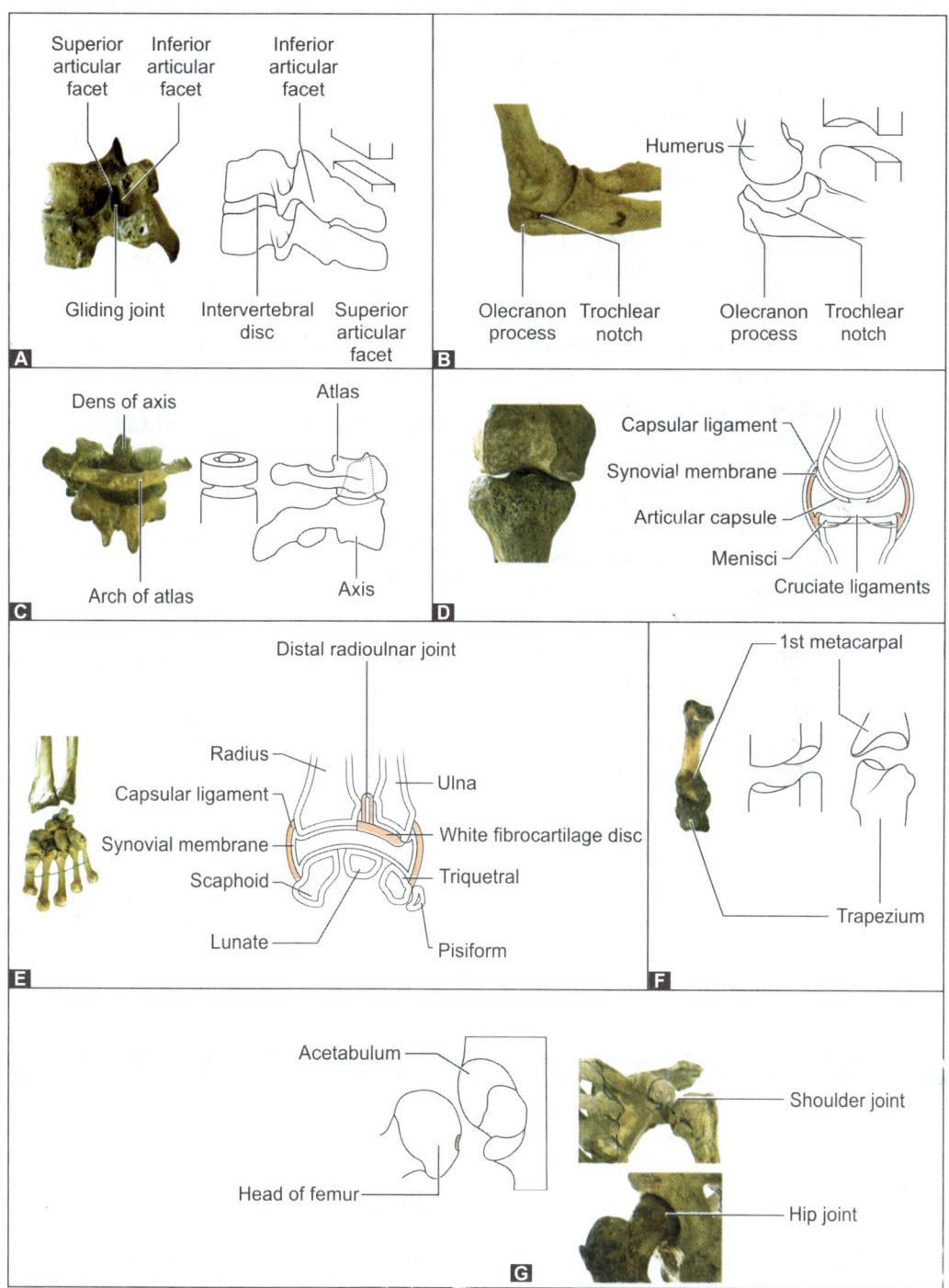

Figs. 6.10A to G: Synovial joint—subtypes. (A) Planner or gliding joint; (B) Hinge joint; (C) Pivot joint; (D) Condylar joint; (E) Ellipsoid joint; (F) Saddle joint; (G) Ball and socket joint.

axis, adduction and abduction along anteroposterior axis and circumduction are possible. Rotation does not take place.
- Examples:
  * Radiocarpal (wrist) joint
  * Metacarpophalangeal joint
  * Metatarsophalangeal joint
  * Atlanto-occipital joint.

4. *Polyaxial joint:*
   - Movement occurs in three axes with a common center.
   - They possess three degrees freedom of movement.
   - Subtypes:
     - *Saddle joint* (**Fig. 6.10F**):
       - Articular surfaces are reciprocally curved, i.e., concavoconvex.
       - Movements are permitted in two axes with addition of some conjugant rotation around a third axis which however cannot occur independently.
       - Example: Carpometacarpal joint of thumb, sternoclavicular joint, joint between incus and malleus (incudo-malleolar joint) of ear.
     - *Ball and socket (spheroidal) joint* (**Fig. 6.10G**):
       - Distal articular surface is globular head which fits into a cup-shaped socket of proximal articular surface.

- Movement occurs around an indefinite number of axes which have one common center.
- Examples:
  * Shoulder joint
  * Hip joint
  * Talocalcaneonavicular joints
  * Articulation between the incus and stapes (Incudo-stapedial joint).

BASIC TERMS USED FOR DESCRIBING MOVEMENTS IN JOINTS

Axes of Movement in a Joint (Tables 6.4 and 6.5 and Fig. 6.11)

An axis is a straight line around which an object rotates. Movement at a joint takes place in a plane about an axis. There are three axes of rotation.

1. *Sagittal/anteroposterior axis*: Passes horizontally from posterior to anterior. It is at the intersection of sagittal and transverse planes.
2. *Frontal/mediolateral axis*: Passes horizontally from left to right. It is at the intersection of frontal and transverse planes.
3. *Vertical axis*: It passes from inferior to superior. It is at the intersection of sagittal and frontal planes.

The movements are called *angular movements* as the angle between adjoining bones is change during movement.

Degrees of freedom: Number of axes at which the bone in a joint can move.

Table 6.4: Axis of rotation and plane of a joint during various movements (**Fig. 6.11**).

Plane of the body	Axis of rotation of joint	Movement	Example
Sagittal plane	Frontal axis	Flexion and extension both in limbs and trunk and inversion and eversion in limbs. Lateral flexion in trunk.	Moving the arm forward and backward from anatomical position
Frontal plane	Sagittal axis	Abduction and adduction	Moving the arm away from the side of trunk and bringing it back to anatomical position
Transverse plane	Vertical axis	Medial and lateral rotation and supination and pronation in limbs. Rotational movements of trunk.	Rotating the arm medially and laterally from the anatomical position

Table 6.5: Various types of joints of the body—location and movements.

Location	Type	Bones articulating	Movements
Head—vault of skull	Fibrous joints—sutural	Between bones of skull cap—frontoparietal, parietooccipital, parietotemporal, and interparietal	No movements
Head—base of skull	Fibrous—sutural	□ Rostrum of sphenoid and vomer □ Between palatine processes of maxilla	No movement
	Primary cartilaginous	Between basiocciput and basisphenoid	
	Synovial—polyaxial—ball and socket	Between incus and stapes	Transfer of vibration
Face	Fibrous joints—gomphosis	Teeth to the upper and lower jaw	No movement
	Synovial—biaxial—condylar	Temporal bone and mandible—temporomandibular joint	Elevation, depression, protraction, retraction, side to side
	Synovial—uniaxial—pivot	Atlas and axis vertebrae	Rotation
Neck	Synovial—biaxial—ellipsoid	Atlas and occipital bone	Flexion and extension (nodding of head) lateral tilting
Trunk	Secondary cartilaginous	Between bodies of vertebrae	Limited movement
	Synovial—plane/gliding	Between articular processes of vertebra	Flexion, extension, lateral flexion, and rotation
	Synovial—plane-modified amphiarthroidal	Sacrum and ilium—sacroiliac joint	Very limited range due to strong ligaments
	Secondary cartilaginous	Manubriosternal joint	Small angular movement
	Synovial—polyaxial—saddle	Sternoclavicular joint—between sternum and clavicle	Anteroposterior and vertical planes and some rotation
	Synovial plane	Acromioclavicular joint	Axial rotation, anteroposterior movement
	Secondary cartilaginous	Symphysis pubis	Slight widening
	Primary cartilaginous	□ 1st chondrosternal □ Ribs with costal cartilages	No movement
Shoulder	Synovial—polyaxial—ball and socket	Humerus, scapula, and clavicle	Flexion, extension, abduction, adduction, rotation, circumduction, elevation, depression, protraction, and retraction
Elbow	Synovial—uniaxial—hinge	Humerus, and ulna	Flexion and extension

Contd...

Chapter 6: Introduction to Arthrology/Joints

Contd...

Location	Type	Bones articulating	Movements
Forearm	❑ Synovial—uniaxial—pivot ❑ Superior and inferior radioulnar joints	Head of radius and radial notch of ulna Ulnar notch of radius and ulnar head	Supination and pronation
	Fibrous joint—syndesmosis—middle	Interosseous membrane	Stability
Wrist	Synovial—biaxial—ellipsoid	Radius, ulna, and proximal row of carpal bones	Flexion, extension, abduction, adduction, and circumduction
Intercarpal	Synovial—plane/gliding	Between carpals	Assist wrist movement
Carpometacarpal	Synovial—polyaxial—saddle	Carpo (trapezio) metacarpal joint of thumb	Flexion, extension, abduction, adduction, rotation, and opposition
	Synovial—biaxial—ellipsoid	Carpometacarpal of other fingers	Flexion, extension, and opposition
Metacarpophalangeal	Synovial—biaxial—ellipsoid	Between metacarpal and proximal phalanx	Flexion, extension, abduction, adduction, and circumduction
Hip	Synovial—polyaxial—ball and socket	Femur and pelvis	Flexion, extension, abduction, adduction, rotation, and circumduction
Knee	Synovial—biaxial—condylar	Femur, patella, tibia, and fibula	Flexion and extension
Leg	Fibrous joints—interosseous membrane and ligaments—syndesmosis	Tibia and fibula	No movement
Ankle	Synovial—uniaxial—hinge	Tibia, fibula, and tarsals	Plantar flexion, dorsiflexion, inversion, eversion, supination, and pronation
	Synovial—polyaxial—ball and socket	Talocalcaneonavicular	
Interphalangeal joints of fingers and toes	Synovial—uniaxial—hinge	Between phalanges	Flexion and extension
Metatarsophalangeal	Synovial—biaxial—ellipsoid	Metatarsal and proximal phalanx	Flexion, extension, abduction, and adduction

- *Uniaxial movement*: Movement of bone at a joint limited to one axis only that is with *one degree of freedom,* e.g., elbow (flexion and extension).
- *Biaxial movement*: Movement of a bone at a joint with *two degrees of freedom,* e.g., wrist (flexion and extension; adduction and abduction).
- *Multiaxial movement*: Movement of a bone at a joint limited to three axes with intermediate positions as well is having *three degrees of freedom,* e.g., shoulder (flexion and extension, adduction and abduction, medial and lateral rotation, and circumduction).

Chapter 6: Introduction to Arthrology/Joints

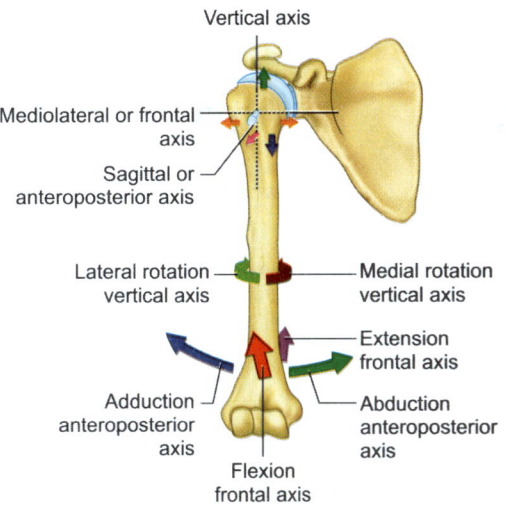

Fig. 6.11: Axes of movement in a joint.

TERMINOLOGY OF BODY MOVEMENTS

Synovial joints allow different range of movements. Movement types are generally paired. The body movements are to be described in relation to anatomical position. The various movements are described in **Table 6.6** and in **Figures 6.12 to 6.19**.

Blood Supply and Nerve Supply of a Joint

- **Blood supply:** The blood supply to a joint is by epiphyseal vessels in a long bone. These vessels enter near the attachment of fibrous capsule and give articular branches that divide into number of branches that form capillary plexus

Table 6.6: Movements at joints.

Paired movements	
Flexion: Decrease the angle of joint—forward bending of vertebral column	*Extension*: Increase the angle of joint—returning of vertebral column to upright position
Hyperflexion: Excessive flexion beyond normal range	*Hyperextension*: Excessive extension beyond normal range
Abduction: Moving the limb laterally away from the body—spreading fingers	*Adduction*: Moving the limb medially toward the body—bringing fingers together
Elevation: Upward movement of mandible or scapula	*Depression*: Downward movement of mandible or scapula
Plantar flexion: Movement at the ankle lifting the heel off the ground	*Dorsiflexion*: Movement at the ankle bringing the dorsum of foot upward
Inversion: Sole of foot turned medially, toward midline	*Eversion*: Sole of foot turned laterally, away from midline
Lateral (external) rotation: Movement of arm (at shoulder joint) or thigh (at hip joint) moving front of arm or thigh away from the midline	*Medial (internal) rotation*: Movement of arm (at shoulder joint) or thigh (at hip joint) moving front of arm or thigh away toward the midline
Supination: Movement to bring forearm so that the palm faces anteriorly (as in anatomical position)	*Pronation*: Movement to bring forearm so that the palm faces backward
Protraction: Anterior movement of mandible or scapula	*Retraction*: Posterior movement of mandible or scapula
Other movements	
Circumduction: Circular movement of arm, hand, thumb or finger that is produced by combination of flexion, abduction, extension, and adduction	
Medial and lateral excursions: Side to side chewing movements of mandible from and toward midline	
Opposition: Movement of thumb that brings tip of thumb in contact with the tip of other finger	
Lateral flexion: Bending the neck or body toward the right or left side	
Rotation: Movement of a bone around its long axis (shoulder joint, proximal radioulnar joint, and hip joint) or along its central axis (atlantoaxial joint) or twisting of vertebral column (summation of small movements between adjacent vertebrae)	

Chapter 6: Introduction to Arthrology/Joints

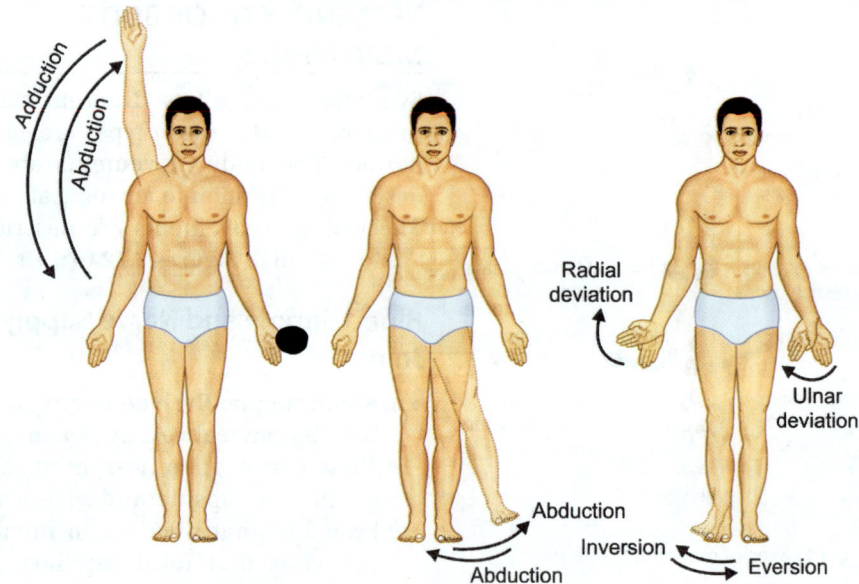

Fig. 6.12: Limbs—paired movements.

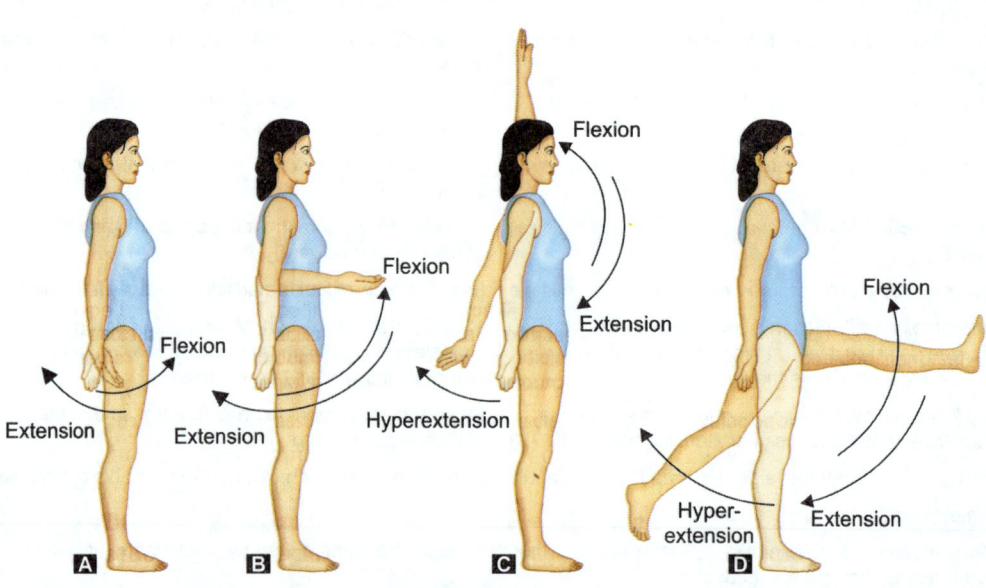

Figs. 6.13A to D: Limbs—paired movements. (A) Movements at wrist; (B) Movements at elbow; (C) Movements at shoulder; (D) Movements at hip.

Chapter 6: Introduction to Arthrology/Joints

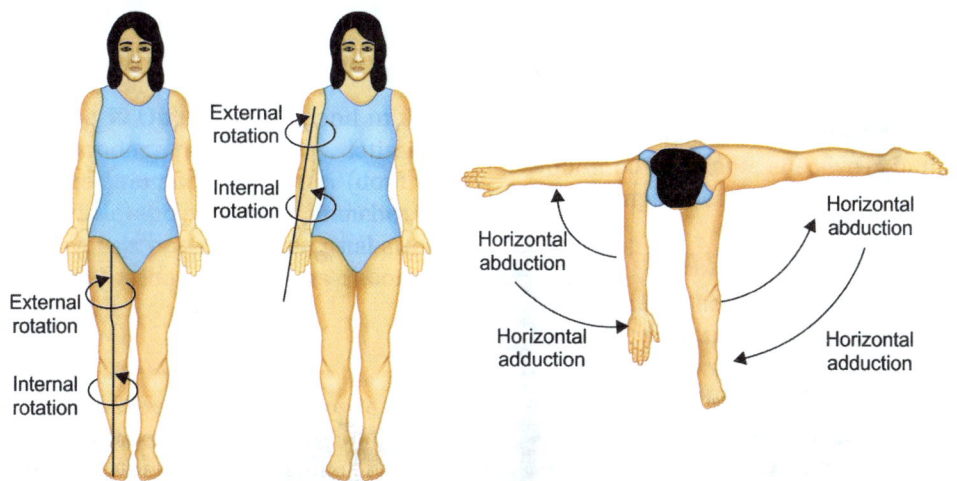

Fig. 6.14: Limbs—paired movements.

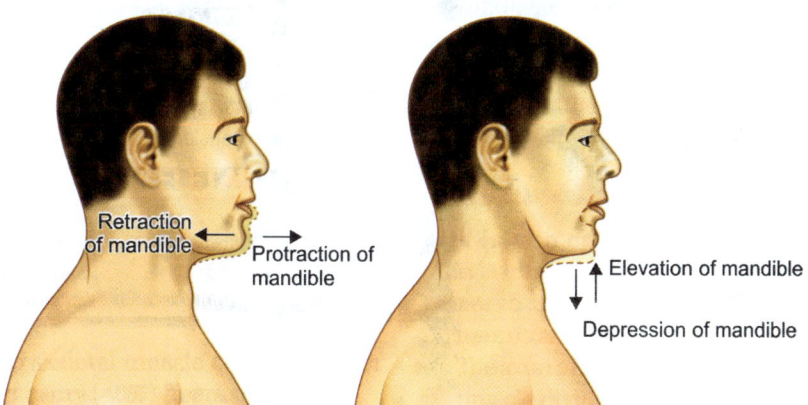

Fig. 6.15: Mandible—paired movements.

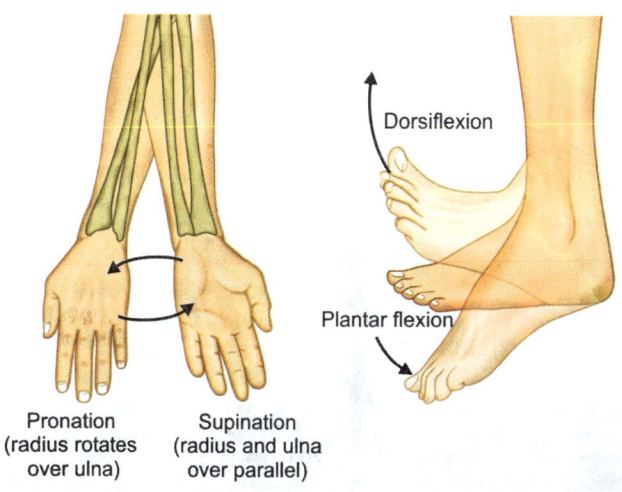

Fig. 6.16: Forearm and ankle—paired movements.

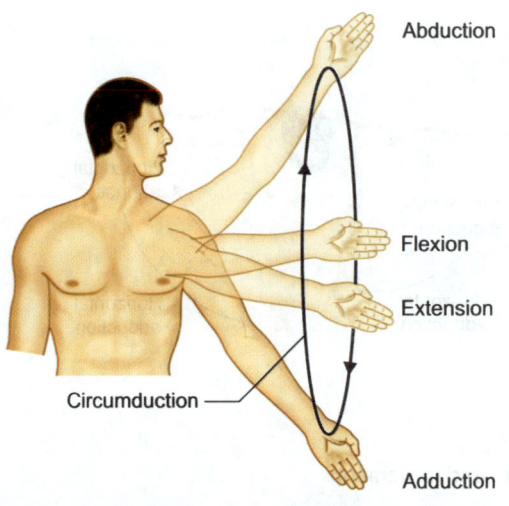

Fig. 6.17: Shoulder—circumduction movement.

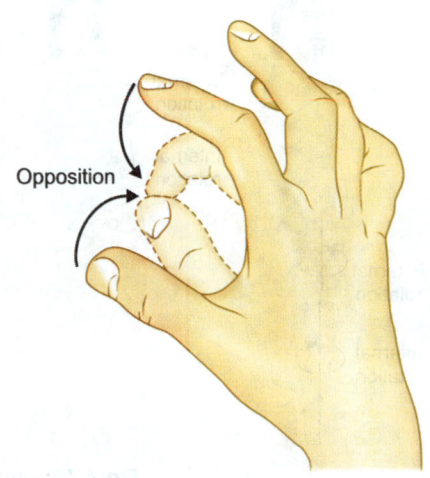

Fig. 6.18: Thumb—opposition movement.

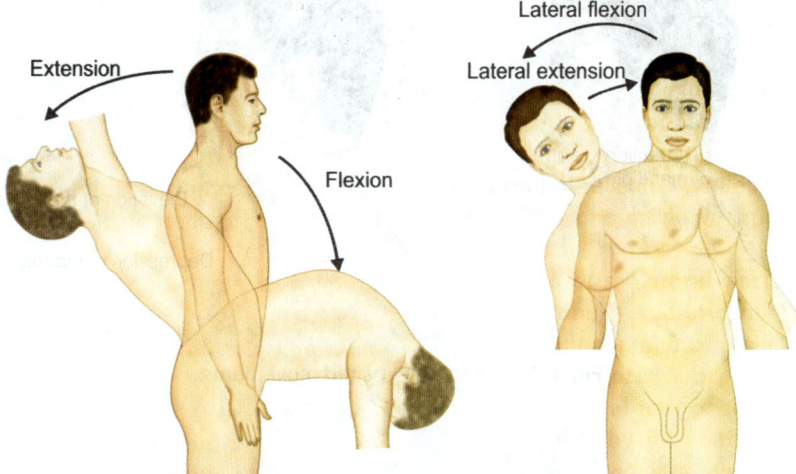

Fig. 6.19: Movements of trunk and neck.

(circulus vasculosus) on the synovial membrane.

AN2.6: Explain the concept of nerve supply of joints and Hilton's law.

- **Nerve supply:** The articular capsule and ligaments in relation to a joint are richly innervated. These nerves contain sensory and autonomic fibers. Sensory fibers are concerned with reflex control of posture, position and movement sense and convey pain sensations from the joint capsule.

AN2.6: Explain the concept of nerve supply of joints and Hilton's law.

Hilton's law: According to Hilton's law the nerves which supply a joint, also give branches to the group of muscles acting on the joint and to the skin over the joint (**Fig. 6.20**).

Example: Axillary nerve—it supplies capsule of shoulder joint, muscles acting on the joint, e.g., deltoid and skin over the upper lateral part of arm as lateral cutaneous nerve of arm.

This law provides explanation for the reflex spasm of muscles in cases of joint disease because of irritation of nerves and the referred pain on the overlying skin of the joint.

Exceptions for Hilton's law: The Hilton's law is obeyed by all the nerves with two exceptions:
1. **Temporomandibular joint**: The sensory innervation for the joint is by mandibular nerve (a division of trigeminal nerve) that also supplies the skin over it. The mandibular nerve is the motor nerve for all the muscles acting on the joint except buccinator. The buccinator muscle is perced by the buccal branch of mandibular nerve but it is supplied by the facial nerve.

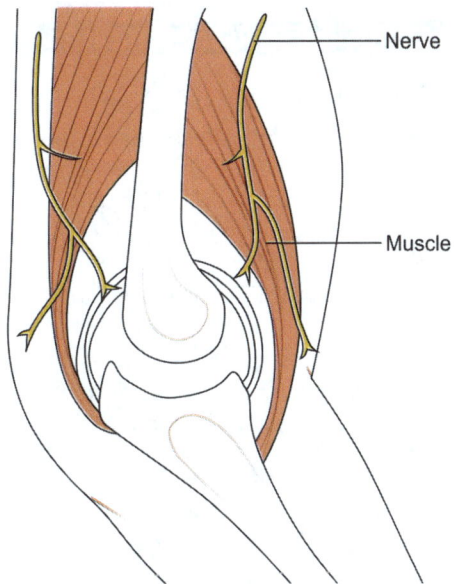

Fig. 6.20: Hilton's law.

Clinical Application of Joints

- *Arthritis:* It is inflammation of joint. There are about 100 different types of arthritis. The most common conditions, rheumatoid arthritis or osteoarthritis (old age), psoriatic arthritis and gout. The involved joints are swollen, painful, and with restricted movement.
- *Arthroscopy:* It is the procedure used for visualization of joint cavity and treating joint problems. A fiberoptic video camera is passed through a small incision into the joint cavity. The image is transmitted to the video-monitor.
- *Arthroplasty*: It is an orthopedic surgical procedure where the articular surface of a joint is replaced or remodeled to restore the function of the joint, e.g., total hip replacement, and total knee replacement.
- *Sprain*: Tear of a ligament causes severe pain due to fluid effusion in the ligament and joint. There will not be any dislocation.
- *Dislocation and subluxation*: Dislocation is loss of contact between the two articulating bones. If the contact is retained it is called subluxation. The common cause for dislocation is trauma and can cause pain, loss of function and deformity. The dislocation is diagnosed by X-ray.
- *Neuropathic joint*: It is caused by leprosy, tabes dorsalis and the joints show painless swelling and bone destruction.
- *Osteotomy*: It is a surgical procedure whereby a bone is cut to shorten or lengthen it or change its alignment if it has healed in an abnormal fashion following a fracture. It is also used to correct deformities of the limb, i.e., coxa vara and valga (deformity of hip), genu valgum (knock knee) and genu varum (bowed legs).

Anatomical Basis for Clinical Condition

Case Scenario

Problem: A sports person had a fall on outstretched arms and comes to the orthopedic surgeon with pain and swelling of the shoulder and restricted movement. It was diagnosed as dislocation of shoulder joint.

Questions:
1. What is the difference between fracture, dislocation, subluxation, and sprain in a shoulder joint?
2. What investigation is required to rule out fracture?
3. What treatment will be advised by the doctor?
4. Why is the shoulder more prone for dislocation?

Anatomical explanation:
1. Dislocation is complete disruption of a joint. It occurs when the two bones are out of place at the joint connecting them. Subluxation is partial dislocation followed by relocation. Fracture is a break in the bone. Dislocation can be associated with a fracture of the bone. A sprain is due to the tear of the ligament.
2. An X-ray of shoulder to be done to rule out fracture.
3. Surgical reduction to be followed by immobilization of the joint. After immobilization exercise for strengthening the joint to be advised.
4. The shoulder joint is a ball and socket joint formed by larger head of humerus and a smaller glenoid cavity of scapula. The range of mobility is more than the stability in the shoulder joint. Hence, it is more prone for dislocation.

2. **Hip joint:** This joint is supplied mainly by femoral, obturator and sciatic nerves mainly and also by nerve to quadratus femoris, superior gluteal nerve. The joints and the skin over it are also supplied by the same nerves. All the muscles acting on the joint are also supplied by the branches from these nerves except pyriformis. The sciatic nerve is closely related to the pyriformis muscle and sometimes few of its fibers pass through the muscle but it will not supply the muscle. The pyriformis

☞ Key Concept

Take Home Message—Joints

- A joint is the connection between two or more bones or cartilages to permit movement.
- Long bones articulate at their ends, flat bones at margins and short or irregular bones at their articular surfaces.
- Joints are classified based on their structure and function into synarthroses (fibrous and immovable), amphiarthroses (cartilaginous and slightly movable) and diarthroses (synovial and freely movable).
- Fontanels are unossified fibrous tissue between the bones of vault of skull in fetus and in the infant.

Contd...

Chapter 6: Introduction to Arthrology/Joints

Contd…

- In a fibrous joint the articulating bones are connected by modification of fibrous tissue, i.e., ligament or interosseous membrane.
- Primary cartilaginous joints are temporary. Secondary cartilaginous joints are midline joints.
- The eight important components of a synovial joint are articulating bones, articulating cartilage, articular capsule, articular disc, joint capsule, accessory ligaments, synovial fluid, and bursa.
- Bursae are small fluid-filled, closed, synovial membrane lined sacs located between bone and muscle or tendon or ligament at the sites of friction and the fluid is called synovial fluid.
- There are five types of bursa—(1) synovial, (2) subcutaneous, (3) subtendinous, (4) submuscular, and (5) adventitious.
- Most of the joints of appendicular skeleton are synovial and are important in the field of medicine.
- The factors contributing to stability of synovial joint are contour of bones, ligaments, muscles, and atmospheric pressure.
- The three axes through which movement takes place in a synovial joint are sagittal, frontal and vertical with each at the intersection of two fundamental planes of the body.
- Depending on the number of axes through which movement of bone takes place the synovial joints are classified as uniaxial with one degree of freedom, biaxial with two degrees of freedom, and multiaxial with three degrees of freedom.

is supplied by branches from sacral plexus.

QUESTIONS

1. Describe the general features of synovial joints.
2. Describe the features of fibrous joints and classify them with examples.
3. Classify synovial joints with examples.
4. Differences between symphysis and synchondrosis.
5. Bursa.
6. What do you understand by axes of movement and degrees of freedom? Give examples.

MULTIPLE CHOICE QUESTIONS

1. **Which of the following joints is biaxial?**
   A. Wrist joint
   B. Sternoclavicular joint
   C. Radioulnar joint
   D. Incudostapedial joint

2. **The joint between vertebra and intervertebral disc is an example of which joint?**
   A. Syndesmoses
   B. Synarthroses
   C. Synchondroses
   D. Symphyses

3. **The joint between tibia and fibula is what type?**
   A. Symphysis
   B. Gomphosis
   C. Syndesmosis
   D. Primary cartilaginous

4. **Example of a wide fibrous joint is:**
   A. Fontanelle
   B. Interosseous membrane of fore arm
   C. Synostosis
   D. Gomphosis

5. A cartilaginous joint has all the features, *except:*
   A. A joint cavity
   B. Hyaline cartilage
   C. Amphiarthroses
   D. White fibrocartilage

6. All the following symphyses are separated by a fibrocartilage, *except:*
   A. Intervertebral discs between the bodies of vertebra
   B. Manubriosternal joint
   C. Symphysis pubis
   D. Symphysis menti

7. Atlanto-occipital joint is an example for one of the following type of synovial variety:
   A. Pivot
   B. Ellipsoid
   C. Condylar
   D. Saddle

8. What type of joint is present at the junction of epiphysis and diaphysis, i.e. at the growth plate?
   A. Fibrous
   B. Primary cartilaginous
   C. Secondary cartilaginous
   D. Plane joint

9. Synovial joints are:
   A. Synarthroses
   B. Bones connected with white fibrocartilage
   C. Bones connected with one another in a fluid-filled cavity
   D. Amphiarthroses

ANSWERS

| 1. A | 2. D | 3. C | 4. B | 5. A | 6. D |
| 7. B | 8. B | 9. C | | | |

CHAPTER 7

Introduction to Blood Vascular System

LEARNING OBJECTIVES

- Purpose and functions
- Types of circulation: Systemic, pulmonary, portal
- Blood vessels: Classification, structure
- Anastomoses
- Collateral circulation
- End-arteries
- Vasa vasorum
- Clinical case with anatomical explanation

PURPOSE AND FUNCTIONS

- In a large complex organism continuous transport of specific components ranging from ions to whole cells to every part of the body for nutrition, respiratory exchange of gases and excretion of waste products of metabolism requires a system that is widespread and has greater capacity.
- This function is carried by *circulatory* or *vascular system*.
- Two types of fluids move through the circulatory system: (1) blood and (2) lymph. Accordingly, it is divided into two parts:
  1. *Cardiovascular system*: It consists of the blood that circulates through heart and blood vessels. Cardiovascular system is one through which nutrition is transported to all the tissues of the body for utilization, waste products of metabolism are received and transported to the appropriate organs for excretion from the body.
  2. *Lymphatic system:* The lymph, lymph nodes, and lymph vessels form the lymphatic system.
     Note: For convenience the lymphatic system is described in a separate chapter.

Difference between Blood Vascular and Lymphatic System

AN5.1: Differentiate between blood vascular and lymphatic system.

The difference between blood vascular and lymphatic system are shown in **Table 7.1**.

Cardiovascular System

The components of cardiovascular system are:
- Heart
- Blood vessels.

Heart and Blood Vascular System

- Heart and blood vessels together make up the cardiovascular system.
- About 5 L (1/11th of body weight) of blood is present in the vascular system.

Heart:
- The heart is the main organ in the cardiovascular system with four muscular chambers and four valves. It pumps blood to various parts of body (**Fig. 7.1**).
- Heart is divided structurally and functionally into two halves, (1) the right and (2) the left. Each half is having a receiving or inflow chamber called *atrium* and a pumping or outflow chamber the *ventricle*.

Chapter 7: Introduction to Blood Vascular System

Table 7.1: Blood vascular system versus lymphatic system.		
Feature	Blood vascular system	Lymphatic system
Definition	Concerned with transportation activity (blood components) and consists of cardiovascular and lymphatic systems	Consists of network of tissues and organs that transport lymph throughout the body
Components	Blood, blood vessels—arteries and veins	Lymph, lymph nodes and lymph vessels
Transportation of fluid	Moves through heart, arteries, veins, capillaries and lungs—circular movement	Moves through lymph nodes, lymph vessels, lymph capillaries—unidirectional movement
Composition of transporting fluid	Red blood cell (RBC), white blood cell (WBC), platelets + fluid plasma (proteins, ions, glucose)	WBC+ interstitial fluid (similar to blood plasma but without proteins)
Fluid moving and its color	Blood—reddish	Lymph—colorless
Flow of fluid	Faster	Slow
Function	Circulation of respiratory gases (oxygen, carbon dioxide) nutrients, hormones, wastes and other toxins	❑ Helps in body defense and is part of immune system ❑ Transport fats (chylomicrons) from digestive system

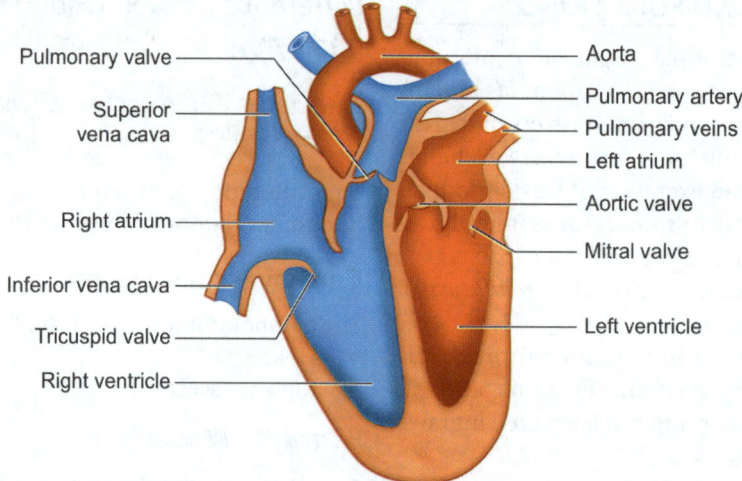

Fig. 7.1: Heart—chambers and major blood vessels connected to heart.

- The right and left atria are separated by *inter atrial septum*. The right and left ventricles are separated by *interventricular septum*. The right atrium communicates with right ventricle through right atrioventricular orifice which is guarded by *tricuspid valve*. The left atrium communicates with left ventricle through the left atrioventricular orifice which is guarded by *mitral valve*. The valves allow flow of blood from atrium to ventricle but not in reverse direction.

- The "right heart" circulates blood through lungs for oxygenation through *pulmonary circulation*. The "left heart" circulates blood to various tissues of the body through *systemic circulation*.

Blood vascular system:

- The blood vascular system consists of vessels of different caliber, structure, and function. They carry blood from the heart to the tissues and then return back to the heart.

- The term "angeion" means a vessel in Greek. It can be blood vessel or lymph vessel. *Angiology* is the medical specialty concerned with the study of diseases of the circulatory and lymphatic system.
- A number of tubes known as *arteries* travel away from the heart and carry oxygenated blood to the peripheral parts of the body, i.e. organs and tissues. From the tissues and organs a system of tubes known as *veins* loop back and reach the heart returning the deoxygenated blood.
- The blood vessels are broadly categorized as follows **(Fig. 7.2)**:
  - *Arteries*: These carry blood away from the heart for distribution to different parts of the body. The largest artery in the body is the *aorta* that arises from the heart. The arteries divide into smaller branches. Large artery is more than 1.0 cm in diameter. Medium-sized arteries are 1–10 mm in diameter.
  - *Arterioles*: Minute branches of arteries that are just visible to the naked eye are called arterioles. They are less than 0.5 mm diameter. These end in a plexus of thin walled capillaries/sinusoids in the tissues.
  - *Capillaries*: Network of microscopic vessels that connect arterioles and venules. These are in intimate contact with tissues for exchange of nutrients

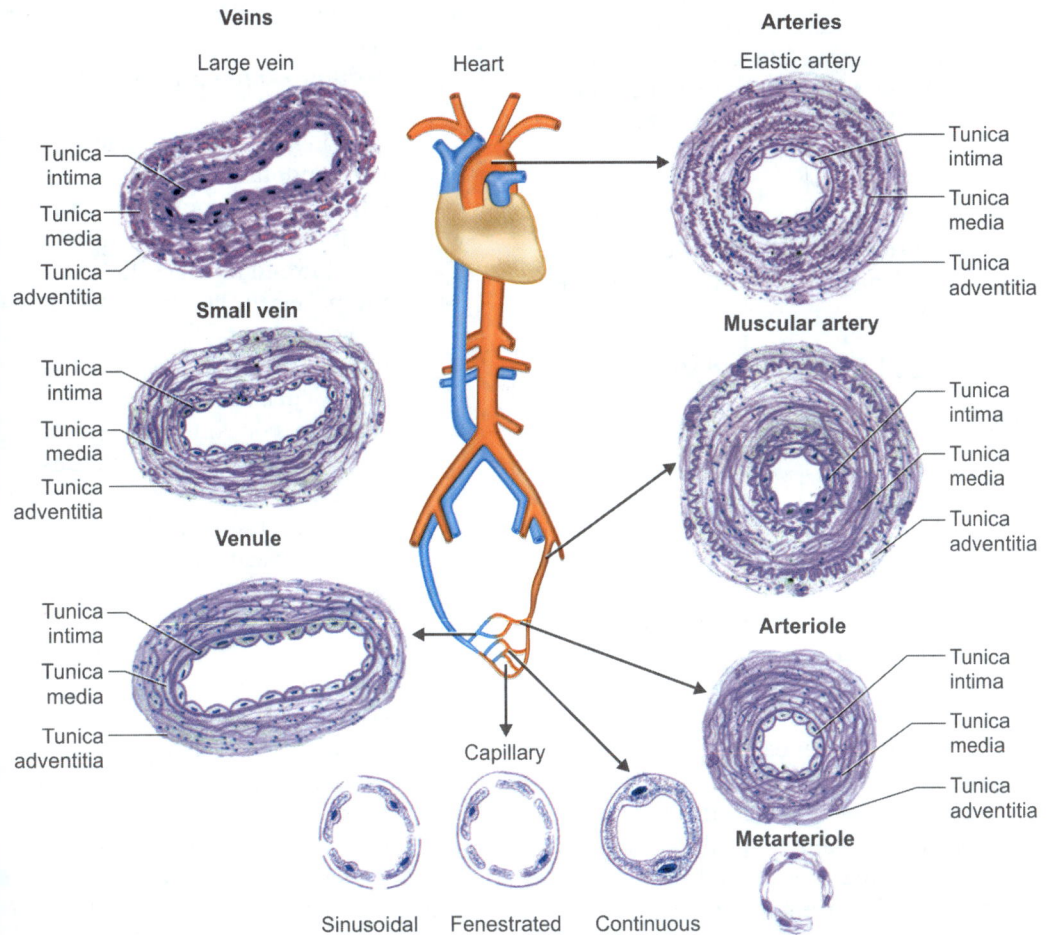

Fig. 7.2: Different types of blood vessels.

and metabolites between blood and tissues. A small part of the metabolites are drained by lymphatics.
- *Sinusoids and cavernous tissues*: Capillaries are replaced by sinusoids in some organs like *liver, spleen* and by cavernous tissue in *penis and clitoris*.
- *Venules and veins*: The veins adjoining capillaries are very small and are called *venules*. These carry blood from different parts of the body to the heart. The veins are formed by union of venules which are called *tributaries*. Venules are 0.5–1 μ in diameter. Medium-sized veins are 1–10 mm in diameter. Large veins are more than 1.0 cm in diameter. Finally two large veins are formed that drain deoxygenated blood from upper half of body (*superior vena cava*) and lower half of body (*inferior vena cava*) to the right atrium of heart.
- A special set of arteries and veins circulate blood through the lungs for oxygenation of blood. They are pulmonary arteries and pulmonary veins.

Structure of Arteries and Veins

> **AN5.3:** List general differences between arteries and veins.

Arteries **(Fig. 7.3)**

- Arteries are thick walled tubes that convey oxygenated blood from heart and distribute it through its branches, to various parts of the body and end as capillaries.
- Increase in number as they move away from heart by repeated division and by issuing side branches in both systemic and pulmonary circulation.
- Decrease in diameter as they move away from the heart. So, blood flow is faster nearer the heart than at the periphery.
- Thickness of wall of the arteries decreases as they move away from the heart although

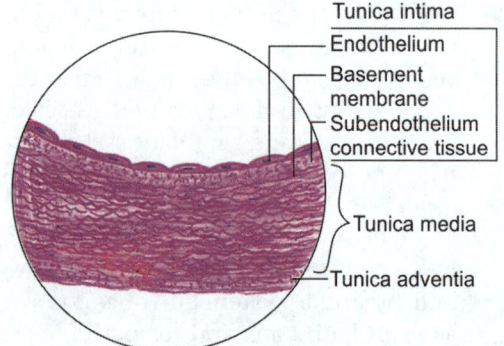

Fig. 7.3: Large artery.

not as substantial as the decrease in diameter.
- Arteries have no valves.
- Microscopically, all arteries consist of three coats:
  1. *Inner tunica intima*: It presents two layers:
     - Endothelial layer—contains flattened endothelial layer
     - Subendothelial connective tissue—longitudinally arranged and supports the endothelial cells
     - Internal elastic lamina—a fenestrated elastic layer.
  2. *Middle tunica media*:
     - Thickest of all coats
     - Contains concentrically arranged alternate layers of smooth muscle and fenestrated elastic tissue in the form of layers (70 layers)
     - External elastic lamina—external layer.
  3. *Outer tunica adventitia*:
     - Thinnest and strongest of the three coats
     - It consists of longitudinally arranged elastic and collagenous tissue
     - Clinical importance: This layer resists the outward pressure of blood and prevents the formation of aneurysm of arteries.

Tunica adventitia and outer part of tunica media are supplied by capillaries of *vasa vasorum*.

Veins (Fig. 7.4)

- Channels carrying blood from capillary bed to heart.
- Capillaries unite to form venules which join to form veins. Smaller veins join to form larger veins which in turn join to form superior/inferior vena cava.
- Lumen is larger than artery.
- Amount of blood conveyed by it is same as that of artery and so lumen becomes large.
- All veins carry deoxygenated blood except pulmonary veins.
- Thin walled. Thickness of wall of the veins is less than that of arteries and the diameter of lumen is more than that of arteries.
- The amount of muscle and elastic fibers are less in veins when compared to arteries.
- Veins are numerous than arteries.
- The pulse pressure is low and blood flow is slow.
- Contraction of abdominal muscles and diaphragm facilitate venous return from the veins of abdomen.
- Structurally three coats—not well-defined like arteries:
  1. Tunica intima: Absence of internal elastic membrane.
  2. Tunica media: Thin, more collagen, few elastic, and smooth muscle fibers. *Exceptions*: Increased smooth muscle in pulmonary veins, deep veins of penis, and uterine veins during pregnancy.
  3. Tunica adventitia: Thickest of all coats. Contains collagen fibers, few elastic fibers and some smooth muscle fibers.
- *Valves* (Fig. 7.5):
  - Interior of the veins are provided with *valves* that prevent reflux of blood thus maintaining unidirectional flow of blood. The blood flows against gravity and prevents back flow.
  - The valves are formed by infolding or reduplication of tunica intima.
  - They have one to three cusps directed toward heart.
  - These are present just distal to the region where a vein undergoes dilatation (sinus).
  - The valves are more in the veins that carry blood against gravity, e.g., lower limb veins. The contraction of muscle increases the venous return by generating pressure and opening up of valves.
  - Usually absent in veins of thorax and abdomen.
  - Absent in very small veins (<2.0 mm diameter) and very large veins (cerebral, spinal, vena cavae, pulmonary, hepatic, renal, uterine, ovarian, testicular, and umbilical).
- *Dead space*: Large veins are surrounded by a *dead space* to allow expansion of

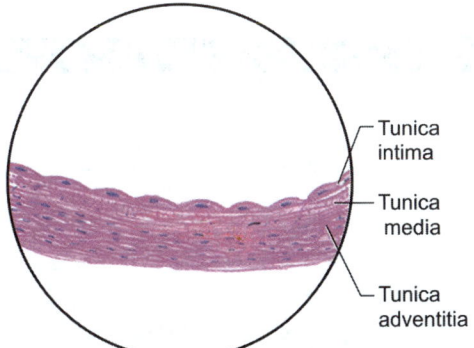

Fig. 7.4: Microscopic structure of large vein.

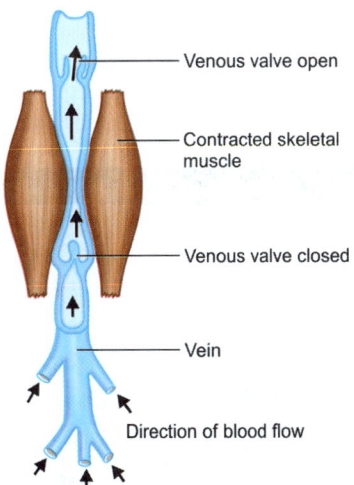

Fig. 7.5: Venous valves.

veins during increased venous return, e.g., femoral vein in femoral sheath, inferior pulmonary vein in pulmonary ligament.
- *Arrangement of veins*: Arranged in two sets—*(1) superficial and (2) deep.*
  1. Superficial veins run in superficial fascia and are not accompanied by corresponding arteries.
  2. Deep veins lie under cover of deep fascia and are accompanied by arteries.

The differences in structure between an artery and a vein are presented in **Table 7.2**.

TYPES OF CIRCULATION OF BLOOD (FIG. 7.6)

AN5.2: Differentiate between pulmonary and systemic circulation.

- There are two types of loops in circulation of blood, (1) the minor or lesser (pulmonary) and (2) the major or greater (systemic).
- Heart pumps blood through a pair of muscular pumps to regulate these two circuits of blood flow. One pump feeds the minor loop, the *pulmonary circulation* which supplies the lungs. Other feeds the major loop, the *systemic circulation* which supplies rest of the body.
- Major loop consists of two circulations the *systemic* and the *portal*. Each loop is a closed system so blood does not leave the circulation.
  - *Pulmonary circulation (lesser)*:
    - Blood flows from right ventricle to lungs via pulmonary trunk and pulmonary arteries. In the lung carbon dioxide is exchanged for oxygen through capillaries.
    - The oxygenated blood reaches left atrium via pulmonary veins.
    - It is *right to left flow in pulmonary circulation*.
  - *Systemic circulation (greater)*:
    - Oxygenated blood flows from left ventricle of heart to various tissues of body through aorta and its branches of arteries.
    - Nutrients and oxygen passes to the tissues through capillaries and waste products of metabolism and carbon dioxide return from tissues to veins.
    - Finally the deoxygenated blood is returned to right atrium through superior and inferior vena cava.
    - The blood flow is from *left to right in systemic circulation*.
  - *Portal circulation*:
    - Here blood flows through two sets of capillaries before reaching systemic vein. The vein draining *first capillary network is called portal vein*.
    - The portal vein branches like an artery to form a *second set of capillaries or sinusoids*, e.g., hepatic, hypophyseal, and renal portal circulations.
  - *Vascular loops*: There are two types of vascular loops in the body.

Table 7.2: Differences between arteries and veins.

Feature	Arteries	Veins
Wall thickness	Thick wall	Thin wall
Muscle fibers	More	Less
Elastic fibers	More	Less
Lumen size and patency	Small and patent	Large and collapsed
TM vs TA thickness	TM < TA	TA > TM
Valves in the lumen	Absent	Present
Number	Less	More than arteries
Oxygen content of blood flowing	Oxygenated except pulmonary arteries	Deoxygenated except pulmonary veins

Chapter 7: Introduction to Blood Vascular System

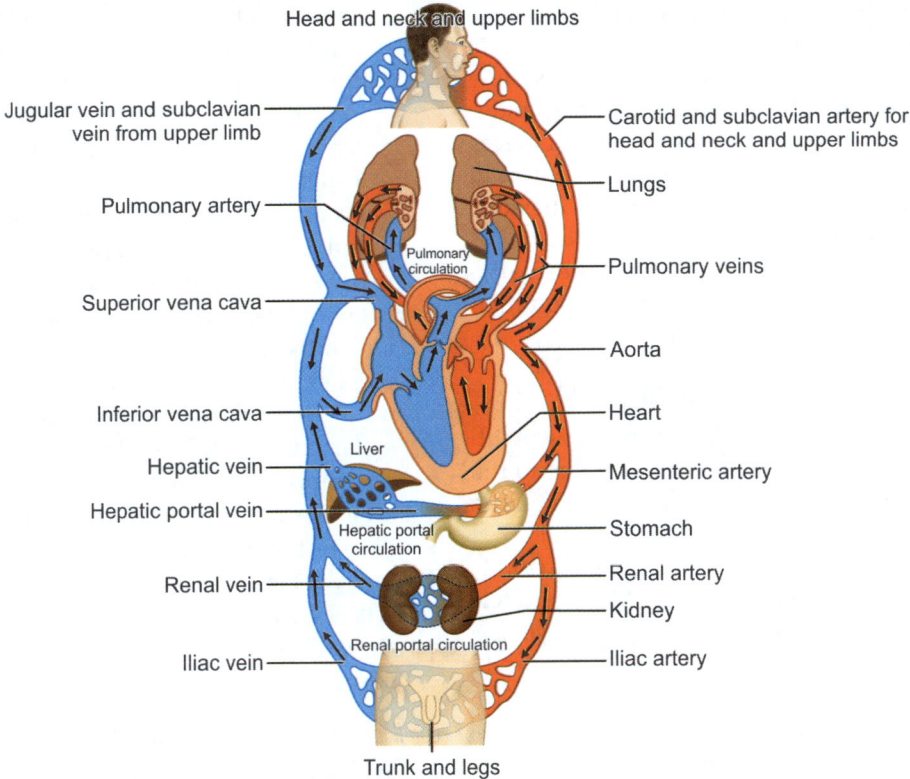

Fig. 7.6: Blood circulation—types.

1. A long loop consisting of heart, large arteries, and veins.
2. A short loop at the periphery consisting of capillaries.

- Distributing vessels
- Resistance vessels
- Exchange vessels
- Capacitance/reservoir vessels.

CLASSIFICATION OF BLOOD VESSELS

Based on structural and functional characters the blood vessels are classified. The two classifications can be correlated (**Table 7.2** and **Fig. 7.2**).
1. *Anatomical classification*: Based on structure
   - Elastic artery
   - Muscular artery
   - Arteriole
   - Capillary/sinusoid
   - Venules
   - Veins
2. *Functional classification*: Based on function
   - Conducting vessels

STRUCTURE OF VASCULAR TREE FROM CENTER TO PERIPHERY

AN5.4: Explain functional difference between elastic, muscular arteries and arterioles.

The relative thickness of the coats, relative proportion of muscular, fibrous and elastic tissues varies in different vessels.

Various Vessels of Vascular Tree (Fig. 7.2)

Large/Elastic Arteries (Conducting Vessels)

- Subendothelial connective tissue is thick.
- Elastic tissue is more in tunica media.

- Tunica externa contains elastic fibers.
- *Functional importance*: Because of elastic fibers the vessel distends during systole when blood enters from the heart under force. Because of elastic recoil it drives the blood to the periphery and returns to normal caliber thus maintains diastolic blood pressure.
- *Examples*: Aorta, brachiocephalic, common carotid, subclavian, common iliac, pulmonary arteries.

Medium/Muscular Arteries (Distributing Vessels)

- Thickness of tunica intima varies with age and is thicker in old age due to the deposition of lipids. The internal elastic lamina is prominent.
- Tunica media contains more of circularly arranged smooth muscle fibers and few scattered elastic fibers. Right side vessels present clockwise direction of muscle fibers and left side vessels in anticlockwise direction.
- Tunica adventitia is thicker than in elastic arteries.
- *Functional importance*: These move the blood forward by muscular contraction that is under the control of autonomic nervous system. The muscle fibers respond to nerve stimuli that regulate the size of lumen.
- *Examples*: Occipital, popliteal, radial, and ulnar arteries.

Arterioles (Resistance Vessels)

- These are smallest divisions of muscular arteries (<1.0 mm in diameter).
- They contain all the three coats.
- Tunica media contains only plain muscle fibers.
- They progressively divide into smaller branches called *terminal arterioles* and *metarterioles*.
  - Terminal arterioles are 50–100 µm in diameter, devoid of internal elastic lamina and covered by a continuous coat of smooth muscle cells.
  - Metarterioles are 15–20 µm in diameter and the smooth muscle is replaced by discontinuous, noncontractile cells called pericytes or Rouget cells. The meta-arterioles terminate in capillaries.
- *Functional importance*: Arterioles regulate blood flow into the capillaries, offer peripheral resistance and there by regulate systolic blood pressure. Thick muscle wall and muscle tone controls the arterial pressure. The tone of the arteriolar smooth muscle is regulated by autonomic nervous system and partly by renin-angiotensin II mechanism. Persistent increased tone of arteriolar wall produces hypertension.
- Rate of blood flow through aorta is 0.5 m/s. Rate of blood flow through arterioles is 0.5 mm/s.
- *Example*: Afferent and efferent arterioles in the glomerulus of kidney.

Capillaries (Exchange Vessels) (*See* **Fig. 7.2**)

- The arterioles terminate in capillaries.
- These are fine channels made of single layer of endothelium resting on a basal lamina of glycoproteins.
- Basal lamina splits at places to enclose pericytes or Rouget cells. These cells are noncontractile, phagocytic, facilitate blood flow and are responsible for formation of new blood vessels.
- Each capillary is 8–10 µm in diameter and 1 mm long. The diameter is larger than RBC that can flow through the capillaries in a single profile.
- These are *smallest* in brain and intestines. *Largest* in skin and bone marrow.
- Total cross sectional diameter of capillaries is 800 times more than that of aorta (30 mm). Total length of capillaries is 60,000 miles.
- Walls of capillaries act as semipermeable membranes for transportation and exchange.
- Increase in number in active tissues—muscles, glands, liver, kidneys, and lungs.

- Decreased number in less active tissues—tendons and ligaments.
- *Avascular structures*: Structures where capillaries are *absent. Examples:* Cornea of the eye; articular hyaline cartilage; epidermis of skin, hairs and nails; epithelial cells resting on basement membrane.
- *Types of capillaries*:
  - *Continuous capillaries*: Endothelium forms continuous barrier, e.g., skin, connective tissue, skeletal and smooth muscles, brain, and lung.
  - *Fenestrated capillaries*: Pores of 0.1 µm or less are present between endothelial cells and extend from inner to outer surface of cytoplasm, e.g., intestinal mucous membrane, pancreas, endocrine glands, and renal glomeruli.
- *Functional importance*: Capillary bed and postcapillary venules provide an area for exchange of nutritive material, metabolites, gases, water between blood and intestinal fluid.

Sinusoids (Exchange Vessels) (Fig. 7.7)

- Minute blood vessels replacing capillaries in some organs like *liver, spleen, bone marrow, suprarenal glands, hypophysis cerebri, etc.*
- Large irregular uneven dilatations or blood spaces.
- Lumen is wider but walls are thin.

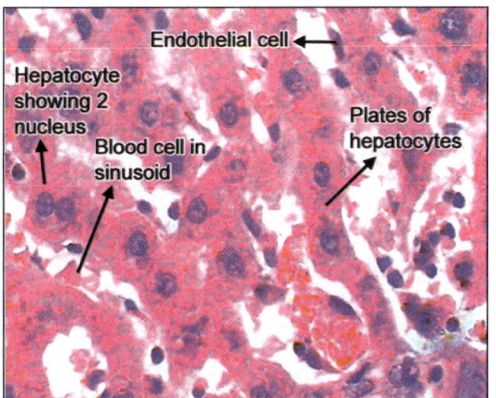

Fig. 7.7: Sinusoids in liver.

- Perithelium is absent. So, some are in direct contact with surrounding tissues.
- Phagocytic cells of macrophage type line the walls of lumen of sinusoids.
- No adventitial support but basal lamina is a thin reticular tissue.
- They may connect venule with a venule (liver) and arteriole with venule (bone marrow and spleen).
- Developed as a result of breaking down of large vein (vitelline vein) in liver.
- *Types*:
  - Discontinuous in red pulp of spleen
  - Closed in brain, thymus, and testis
  - Fenestrated in endocrine glands.

Cavernous Tissues

- Blood filled spaces lined by endothelium and surrounded by trabeculae containing smooth muscle cells.
- Arterioles and venules directly open into these spaces.
- *Examples*: Erectile tissue of penis, clitoris, and in nasal mucous membrane.

Small and Large Veins (Capacitance/Reservoir Vessels)

- These are the vessels that hold major portion of blood volume (70–80%).
- They are capable of holding and storing blood.
- Muscular tissue is *absent* in dural venous sinuses, retinal veins, and veins in erectile tissue of penis.
- *Examples*: Cephalic vein, popliteal vein, saphenous vein, inferior vena cava, and superior vena cava.

Venae Comitantes (Fig. 7.8)

- These are pair of veins that accompany an artery.
- Above elbow and below knee the deep veins are arranged in pairs along the sides of arteries and are known as venae comitantes.
- These help in return of blood toward the heart by transmitted pulsation of arteries. They also help in counter current heat exchange between arteries and veins.

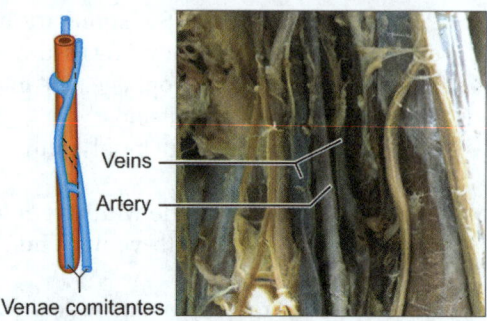

Fig. 7.8: Venae comitantes.

Factors that facilitate venous flow:
- *Gravity*: It helps in venous return from upper part of body. Pressure nearing heart is little more than zero.
- *Vis-a-tergo*: It is the overflow from the capillaries because of the pressure from the arteries that pushes the blood.
- *Negative pressure within thorax*: Because of this the blood is pulled (sucked) into the heart.
- *Transmitted arterial pulsations*: These exert intermittent pressure on the venae comitantes and facilitate movement of venous blood toward the heart.
- *Venous valves*: These prevent backflow.
- *Contraction of muscles*: The muscle acts as a pumping organ, e.g., calf muscle, the soleus is called the peripheral heart.
- *Tight sleeve of deep fascia*: The deep fascial sleeve around the lower limb muscles facilitate calf muscle pump.

Venous Systems in Human Body

AN5.5: Describe portal system giving examples.

There are four types of venous systems:
1. *Caval system*: It drains blood into right atrium from upper and lower parts of body through superior and inferior vena cava. Special veins of caval system are:
   - *Emissary veins* that pass through various foramina in skull and connect intracranial dural venous sinuses with extracranial veins. They are devoid of valves.
   - *Intracranial venous sinuses*: Devoid of muscular coat and wall.
   - *Coronary sinus*: It returns 60% of venous blood to right atrium. Some of its tributaries establish arteriovenous anastomosis with branches of coronary arteries. In occlusion of coronary artery the coronary sinus provides nutrition to cardiac muscle through this anastomosis.
   - *Bronchial veins*: Drains venous blood from lungs and consists of two sets. The superficial set drains to right atrium through azygos veins, the deep veins join with pulmonary veins and drain into left atrium.
2. *Portal system*: It consists of blood vessels that connect two sets of capillaries at their ends. These are found in liver, kidney, suprarenal and hypophysis cerebri (*see* **Fig. 7.6**).
   - *Hepatic portal system*: Extends from capillary plexus of gut to wall to hepatic sinusoids.
   - *Renal portal system*: Connects glomerular plexus with peritubular plexus through efferent arterioles.
   - *Hypophyseal portal system*: Connects capillary plexus of median eminence and infundibular stem of hypothalamus with sinusoids of adenohypophysis.
   - *Suprarenal portal system*: Connects cortical sinusoids with medullary sinusoids.
3. *Azygos system*: These communicate with caval system in front and with vertebral venous plexus behind.
4. *Paravertebral veins of Batson*: These are valve less veins within vertebral canal that communicate with azygos, portal and caval systems. Venous blood from thyroid, mammary gland and prostate drains into this system in addition to caval system. In cases of increased intrathoracic or intra-abdominal pressure, the venous blood from these organs bypasses systemic veins and drains directly into this system. This gives

explanation for secondaries in vertebra in carcinoma breast, pelvic organs like rectum and prostate.

ANASTOMOSES (FIG. 7.9)

> **AN5.6:** Describe the concept of anastomoses and collateral circulation with significance of end-arteries.

- *Definition*: Anastomoses are communication between adjacent vessels.
- Arteries do not always end in arterioles and capillaries. They may unite forming anastomoses.
- Anastomoses between arteries of equal caliber are seen in brain—between vertebral and anterior cerebral arteries, in limbs around joints and in intestines.
- Increase in frequency in those vessels away from heart.
- Smaller branches of arteries anastomose more frequently than larger ones.
- Anastomoses equalize pressure differences.
- They are alternative routes of blood flow.
  - Examples:
    - In periarticular sites where circulation may be temporarily impeded by joint movements.
    - Where arteries join end-to-end—palmar, plantar, intercostal, gastrointestinal arteries.

- Section of the vessel participating in anastomosis results in bleeding from both ends.

COLLATERAL CIRCULATION

> **AN5.6:** Describe the concept of anastomoses and collateral circulation with significance of end-arteries.

- *Definition*: Circulation of blood through anastomosis.
- *Cause*: In case of restricted blood flow through an artery an anastomotic channel may become enlarged providing collateral circulation, e.g., when a vessel is interrupted by accident, disease or ligation.
- This often develops rapidly.
- If the increased flow and pressure in the collateral channel are maintained vessels enlarge, often tortuously and finally provide a new arterial route but never in excess of functional needs.
- In some sites *sudden occlusion* causes death of the region supplied. But, a *gradual occlusion* may allow the adequate dilatation of anastomosing channels.
- The collateral circulation develops rapidly in young.
- Mechanism—not properly understood. Hemodynamic changes consequent on:
  - Fall of peripheral resistance
  - Anoxia
  - Neural factors
  - Accumulating metabolites.
- *Types*: They are three types:
  1. *Interarterial anastomosis*: Anastomosis between arteries of equal caliber, e.g., brain—vertebral and anterior cerebral, intestines, and in limbs around joints.
     - *Actual (end-to-end meeting of arteries)*: Blood flows in both directions from cut end of anastomotic vessels, e.g., between right and left gastric arteries, plantar arch, palmar arch, circle of Willis, labial branches of facial artery, and uterine and ovarian arteries **(Fig. 7.9)**.

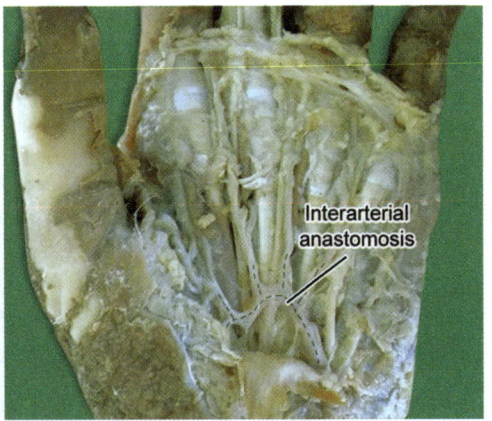

Fig. 7.9: Interarterial anastomosis.

- *Potential (between terminal arterioles)*: Collateral circulation cannot occur but gradual dilatation of arterioles occurs to save the part. So, it cannot compensate the loss due to occlusion. Blood flows in one direction only from the cut end, e.g., anastomosis between right and left coronary arteries and between cortical branches of cerebral arteries.
2. *Venous anastomosis*—communications between veins and their tributaries, e.g., dorsal venous arches of foot and hand **(Fig. 7.10)**.
3. *Arteriovenous anastomosis (vascular shunts)*:

> **AN5.7:** Explain function of meta-arterioles, precapillary sphincters, arterio-venous anastomoses.

It is communication between an artery and a vein. When the organ is active these shunts are closed and the blood circulates through capillaries. When the organ is at rest the blood bypasses the capillary bed and is shunted through arteriovenous anastomosis. Arterioles directly communicate with venules by number of anastomotic channels in addition to the capillary bed **(Fig. 7.11)**.
- *Preferential through fare channels*: In many tissues true capillaries arise not only as direct side branches of terminal arterioles but also as side branches of main or thorough fare channel connecting terminal arteriole and venule. This channel has a large caliber than true capillary. Each capillary side branch has a precapillary sphincter. When functional demand is low precapillary sphincter is closed. With increased demand blood flow increases following opening of many sphincters.
- *Simple arteriovenous anastomoses*: Small arteries directly communicate with surrounding veins. So, during active stage under sympathetic stimulation shunting vessels contract and become closed and blood passes through capillaries. During rest blood directly passes to venules from the arteries by passing capillaries through shunts, e.g., skin of nose, lips, and external ear. Mucous membrane of nose, GIT, coccygeal body, erectile tissue of sex organs, and thyroid.
- *Specialized arteriovenous anastomoses (GLOMUS)*: It forms a

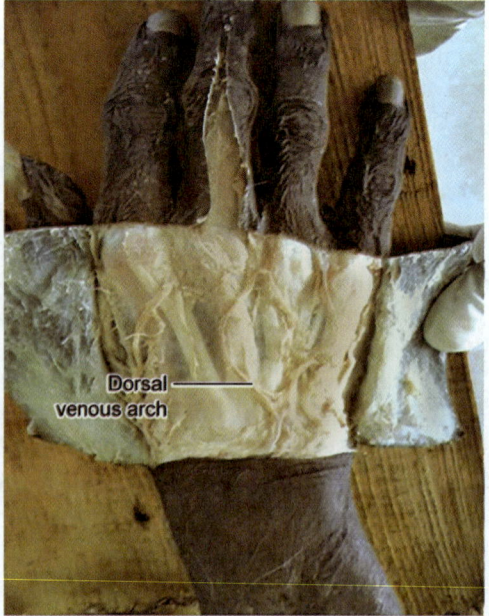

Fig. 7.10: Venous anastomosis—dorsal venous arch.

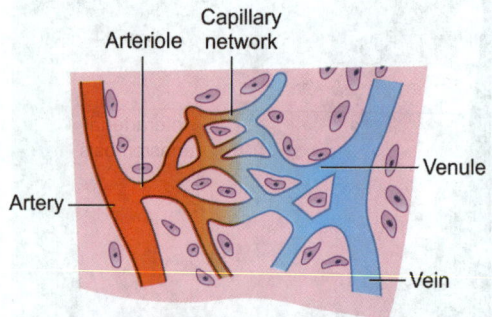

Fig. 7.11: Arteriovenous anastomosis.

number of small units called glomera. Each unit has one or more afferent arterioles which give fine branches and the glomus becomes dilated and becomes "S" shaped and tortuous before it enters into a venule and the vein begins from the deep aspect of the glomus, e.g., digital pads, nail beds.

- *Functional importance*:
  - Regulation of blood flow by capability of contraction and narrowing of lumen—menstruation and erection.
  - Regulation of temperature—thermoregulation by regulating flow of blood in lower or high temperature surfaces.
  - Regulation of blood flow in intestine during stage of absorption or resting.
  - Regulates blood pressure.

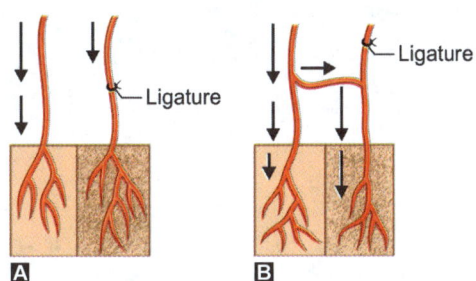

Figs. 7.12A and B: End-arteries. (A) Anatomic end-artery; (B) Functional end-artery.

END-ARTERIES

AN5.6: Describe the concept of anastomoses and collateral circulation with significance of end-arteries.

- In some regions the arteries do not anastomose with neighboring arteries. Such arteries are called end-arteries.
- These are arteries which do not anastomose with any other adjacent arteries in capillary or precapillary stage.
- *Anatomical end-arteries*: Anatomical end-arteries are those vessels whose terminal branches do not anastomose with branches of arteries supplying adjacent areas. Examples: Central artery of retina, splenic artery, renal arteries, arteries of lungs, metaphyseal arteries of long bone, central branches of cerebral arteries, and vasa recta of mesenteric arteries (**Fig. 7.12A**).
- *Functional end-arteries*: Functional end-arteries are those vessels whose terminal branches do anastomose with branches of adjacent arteries supplying the area but the caliber of the anastomosis is insufficient to keep the tissue alive if one of the arteries is blocked, e.g., the branches of coronary arteries are not true end-arteries anatomically as there are numerous anastomoses between branches of right and left coronary arteries and also between branches of each of them. These communications are small and are ineffective for providing collateral circulation in cases of occlusion of one coronary artery. Hence, the coronary arteries are called functional end-arteries (**Fig. 7.12B**).

Clinical Importance

Blocking of an end-artery causes serious disturbances in nutrition and results in necrosis or death of tissue, e.g., occlusion of central artery of retina leads to blindness. Central arteries in the substance of brain though large, communicate only through capillaries. Coronary artery branches, though they anastomose to some extent insufficient to provide adequate collateral circulation.

VASA VASORUM (FIG. 7.13)

- The term "vasa vasorum" is derived from Latin which means the vessels of the vessels. These are minute blood vessels that supply nutrition to the walls of large blood vessels (nutrient vessels to vessels) like the elastic arteries (e.g. aorta) and large veins (e.g. vena cavae).

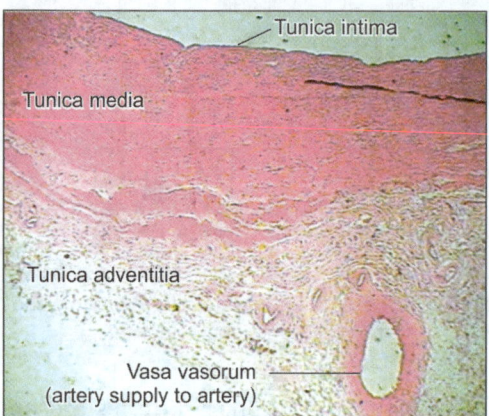

Fig. 7.13: Vasa vasorum in elastic artery.

- These supply tunica adventitia and outer part of tunica media of large arteries and veins. Inner part of tunica media and tunica intima receive nutrition by diffusion of blood circulating in the lumen.
- The arterial blood is derived from the branch of same artery or from neighboring arteries.
- The branch of artery breaks up into capillary plexus in tunica adventitia.
- Venous blood from the plexus drains into the veins that accompany the artery.

- The vasa vasorum are present in the walls of vessels up to 1 mm diameter. Best example is coronary arteries of heart arising from ascending aorta.

> **Clinical Importance**
>
> Vasa vasorum are more abundant in veins than arteries. Because of low venous pressure vasa vasorum in veins are close to intimal wall. Because of this, lymphatic capillaries ramify in the venous wall more closely than that of arteries. This explains the reason for invasion of venous wall by malignant tumor spreading by lymphatics.

Nerve Supply of Blood Vessels

The blood vessels are supplied by autonomic nerves that are mostly nonmyelinated. The sympathetic fibers mainly cause vasoconstriction. The parasympathetic causes vasodilatation. Sympathetic stimulation increased heart rate and blood pressure whereas parasympathetic decreases heart rate and blood pressure.

> **Clinical Application of Blood Vascular System**
>
> ❑ *Palpable arteries*: Some arteries can be palpated through the skin in areas where they can be compressed. They are carotid artery in the neck, facial artery at the lower border of mandible, brachial artery in the arm, radial artery at the wrist, femoral artery at the groin, popliteal artery behind the knee, and dorsalis pedis artery in the foot.
> ❑ *Visible veins*: With age the veins become prominent because of thinning of fat underneath the skin.
> ❑ *Varicose veins*: These are large, swollen veins. Any vein can become varicose but commonly these are seen in legs and feet. Because of prolonged standing, obesity and pregnancy the valves in these veins become weak and do not work effectively and slows the blood flow. The blood collects in legs and pressure in the veins of legs increases. They cause throbbing pain and swelling of legs.
> ❑ *Venesection (phlebotomy)*: It is the process of drawing or removing blood through an incision or puncture of superficial vein for the purpose of drawing blood for analysis or for blood transfusion or injecting fluids or medicines as part of treatment. The common veins that are used are median cubital, cephalic or basilic vein.

- *Spider veins/telangiectasis*: These are small aggregations of minute blood vessels on the surface of skin that results from backed up blood. They are commonly seen on face and legs. They can be blue, red or purple in color. These are due to reduced venous efficiency.
- *Phlebitis*: It is inflammation of a vein.
- *Thrombophlebitis* is presence of blood clots in the vein causing inflammation and usually occurs in leg veins. The thrombus causes pain and irritation and can block the blood flow in vein.

> **AN5.8:** Define thrombosis, infarction and aneurysm.

- *Thrombosis:* Clotting of blood within an injured blood vessel due to aggregation of platelets and fibrin is called thrombosis. Formation of thrombus is a mechanism to prevent blood loss. Thrombosis of a vital vessel reduces blood flow to the organ and is fatal. For example, thrombosis of vessels (coronary arteries) supplying cardiac muscle results in myocardial ischemia. A thrombus in cerebral blood vessel results in stroke.

> **AN5.8:** Define thrombosis, infarction and aneurysm.

- *Infarction:* Obstruction to the flow of blood in an organ or an area of tissue due to thrombus or embolus or atheromatous plaque or narrowing of the vessel or compression of the vessels from a tumor resulting in death of the tissue. The dead tissue is called infarct. Examples are myocardial infarction (MI) due to occlusion of coronary arteries resulting in death of myocardium. Cerebral infarction results from obstruction to blood supply to vital areas of cerebrum.

> **AN5.8:** Define thrombosis, infarction and aneurysm.

- *Aneurysm:* Outward bulging or ballooning of wall of a blood vessel due to localized weakness is known as aneurysm. It can be hereditary or acquired. The aneurysms are more prone for rupture resulting in uncontrolled bleeding. It can occur in any blood vessel. Examples are cerebral artery aneurysm, aneurysm of thoracic or abdominal aorta, aneurysm of external or internal jugular veins, popliteal artery aneurysm in leg, renal artery aneurysm.
- *Deep vein thrombosis*: It is a blood clot in a deep vein usually the leg or thigh vein. The thrombus can get dislodged and can cause serious problems in the lung called pulmonary embolism.
- *Angiography*: It is an imaging technique to visualize lumen of blood vessels. Angiogram is the X-ray image of blood vessel. An angiogram of the heart is called coronary angiogram carried for evaluation of coronary artery disease.
- *Hemangioma*: It is a benign tumor made up of blood vessels. They can occur in skin, muscle, bone or internal organs. Most of them are *seen* on the surface of the skin or just beneath it **(Fig. 7.14)**.
- *Arteriosclerosis and atherosclerosis*: Arteriosclerosis is hardening and stiffening of arterial wall. Atherosclerosis is narrowing of the artery because of formation of an atheromatous plaque.
- *Thromboangiitis obliterans*: It is also known as Buerger's disease. It results from recurrent inflammation and clotting of blood in small and medium-sized arteries and veins of the hands.
- *Occlusive arterial diseases*: These are due to occlusion of end-arteries. The effect of the occlusion of artery varies for each artery:
  - Cerebral artery—occlusion causes paralysis
  - Central artery of retina—results in blindness
  - Renal, splenic arteries—can cause death
  - Gut arteries—causes gangrene
  - Coronary arteries—result in myocardial infarction and heart attack.

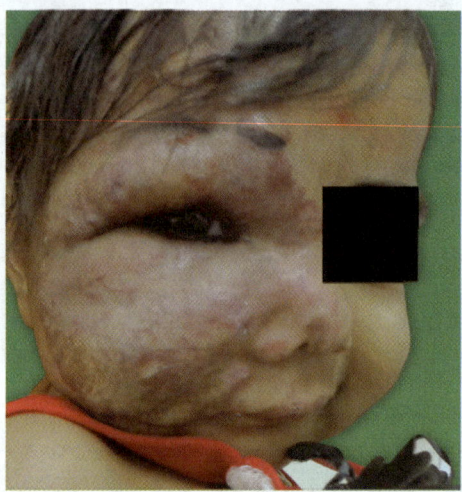

Fig. 7.14: Hemangioma.

Anatomical Basis for Clinical Condition

Case Scenario

Problem: A 55-year-old executive of a multinational company was brought to the emergency room in an ambulance when, he has suddenly collapsed in his office and with no pulse or respiration. With the first aid, the cardiopulmonary resuscitation (CPR) administered by paramedics in the ambulance, the pulse rate and blood pressure returned to normal and the patient was conscious and his breathing was normal. The patient gave a history of smoking, hypertension, diabetes, and sedentary lifestyle. After the investigation of ECG and blood work for cardiac enzymes and blood sugar it was diagnosed as a case of acute myocardial infarction (MI).

Questions:
1. What is acute myocardial infarction?
2. What is coronary artery disease?
3. What is the cause for damage to coronary arteries?
4. Are coronary arteries end-arteries?

Anatomical explanation:
1. Acute myocardial infarction is the medical term for heart attack. A myocardial infarct is an area of necrosis of heart muscle that results from a sudden insufficiency of blood supply.
2. Coronary artery disease (CAD) is hardened and narrowed coronary vessels resulting from blockage of one or more coronary arteries that supply the heart. It is a life-threatening condition as the blood flow to the cardiac muscle is abruptly stopped and leads to oxygen starvation of the muscle and is called myocardial ischemia. If it persists for a longer period it causes death of the starved cardiac muscle.

Contd...

Contd...

3. Damage to the coronary arteries is due to the formation of atheromatous plaques that can cause narrowing of the vessels and is known as atherosclerosis. Reduction in coronary arterial blood flow can cause progressive atherosclerosis with occlusion of coronaries leading to loss of blood supply to the myocardium and its necrosis. In the present case the adverse lifestyle is the cause for atherosclerosis, CAD, and MI.
4. End-arteries are arteries that do not anastomose with other arteries or arterial branches. Obstruction of an end-artery interferes with the blood supply to that part of the organ supplied by the artery. The coronary arteries are functional end-arteries and if they are blocked the tissue which they supply undergoes necrosis.

☞ Key Concept

Take Home Message—Blood Vessels

- The blood vascular system consists of vessels of different caliber, structure and function.
- The blood vessels are broadly categorized into arteries and veins.
- The walls of the arteries and veins contain three tunics: (1) tunica intima, (2) tunica media, and (3) tunica adventitia. Depending on the difference in the components of tunics, luminal size and function the blood vessels are further classified into different types.
- As they move away from the heart the number of arteries increases, their diameter and thickness of wall decrease. Arteries have no valves.
- Veins are more in number than arteries, have less amount of muscle and are thin walled. The diameter of lumen is more and the amount of muscle and elastic fibers are less in veins when compared to arteries.
- There are two loops in circulation of blood a lesser and a greater. The lesser loop is pulmonary circulation. The major loop consists of systemic and portal circulations.
- Venae comitantes are a pair of veins accompanying an artery.
- Anastomoses are communication between vessels. They are interarterial, venous and arteriovenous. Collateral circulation is important in regulation of blood flow, temperature, blood pressure, and intestinal absorption.
- Vasa vasorum is the minute blood vessel that is supplying nutrition to a larger artery and larger vein.
- End-arteries are those that do not anastomose with neighboring arteries in capillary or precapillary stage.

QUESTIONS

1. Classification of blood vessels.
2. Types of blood circulation.
3. End-arteries.
4. Collateral circulation.
5. Vasa vasorum.
6. Name the factors that help in venous return of blood.
7. Sinusoids.
8. Venae comitantes.

MULTIPLE CHOICE QUESTIONS

1. **The word tributaries is used for:**
    A. Arteries
    B. Arterioles

C. Lymphatics
D. Veins

2. **All the following statements are true about vasa vasorum,** *except:*
   A. These are nutrient vessels of the vessels
   B. The vessels are seen in tunica media
   C. Present in coronary arteries
   D. More abundant in veins

3. **All the following are correct about venae comitantes,** *except:*
   A. Pair of veins accompanying superficial artery
   B. These are deep veins
   C. Help in venous return of blood
   D. Help in counter current heat exchange

4. **In which of the following organs sinusoids are present?**
   A. Red pulp of spleen
   B. Endocrine gland
   C. Liver
   D. Lymph node

5. **Which one of the following is an example for capacitance vessel?**
   A. Elastic artery
   B. Muscular artery
   C. Arteriole
   D. Large vein

6. **All the following are end arteries,** *except:*
   A. Central artery of retina
   B. Splenic artery
   C. Renal arteries
   D. Radial artery

7. **Arteriovenous anastomosis is found in all the following sites,** *except:*
   A. Skin of nose
   B. Spleen
   C. Coccygeal body
   D. Thyroid

8. **Which one of the following is not a portal circulation?**
   A. Hepatic circulation
   B. Hypophyseal
   C. Renal circulations
   D. Pulmonary circulation

ANSWERS

1. D
2. B
3. A
4. D
5. D
6. D
7. B
8. D

CHAPTER 8

Introduction to Lymphatic System

LEARNING OBJECTIVES

- Defense mechanisms of the body
- Tissue fluid and lymph
- Components of lymphatic system
- Functions of lymphatic system
- Structure of lymphatic system components
- Circulation of lymph
- Lymphoid organs—description, functions
- Clinical case with anatomical explanation

INTRODUCTION

- *Synonym: Lymphoid system; immune system.*
- It consists of closed system of vessels that are formed from minute capillaries in the tissue spaces in and around blood capillaries. These convey tissue fluid into the blood vascular system. It acts as an alternate to venous system **(Fig. 8.1)**.
- *Tissue fluid:* As the blood flows through the capillaries small amount of the fluid enters the interstices of tissue and this fluid is called *interstitial/tissue fluid*. Tissue fluid is plasma without plasma proteins. Most of the fluid reenters the capillaries. Some amount of fluid stays in the tissue spaces.
- *Lymph:* The excess fluid that is staying in the interstices of tissue is taken up by lymph capillaries and is returned to the bloodstream. This tissue fluid that is entering the lymphatic system is called *lymph*. Lymph is a milky liquid made up of tissue fluid, fatty substances, and lymphocytes.
- *Transportation of lymph:* From the lymph capillaries it is transported through larger lymphatic vessels. During their passage the lymph vessels are interrupted by chains of lymph nodes that filter the lymph and add lymphocytes to the circulating lymph that is ultimately emptied into the right or left subclavian vein **(Fig. 8.1)**.
- The lymphatic system consists of tissues and organs concerned with protection of internal environment of the body from invasion by microorganisms.
- The cardiovascular system has the heart that acts as a pump, but the lymphatic system lacks that pump. Like in the venous return of blood contraction of skeletal muscle causing compression of the lymph vessels (muscle pump), pressure changes in the lymph vessels associated with respiration (respiratory pump), the unidirectional valves in lymph vessels that prevent reverse flow of lymph, and the contraction of smooth muscle in the walls of lymph vessels facilitate the flow of lymph.

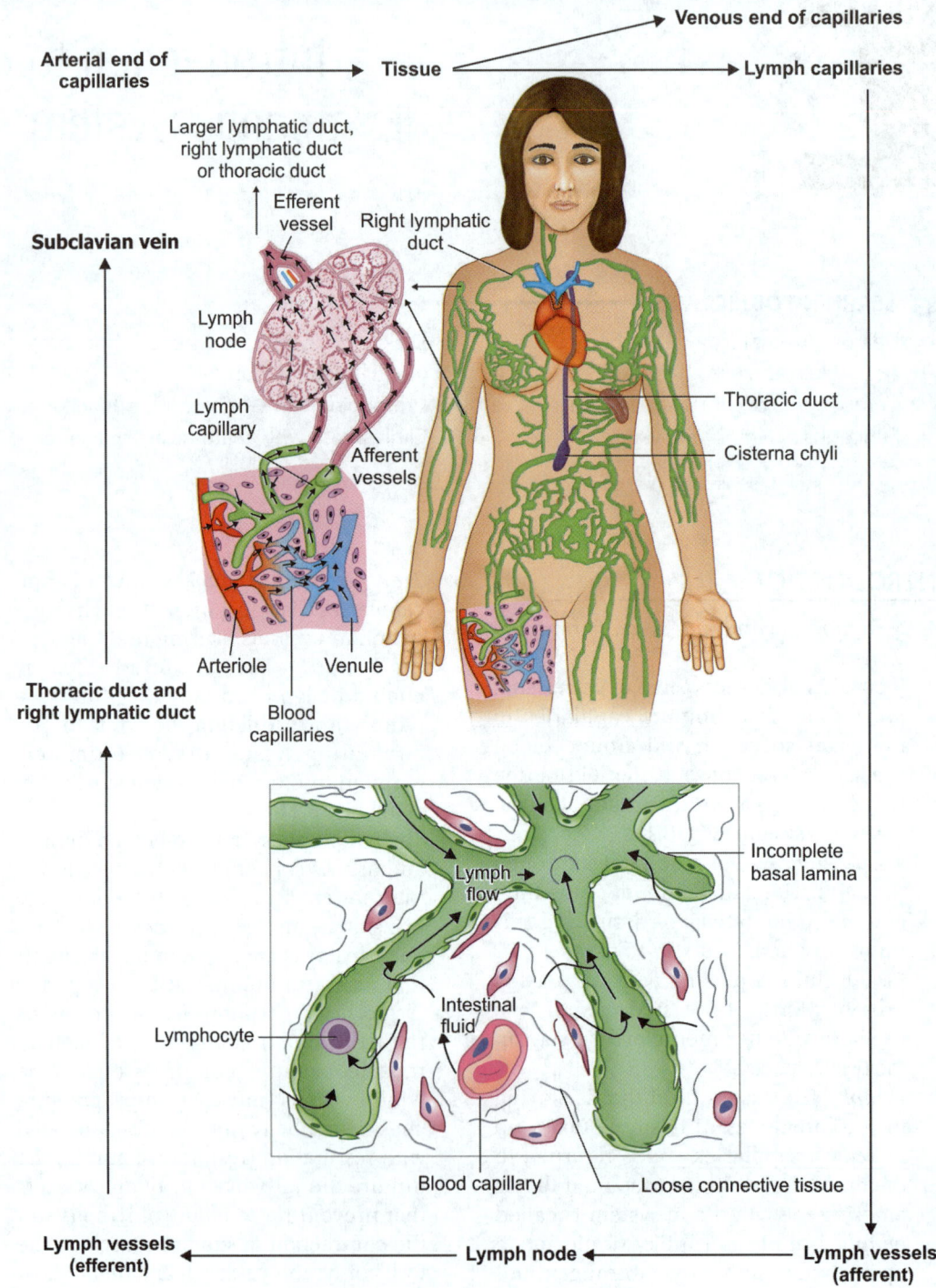

Fig. 8.1: Lymphatic system and lymph flow.

Chapter 8: Introduction to Lymphatic System

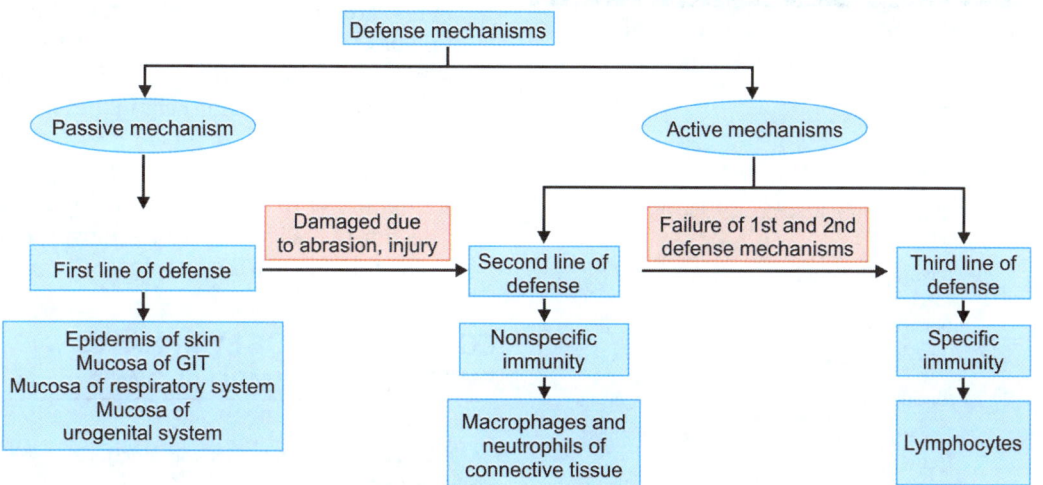

Flowchart 8.1: Defense mechanisms of the body.

DEFENSE MECHANISMS OF THE BODY (FLOWCHART 8.1)

There are three lines of defense mechanisms in the body:

1. *First line of defense:* This is provided by *surface epithelia,* i.e., epidermis of skin, mucosa of gastrointestinal, respiratory, urogenital system, etc. that are in contact with external environment and exposed to various types of microorganisms.
2. *Second line of defense:* This comes into action when the first line of defense is damaged due to abrasion, injury, etc. and the organisms invaded the epithelia. This is provided by *macrophages* and *neutrophils* of connective tissue present in lamina propria of mucosa and dermis of skin. The nonspecific immune response provided by these cells destroys the pathogens by phagocytosis.
3. *Third line of defense:* When first and second lines of defense fail to check the invasion of microorganisms this gets activated. This is a specific immune response evoked by lymphocytes.

FUNCTIONS OF LYMPHATIC SYSTEM

- *Mechanism of formation of tissue fluid:* There is a gradient of blood pressure in different vessels. This facilitates formation of tissue fluid and drainage of fluid. As the blood flows through the arterial end of capillaries fluid continuously gets filtered into the tissue spaces. But nearly 85% of it is reabsorbed by venous ends of blood capillaries. About 15% of it containing water and plasma proteins is not reabsorbed because of the pressure gradient and enters the interstices of tissue and is called interstitial fluid **(Fig. 8.1)**.

  The pressure gradients in various vessels of vascular tree are represented in **Table 8.1**.

- *Accessory drainage system to the venous system* **(Fig. 8.1)**:
  - Because of the pressure gradient micromolecules, crystalloids, and carbon dioxide getting filtered at the arterial end of the capillary bed get reabsorbed at the venous end of capillaries that amounts to about 27 liters. However, this amount of reabsorption is not sufficient even on a daily basis.
  - As much as 3 liters of fluid (tissue fluid) is left to be reabsorbed in the extracellular spaces of the body everyday. In addition, some proteins leak into the extracellular spaces.

Table 8.1: Pressure gradient in various vessels.

Vessel	Pressure (mm of Hg)
Arteries	120 mm of Hg
Arterioles	60 mm of Hg
Capillaries	
❑ At arterial end	
➢ Outward driving force of blood	30 mm of Hg
➢ Inward driving force (osmotic tension of plasma proteins)	25 mm of Hg
➢ Filtration pressure	5 mm of Hg
❑ At venous end	
➢ Inward pulling force (protein osmotic tension)	25 mm of Hg
➢ Outward driving force of blood	12 mm of Hg
❑ Large veins	5 mm of Hg

Further, some more material which cannot enter the capillary bed gets accumulated in the extracellular area. This excess tissue fluid containing colloids and particulate matter is absorbed and transported by lymphatic system back into the blood.

- If all this fluid is left behind, it would lead to a dangerous situation. Reverse osmosis would occur and more fluid will flow into the already loaded extracellular space causing *edema* (excessive interstitial fluid).
- The lymphatic system maintains low protein concentration of tissue fluid by returning the excess protein to the circulatory system.

♦ *Contribution for maintaining fluid balance:* In normal life, the fluid balance is well maintained. Amount of interstitial fluid remains fairly constant and unwanted material does not accumulate in the extracellular space. All these proper balances are possible due to the action of the lymphatics and the lymphatic system.

♦ *Absorption of fat from intestines:* It helps in absorption of fat from the intestines into the cisterna chyli.

♦ *Production of lymphocytes:* The lymphocytes are produced in the lymphatic follicles.

♦ *Production of antibodies:* These are produced by the plasma cells in the lymph nodes.

♦ *A channel for spread of infection or malignancy:* In disease conditions the infection or malignant cells are transported via lymphatics to a distant place.

COMPONENTS OF LYMPHATIC SYSTEM AND LYMPH FLOW

AN6.1: List the components and functions of the lymphatic system.
AN6.2: Describe structure of lymph capillaries and mechanism of lymph circulation.

It consists of:
♦ Lymph
♦ Lymph capillaries
♦ Lymphatic vessels
♦ Lymphatic tissue and organs.

Lymph

♦ The part of circulating blood from arterial end of capillaries that passes into the tissues is called *tissue fluid* (30 liters). Most of this fluid (27 liters) reenters the circulation at the venous end of capillaries. Part of tissue fluid containing particulate matter and colloid material (3 liters) returns to the circulation through separate vessels called *lymph vessels* (lymphatics). The fluid passing through lymphatics is called *lymph*.

♦ The lymph is similar in composition to that of blood plasma *except* that it transports plasma proteins and contains more of white blood cells. In particular the lymph that leaves lymph node is rich is lymphocytes.

♦ The lymph that is leaving the digestive system is called *chyle* and is rich in triglycerides (fat) absorbed from small intestine and looks milky white in

appearance because of the lipid content. The lymph vessels collecting chyle are called lacteals.
- The lymph also carries bacteria, dust, carbon, malignant cells, etc. and brings them to lymph node where they are filtered and destroyed. Metastatic cancer cells also travel through lymph to distant places.

Lymph Capillaries (Fig. 8.1)

- Smaller lymph vessels are called *lymph capillaries* which join to form larger *lymphatic vessels*.
- Extensive networks of thin lymphatic capillaries occur in the extracellular spaces. These are the lymphatic plexuses and drain surplus tissue fluid, proteins, bacteria, debris, and all that which accumulates in the spaces.
- When compared to blood capillaries, much larger molecules can pass through the walls of lymph capillaries. It is believed that these substances pass into lymph capillaries through gaps between endothelial cells lining the capillary, or by pinocytosis.
- Lymph capillaries are *absent* in the following locations:
  - *Avascular structures:* Epidermis, cornea, articular cartilage, hair and nails
  - Splenic pulp
  - Bone marrow
  - Brain and spinal cord
  - Liver lobule
  - Lung units.
- Differences between lymph capillaries and blood capillaries are presented in **Table 8.2**.

Lymphatic Vessels (Fig. 8.1)

- These are found in all parts of the body except—teeth, bone, bone marrow, splenic pulp, hair, nails, cornea, and brain.
- *Structure of a medium-sized lymph vessel:* As in blood vessel there are the tunica intima, media and adventitia from within outward. Tunica intima is lined by endothelium. In tunica media the smooth muscle fibers are arranged circularly. Tunica adventitia contains fibrous tissue.
- These vessels have valves and so have a *beaded appearance*. The vessels are provided with valves that are semilunar in shape. Their free edges are directed along the direction of lymph flow. The walls of lymph vessels are dilated proximal to the valves giving beaded appearance.
- *Categorization:* The vessels are divided into superficial and deep sets. Superficial vessels draining the skin, superficial and deep fascia are subcutaneous in location, and accompany superficial veins. The deep vessels are located under the cover of deep fascia and accompany arteries.
- As the lymphatic vessels run proximally, they merge and become larger. Larger lymph vessels drain into lymphatic trunks

Table 8.2: Differences between lymph and blood capillaries.

Features	Lymph capillary	Blood capillary
Beginning	Intercellular space	In between arteriole and venule
Lumen	Wide, irregular	Narrow, more regular
Basal lamina and pericytes	Absent	Present
Valves	Flap valves between endothelial cells to allow entry of tissue fluid into the capillary but not in reverse direction	Absent
Permeability	Macromolecules—colloid material, fat droplets, cell debris, and microorganisms (bacteria)	Smaller molecules—crystalloids
Effect of increased tissue fluid pressure	Lumen patent allowing entry of bacteria	Collapses the lumen

which ultimately unite to form the *right lymphatic duct* on the right side and the *thoracic duct* on the left side. The thoracic and right lymphatic ducts open into the left and right brachiocephalic veins, respectively.

- The lymph vessels on their way pass through lymph nodes where the lymph is filtered on exposure to lymphocytes present in lymph nodes.
- *Peculiarities:* Lymph flow is unidirectional. The valves guide the lymph flow. Retrograde flow occurs when the vessels are obstructed.

Thoracic Duct *(Fig. 8.1)*

- The lymphatics collecting lymph from the lower parts of the body merge in the abdomen to form the *cisterna chyli*. From this starts the thoracic duct.
- The *thoracic duct* drains lymph from both lower limbs, abdomen, left half of thorax, left upper limb, and left half of head and neck of the body. It drains the lymph into the vascular system by ending at the junction of left subclavian vein and internal jugular vein **(Fig. 8.2)**.

Right Lymphatic Duct *(Fig. 8.1)*

On right side, the *right lymphatic duct* terminates similarly and drains lymph from right half of head and neck, thorax, and right upper limb. Its termination is similar to thoracic duct but on right side **(Fig. 8.2)**.

Factors regulating flow of lymph in the thoracic and right lymphatic ducts:

- Filtration pressure of tissue fluid.
- Skeletal muscle contraction acting as a massage for the lymph vessels.
- Pulsations of arteries that are transmitted to lymph vessels.
- Valves converting the vessels into small segments and directing the flow.
- Gravity.
- Suction movement generated by diaphragm.
- Negative pressure in brachiocephalic veins.

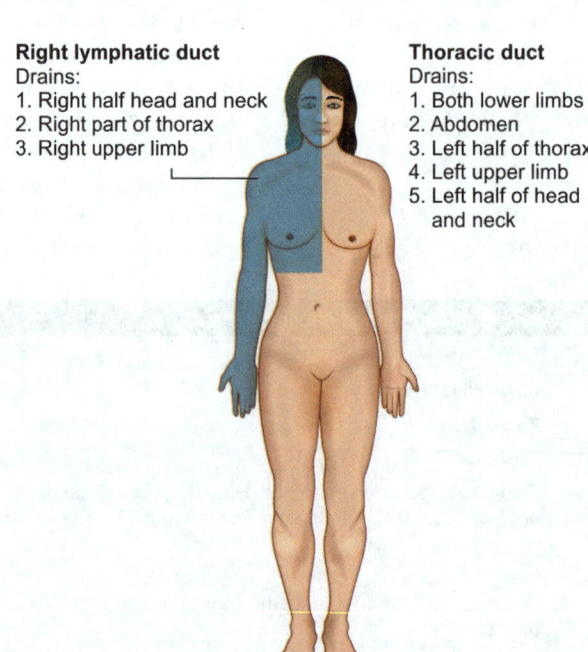

Fig. 8.2: Lymphatic drainage area of thoracic and right lymphatic ducts.

Lymphoid Tissue

- *Components:* The lymphatic tissue is composed of *two* principle components—(1) *Free cells* the lymphoblasts, lymphocytes and plasma cells and (2) A supporting framework of reticular fibers.
- *Lymphocytes:* There are *two* types of lymphocytes—(1) *T lymphocytes* and (2) *B lymphocytes*. Both are similar in structure but differ in their response to antigen or foreign body (defensive mechanism).
- *Antigens* are foreign substances that gain access into the body and produce immunological response. *Antibodies* or *immunoglobulins* are circulating plasma proteins produced by plasma cells (derived from B lymphocytes).
- The defense mechanism initiated by B lymphocyte is called *humoral immunity*. The B lymphocytes are derived from bone marrow. They become active on exposure to antigen and get differentiated into plasma cells that secrete specific antibodies (immunoglobulins) against the antigen that is released into the blood or lymph. Example for humoral immunity is tetanus toxoid.
- The T lymphocytes along with macrophages cause destruction of antigen and this type of response is called *cell-mediated immunity*. The T lymphocytes are produced in bone marrow but mature in thymus from where they migrate to the other lymphoid organs via blood circulation. The T lymphocytes kill the microbes by releasing substances called lymphokines which attach T lymphocyte to the surface of the microbe. Example for cell-mediated immunity is polio vaccination.
- The cells of immune system are:
  - B and T lymphocytes
  - Natural killer (NK) cells
  - Macrophages
  - Antigen presenting cells (APCs)
  - Neutrophils
  - Mast cells and eosinophils.
- *Classification of lymphatic tissue:*
  - *Diffuse lymphoid tissue:* This includes the diffusely arranged lymphocytes and plasma cells in the lamina propria of digestive, respiratory, and urogenital systems.
  - *Dense lymphoid tissue:* This contains large aggregations of lymphocytes, few macrophages, and plasma cells called lymphatic nodules. These can be seen as *nonencapsulated* or as *encapsulated* structures in association with viscera [mucosa-associated lymphoid tissue (MALT)] or as discrete (encapsulated) organs.
    - *Mucosa-associated lymphoid tissue:* These are nonencapsulated lymphoid tissue in the mucosa of digestive and respiratory systems. These include the:
      » Solitary nodules in mucosa.
      » Aggregated nodules in ileum (Peyer's patches) of small intestine **(Fig. 8.3)**.
      » Lymphatic nodules in vermiform appendix (abdominal tonsil) **(Fig. 8.3)**.
      » *Waldeyer's lymphatic ring at the entrance into pharynx:* Composed of anteriorly located lingual, posteriorly placed nasopharyngeal, bilateral palatine, and tubal tonsils **(Fig. 8.3)**.
    - *Encapsulated lymphoid organs:* These are categorized into:
      » *Primary/central lymphoid organs:* Examples are thymus and bone marrow. These contain 100% T lymphocytes.
      » *Secondary/peripheral lymphoid organs:* Examples are lymph node and spleen. These contain 60% T lymphocytes.

Lymph Nodes (Fig. 8.4)

- Lymph nodes are usually present in groups especially in the axilla, groin, and root of lung. There are about 450–500

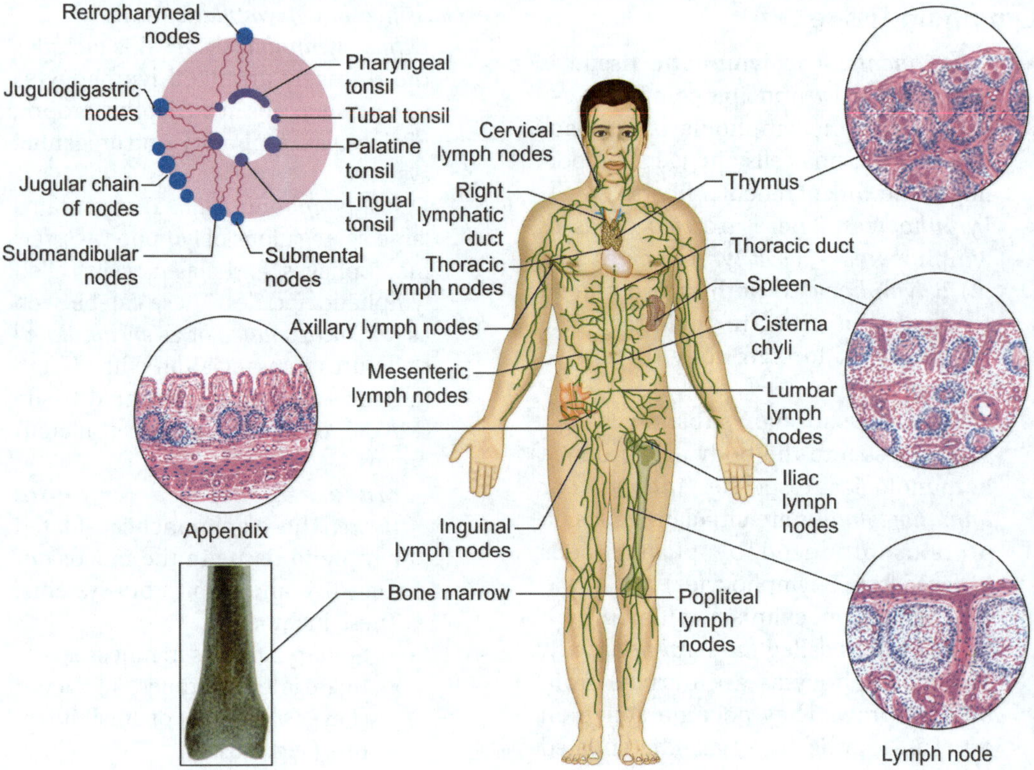

Chapter 8: Introduction to Lymphatic System

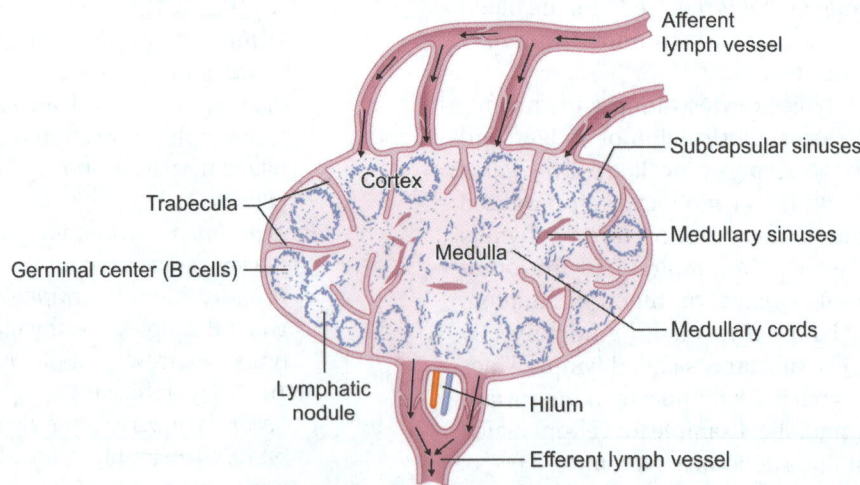

Fig. 8.3: Lymphatic tissue.

Fig. 8.4: Lymph node and flow of lymph.

lymph nodes in the body. Their size varies from few millimeters to centimeters.
- Lymph, the fluid that flows through the lymphatic capillaries and vessels, is filtered by the lymph nodes that are present along the course of the lymphatics. The lymph vessels on their way pass through lymph nodes. When

foreign protein or foreign material drains from an area, the lymph nodes filter them and attempt to eliminate them from the body. Also, antibodies (molecules to fight the foreign substance) are produced by the lymphatic system.
- The lymph nodes are oval or kidney-shaped structure with a convex surface and a slight indention on one side called the hilum where blood vessels, lymph vessels, and nerves enter and leave the organ.
- Numerous afferent lymph vessels enter the node at many places over its convex surface but one or two efferent vessels leave it only at the hilum.
- Various regional lymph nodes of the body and their lymph vessels of drainage are presented in **Table 8.3**.

Structure of Lymph Node

- *Capsule:* The lymph node is covered by a connective tissue capsule.
- *Trabeculae:* From the capsule there are extensions into the substance of lymph node dividing into compartments.
- *Subdivisions of the substance:* The substance of lymph node presents outer darkly stained cortex and inner lightly stained medulla.
- *Subcapsular sinus:* Underneath the capsule is the subcapsular lymph sinus into which numerous afferent lymph vessels open. The subcapsular sinus is continuous with trabecular sinus that is found along the trabeculae. The trabecular sinuses are continuous with medullary sinuses in the parenchyma of lymph node.
- *Cortex:* Cortex is darkly stained and contains lymphatic nodules with or without pale germinal center. It is mainly formed by B lymphocytes.
- *Medulla:* Medulla presents *medullary cords* and *medullary sinuses*. Medullary cords are darkly stained and contain branching and anastomosing cords of lymphoid tissue. They contain B lymphocytes, plasma cells, and macrophages. Medullary sinuses are lightly stained and are extensions of trabecular lymph sinuses. They drain into the efferent lymph vessels at the hilum. The sinuses are traversed by reticular fibers.
- *Functions:*
  - *Defensive*: Filter microorganisms of lymph, localizing the infection.
  - Production of lymphocytes and antibodies.

Spleen (Fig. 8.3)

- It is a large encapsulated lymphoid organ located in the left hypochondrium of abdomen. At the hilum of spleen, splenic vessels and nerves enter and leave. It receives blood from splenic artery and is drained by splenic vein into the hepatic portal system. The circulating blood is filtered through spleen.
- *Structure of spleen:*
  - Spleen is covered by dense connective tissue capsule that sends trabeculae into the substance (pulp).
  - Substance of spleen is arranged in the form of white pulp and red pulp.
  - The white pulp contains Malpighian corpuscles or splenic nodules. These are lymphatic nodules with an eccentrically placed arteriole and contain lymphocytes.
  - Red pulp is found around the white pulp. It contains thin-walled venous sinusoids (splenic sinuses) and intervening cords of cells (splenic cords of Billroth).
- *Functions:*
  - During early fetal life, it is a temporary organ of hematopoiesis.
  - It filters blood and clears the infectious organisms, particulate matter, aged, and defective erythrocytes and platelets.

Thymus (Fig. 8.3)

- It is a flattened, bilobed lymphoepithelial organ that produces lymphocytes.
- It is located in the lower neck and extends into the superior mediastinum of thorax.

Table 8.3: Regional lymph nodes of the body and their lymph vessels.

Regions	Lymph nodes	Lymph vessel
Head and neck	❑ *Superficial:* ➢ Occipital ➢ Mastoid ➢ Parotid ➢ Facial ➢ Waldeyer's ring ➢ Submental ➢ Submandibular ➢ *Superficial cervical*: Anterior and lateral groups ❑ *Deep*: ➢ Pretracheal ➢ Prelaryngeal ➢ Retropharyngeal ➢ Jugulodigastric ➢ Jugulo-omohyoid ➢ Supraclavicular	❑ Left jugular lymph trunk joins thoracic duct at the root of neck ❑ Right jugular lymph trunk empties into the right lymphatic duct at the root of neck
Thorax	❑ *Parietal*: ➢ Parasternal ➢ Intercostal ➢ Diaphragmatic ❑ *Visceral:* Pleura, lungs, and mediastinum ➢ Bronchial ➢ Bronchopulmonary ➢ Tracheobronchial ➢ Hilar ➢ Mediastinal	❑ Thoracic duct ❑ Right lymphatic duct ❑ Bronchomediastinal lymph trunk
Abdomen	❑ *Parietal*: ➢ Lumbar ➢ Aortic ➢ Caval ➢ Inferior epigastric ➢ Iliac ➢ Lumbar ➢ Sacral ❑ *Visceral*: Along big vessels originating from aorta ➢ Celiac ➢ Right/left gastric ➢ Right/left gastroepiploic ➢ Pyloric ➢ Pancreatic ➢ Splenic ➢ Pancreaticoduodenal ➢ Hepatic ➢ Superior mesenteric ➢ Inferior mesenteric	❑ Lumbar lymph trunk ❑ Intestinal lymph trunk ❑ Cisterna chyli
Upper limb and axilla	❑ Axillary ❑ Pectoral ❑ Brachial	❑ Subclavian lymph trunk
Lower limb	❑ Inguinal ❑ Femoral ❑ Popliteal	❑ Lumbar lymph trunk

- This is the only lymphatic organ that is fully developed at the time of birth. Other lymphatic organs reach their full development in postnatal life.
- It is active during childhood and later undergoes involution. From middle age to old age the thymic tissue is gradually replaced with lymphoid and adipose tissues.
- *Structure:*
  - It is covered by connective tissue capsule from which trabeculae extend into its substance.
  - Thymus is divided into number of lobules with each having a peripheral darker cortex capping the central pale medulla.
  - Cortex consists of mainly densely packed small T lymphocytes also called thymocytes.
  - In medulla the lymphocytes are less densely packed and contain lamellated Hassall's corpuscles which are concentrically arranged epithelial reticular cells. With increasing age their number increases.
  - In addition to lymphocytes macrophages are seen in both cortex and medulla.
- *Function*: It produces the hormones thymosin and thymopoietin that stimulate the development and cell differentiation of T lymphocytes.

Clinical Application of Lymphatic System

AN6.3: Explain the concept of lymphoedema and spread of tumors via lymphatics and venous system.

- *Lymphedema:* Obstruction to flow of lymph in the lymphatic trunk causes swelling of the body tissues. It can affect any part of the body but is commonly seen in arms and legs. It can be due to injury, infection, or cancer affecting the lymphatic system. It can be due to the cancer treatment by radiotherapy or removal of lymph nodes that can damage the lymphatic system and cause obstruction to flow of lymph **(Fig. 8.5)**.
- *Lymphangitis:* Inflammation of lymph vessels is called lymphangitis. The lymph vessels are seen as red streaks on the skin and are painful.
- *Lymphadenitis:* Inflammation of lymph nodes is called lymphadenitis.
- *Lymphoma:* It is a malignant growth of lymphocytes. There are two types of lymphomas: (1) Hodgkin's and (2) Non-Hodgkin.
- *Splenomegaly:* It is enlargement of spleen due to accumulation of infectious microorganisms.
- *Tonsillitis:* It is inflammation of tonsils due to bacterial infections.
- *Elephantiasis:* Blockage of lymphatics of lower limbs due to filarial infection (parasitic roundworms infection).
- *Lymphangiography:* It is a procedure to visualize lymphatic channels and lymph nodes using contrast medium. This is used for observing blockage to lymphatic drainage or diseases of lymphatic system.
- *Lymphoscintigraphy:* It is the procedure of introducing radiotracer substance into the lymph channels to observe lymph flow, obstruction to lymph flow, and to locate sentinel lymph nodes.
- *Lymph node biopsy:* It is a minor surgical procedure of removal of a lymph node for observing its microscopic structure for signs of infection or staging the grade of cancer.
- *Sentinel node biopsy:* The sentinel nodes are the first few lymph nodes into which the tumors drain, for example, in carcinoma breast to axillary nodes. This procedure involves injecting tracer material for locating the sentinel node during surgery followed by its removal and microscopic analysis to find out whether the cancer cells are present or not.

Contd...

Contd...

Absence of cancer cells indicates that the disease has not spread to the regional lymph nodes or other organs.

❑ **Spread of tumors via lymphatics and blood vessels (Fig. 8.6):**

> **AN6.3:** Explain the concept of lymphoedema and spread of tumors via lymphatics and venous system.

- The tumor cells from the initial or primary site can penetrate the walls of lymphatic vessels (lymphatic spread) or blood vessels (hematogenous spread) and then circulate through blood to other sites and tissues of the body producing metastatic or secondary tumor.
- In a case of carcinoma of breast the tumor cells from breast at first reach the regional nodes, i.e., axillary lymph nodes (sentinel nodes) and later they can metastasize in the lungs. From the regional lymph nodes the tumor cells travel to thoracic duct/right lymphatic duct and then into the venous system via the brachiocephalic veins.
- The mode of spread of cancers is usually lymphatic. The mode of spread of sarcomas and certain types of cancers, e.g., renal cell carcinoma is by hematogenous route. The veins are more commonly invaded by tumor cells than arteries because of their thin wall.

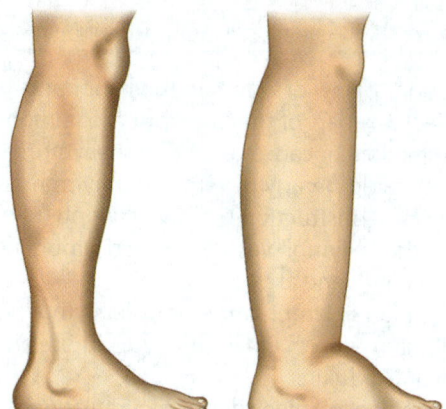

Fig. 8.5: Lymphedema.

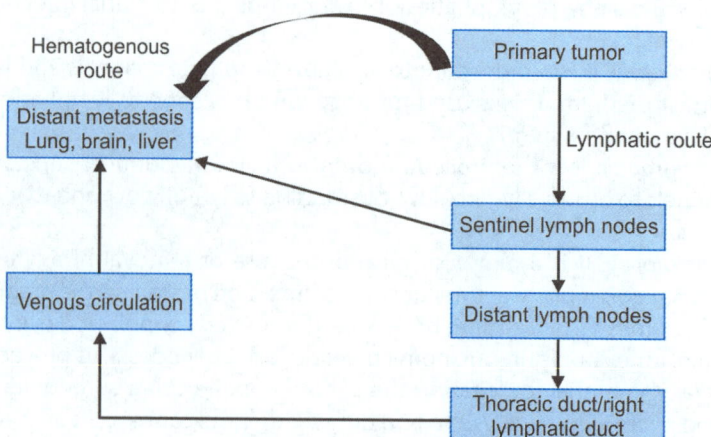

Fig. 8.6: Spread of cancer cells.

Chapter 8: Introduction to Lymphatic System

Anatomical Basis for Clinical Condition

Case Scenario

Problem: A woman aged 45 years came to the surgeon with a palpable, painful lump in her right breast. The surgeon enquired history of similar instances in the family. It was found that there is a family history of breast malignancy causing death of her mother and sister. The surgeon palpated the breasts, axilla, and the neck. The patient was advised mammography, ultrasound scanning of breast, and fine-needle aspiration cytology (FNAC) of breast. Based on the investigations mastectomy with removal of axillary lymph nodes on right side was performed after sentinel biopsy of an axillary lymph node. Postsurgical radiotherapy was given. After 1 year the patient came with a swollen right arm.

Questions:

1. What is the importance of family history in the present case?
2. Why the breasts, axillae, and neck were palpated?
3. What information do the investigations ordered by the surgeon provide?
4. What is the purpose of sentinel biopsy before surgery?
5. What is the cause for swelling of right arm after surgery?

Anatomical explanation:

1. Women with a family history of a close relatives having breast cancer are at a higher risk of developing breast cancer. A strong family history of breast cancer is linked with an abnormal gene for breast cancer *BRCA1* or *BRCA2* gene.
2. Both the breasts to be examined for the presence of a palpable lump and for comparison. Both axillae are to be examined for palpable axillary lymph nodes. Palpation of neck is for enlarged supraclavicular and cervical lymph nodes. As the lymphatics are connected the malignancy can extend to the other groups of lymph nodes.
3. The investigations ordered by the surgeon provide the information about the breast lump. Mammogram diagnoses small areas of calcification in the breast when compared to ultrasound. Ultrasound is used in cases of dense breast parenchyma to assist mammography for demarcating the mass, to guide for FNAC biopsy of breast, and assists in radiotherapy planning.
4. Sentinel node biopsy is done to see the extent of cancer beyond the primary site (breast) into lymphatic system. Sentinel lymph node mapping and biopsy are performed as part of breast cancer surgery.
5. Swelling of right arm after surgery and radiation is due to lymphedema. The cause for this swelling is disruption of lymph flow following lymph node removal and blockage of lymph flow.

Chapter 8: Introduction to Lymphatic System

> ### ☞ Key Concept
>
> ### Take Home Message—Lymphatic System
>
> - It is an accessory drainage system to the venous system in the drainage of tissue fluid.
> - Lymph is the excess tissue fluid that is taken up by lymph capillaries and is returned to the bloodstream.
> - It is a closed system of vessels that start as minute capillaries in the tissue spaces and convey tissue fluid into the blood vascular system.
> - The components of lymphatic system are lymph, lymph capillaries, lymph vessels, lymphatic tissue, and organs.
> - The lymph vessels are absent in teeth, bone, bone marrow, splenic pulp, hair, nails, cornea, and brain.
> - The larger lymphatic ducts are thoracic duct and right lymphatic duct.
> - The *thoracic duct* drains lymph from both lower limbs, abdomen, left half of thorax, left upper limb, and left half of head and neck of the body.
> - The thoracic duct ends at the junction of left subclavian vein and internal jugular vein.
> - Right lymphatic duct drains lymph from right half of head and neck, thorax, and right upper limb. Its termination is at the junction of right subclavian and internal jugular veins.
> - Sound knowledge of regional lymph nodes is important in diagnosis as, it serves as a guide for origin of the problem (from which organ), for predicting the progress of the disease, and treatment outcome.

QUESTIONS

1. Describe the components of lymphatic system.
2. Classification of lymphatic tissue with examples.
3. Describe the flow of lymph.
4. Structure of lymph node.
5. Lymphedema.
6. Lymphatic and hematogenous spread of tumor cells.

MULTIPLE CHOICE QUESTION

1. **Lymph capillaries are absent in the following locations,** *except:*
   A. Epidermis
   B. Hair
   C. Bone marrow
   D. Pancreas

ANSWER

1. D

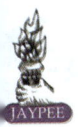
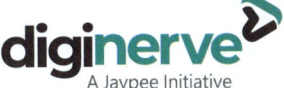

**TOP DOC BANE WOHI
JISKA GUIDE HO SAHI**

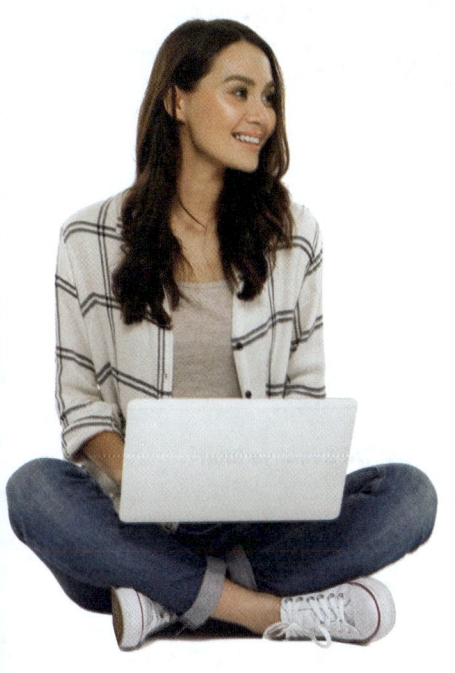

YOUR GUIDE AT EVERY STEP

Expert Knowledge Anytime, Anywhere

SCAN QR CODE
FOR MORE DETAILS

WHY CHOOSE US

Video Lectures

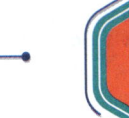

Self-Assessment Questions

Top Faculty

New CBME Curriculum

Clinical Case Based Approach

NEET Preparation

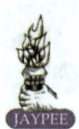 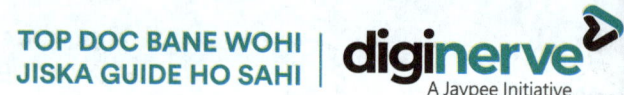

TOP DOC BANE WOHI JISKA GUIDE HO SAHI

Video Lectures | Notes | Self-Assessment
UnderGrad Courses Available

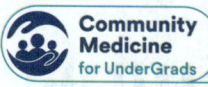 by Dr. Bratati Banerjee

 by Dr. Gautam Biswas
(Forensic Medicine & Toxicology for UnderGrads)

 by Dr. Archith Boloor
(Medicine for UnderGrads)

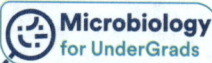 by Dr. Apurba S Sastry, Dr. Sandhya Bhat & Dr. Deepashree R
(Microbiology for UnderGrads)

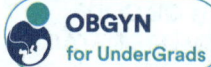 by Dr. K. Srinivas
(OBGYN for UnderGrads)

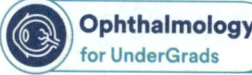 by Dr. Parul Ichhpujani & Dr. Talvir Sidhu
(Ophthalmology for UnderGrads)

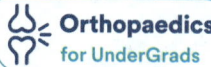 by Dr. Vivek Pandey
(Orthopaedics for UnderGrads)

 by Prof. Harsh Mohan, Prof. Ramadas Nayak & Dr. Debasis Gochhait
(Pathology for UnderGrads)

 by Dr. Santosh Soans & Dr. Soundarya M
(Pediatrics for UnderGrads)

 by Dr. Sandeep Kaushal & Dr. Nirmal George
(Pharmacology for UnderGrads)

 by Dr. Sriram Bhat M (SRB)
(Surgery for UnderGrads)

 Download the App.

*T&C Apply

Contact
+91 8800 418 418
marketing@diginerve.com

CHAPTER 9

Introduction to Nervous System

LEARNING OBJECTIVES

- Subdivisions of nervous system
- Classification of nervous tissue
- Structure of neuron
- Classification of neurons with examples
- Synapse and types
- Classification of neuroglia
- Nerve ganglia
- Blood-brain barrier
- Spinal segment and course of a typical spinal nerve
- Formation of nerve plexuses
- Receptors and their classification
- Reflex arc components
- Process of myelination
- Structure of peripheral nerve and its functional components
- Injury to nerve, its degeneration and regeneration
- Autonomic nervous system
- Clinical case with anatomical explanation

INTRODUCTION

Nervous system is the most highly specialized system of the body. It is concerned with control and coordination of various body activities like movements of joints, contraction of muscles, various visceral sensations, such as hunger, thirst, pain, etc., It has got the properties of conductivity and elicitation of appropriate reflex in response to the stimulus either from environment or within the body.

SUBDIVISIONS OF NERVOUS SYSTEM (FLOWCHART 9.1 AND FIG. 9.1)

> **AN7.1:** Describe general plan of nervous system with components of central, peripheral and autonomic nervous. systems.

Anatomical Subdivision

The nervous system is divided into two parts:
1. *Central nervous system (CNS)*—consisting of brain and the spinal cord located in the cranial cavity and vertebral canal respectively.
   - *Brain or encephalon*: It is located in the cranial cavity. The brain contains higher *controlling centers* (decision making, thinking, analysis, judgment, etc., based on the information received).
   - *Spinal cord*: It is located in the vertebral canal. It contains *reflex centers* [initiating appropriate movements of joints, contraction of muscles (skeletal, cardiac, and smooth), secretion of glands, etc.] for requisite response.
2. *Peripheral nervous system (PNS)*: It consists of nervous tissue lying outside the brain and spinal cord. It is composed of nerve *fibers* and small aggregates of nerve cells called "nerve ganglia".
   - *Nerve fibers*:
     - Twelve pairs of cranial nerves
     - Thirty-one pairs of spinal nerves
     - Splanchnic nerves

Flowchart 9.1: Divisions of nervous system.

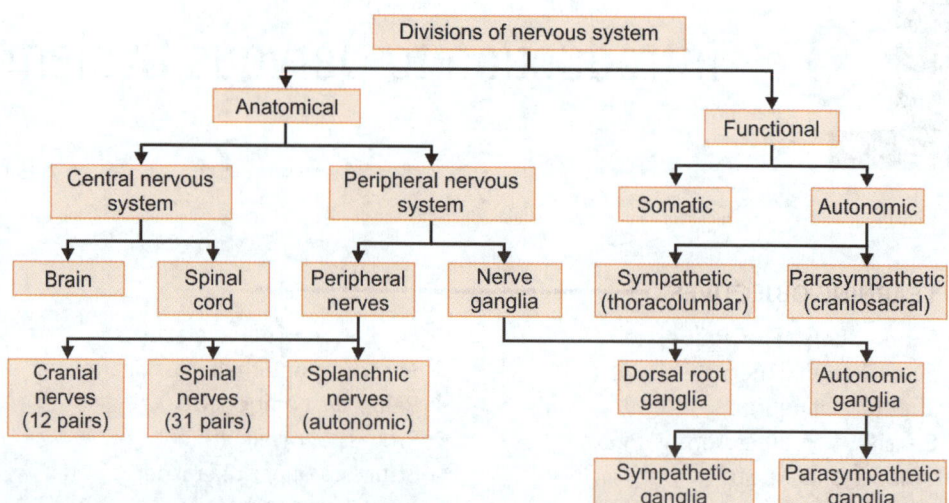

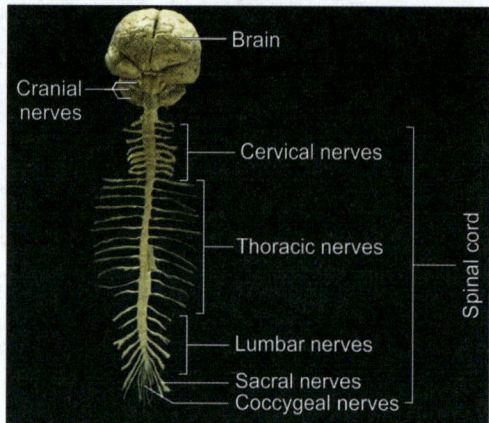

Fig. 9.1: Divisions of nervous system.

- *Ganglia*:
  - Sensory/dorsal root ganglia
  - Autonomic ganglia
    - Sympathetic
    - Parasympathetic.

Functional Subdivision

It is divided into *somatic* and *visceral* components with each in turn having afferent and efferent components.
1. *Somatic nervous system*: It is composed of:
   - *Afferent or sensory nerves*—concerned with transmission of sensory formation from various parts of body to the CNS.
   - *Efferent or motor nerves*—concerned with innervation of skeletal muscles of the body.

   It is further divided into spinal nerves and cranial nerves. This system is responsible for voluntary activities.
2. *Visceral/autonomic nervous system (ANS)*: This is concerned with innervation of various visceral muscles (cardiac and smooth) and glands. The activities of ANS are involuntary.

NERVOUS TISSUE (FLOWCHART 9.2)

AN7.2: List components of nervous tissue and their functions.

Nervous tissue is one of the four basic tissues of the body. Nervous tissue consists of two cell types. They are *neurons and neuroglia*.

Neurons

AN7.3: Describe parts of a neuron and classify them based on number of neurites, size and function.

- These are intercommunicating network of specialized cells containing cell bodies (perikaryon) and their processes.

Chapter 9: Introduction to Nervous System

Flowchart 9.2: Classification of nervous tissue.

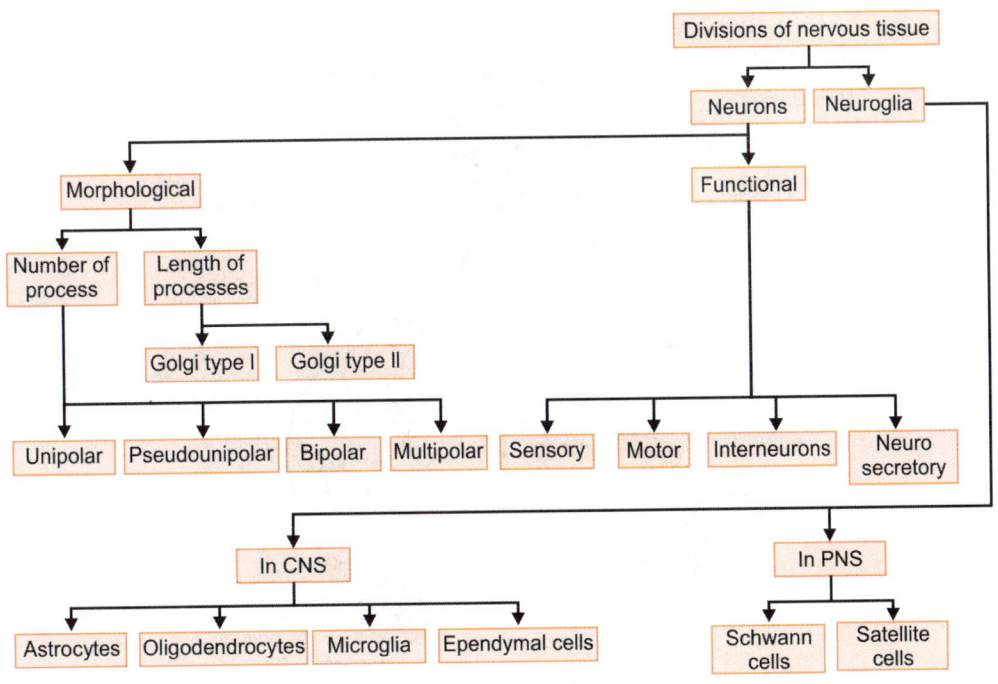

(PNS: peripheral nervous system; CNS: central nervous system)

- These are anatomical and functional units of the nervous system.
- The human nervous system consists of at least 10 billion neurons.
- The neurons are highly differentiated and do not undergo mitosis after birth. Hence, *no regeneration of neurons in postnatal life*.

Note: If the neurons increase in number in postnatal life one will have fleeting memories.

- The neurons are excitable cells and are specialized to respond and transmit the signals to activate other neurons.
- The neurons receive information from external and internal environment and transmit it to the CNS for processing and for making a decision on appropriate action.
- They convey the decision to the effector tissue for implementation.
- The neurons exhibit the property of irritability and conductivity.

Structure of Neuron

The neuron has two main parts **(Fig. 9.2)**:
1. *Cell body* (*soma/perikaryon*)
2. *Processes* (*neurites*): There are two types of processes.
    i. *Dendrites*: Numerous in number and are short.
    ii. *Axon*: Single long process.

Perikaryon (soma/cell body):
- It is the expanded portion of the neuron.
- Cell bodies of most of the neurons are situated in the gray matter of the brain and spinal cord with the exception of cell bodies of spinal ganglia that are located outside the CNS.
- They are 5–100 µ in diameter.
- They are of different shapes—pyramidal, fusiform, stellate, flask-shaped, etc.,
- The cell body presents the following features:
    - *Cell membrane*: Trilaminar with inner and outer phospholipid bilayer and an intermediate lipid layer.

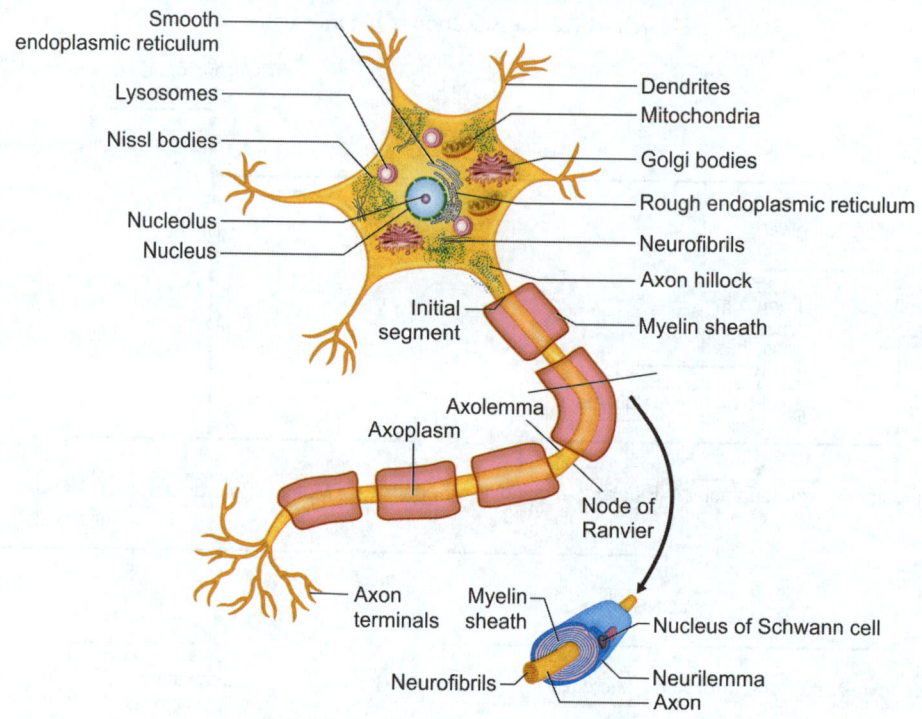

Fig. 9.2: Structure of neuron.

- *Nucleus*: It is large, vesicular and centrally placed with prominent nucleolus. The nucleus is eccentric in position in cases of injury or fatigue of the neuron. It is eccentric in healthy sympathetic ganglia. In females a planoconvex heterochromatin mass known as sex-chromatin or Barr body is present close to the nuclear membrane.
- *Cytoplasm*: It contains the following organelles:
  - Nissl bodies: These are deeply stained (basophilic) bodies of rough endoplasmic reticulum studded with abundant ribosomes. These are distributed throughout the cytoplasm and also extend into the dendrites. They are *absent in axon hillock and axon*. They are active in protein synthesis. They are more in number in motor neurons than in sensory.

> **Clinical Importance**
> In case of injury (mechanical or chemical) or fatigue of the nerve cell the Nissl bodies disappear and the nucleus moves to the periphery (eccentric) and this process is known as *chromatolysis*. When the nerve cell is recovering from stress in a reasonable time the Nissl bodies reappear.

  - Golgi bodies: These are located close to the nucleus and extend into the dendrites.
  - Mitochondria: These are present in cytoplasm and extend into all the processes.
  - Smooth endoplasmic reticulum: It is an extensively folded membrane without ribosomes. It is the site of lipid synthesis.
  - Lysosomes: These are thick-walled membranous vesicles and contain hydrolytic enzymes and acid phosphatase.

Chapter 9: Introduction to Nervous System

Clinical importance: They phagocytose the foreign particles and hydrolyze the Nissl granules during chromatolysis.
- Neurofibrils—filaments of protein that form a network.
- Lipofuscin: A golden brown pigment seen in cell bodies of aged neurons. It is a wear and tear pigment.

Note: Centrosomes and centrioles are absent in neuron and is responsible for the inability of the neuron to divide. In case of damage to the neuron the neuroglial cell replaces it.
Nuclei: Collections of nerve cell bodies within the CNS.
Ganglia: Collections of nerve cell bodies outside the CNS. Examples: Dorsal root ganglia of spinal nerves, ganglia in relation with certain cranial nerves (facial), ganglia in the autonomic nervous system (ANS).

Dendrites:
- Short multiple processes arising from the cell body and each of it presents extensive branching forming dendritic tree.
- They contain all the cytoplasmic contents of the cell body.
- They provide structural support for the neurons in CNS.
- The terminal arborizations of dendrites are thorn-like and are called dendritic spines or gemmules. The dendrites convey the nerve impulse from periphery to cell body.

Axon (Fig. 9.2):
- Each neuron has a single axon which is a long process.
- The length of axons is variable. The diameter of the axon is constant.
- Axons originate at a short pyramid-like structure, the axon hillock, which lacks Nissl substances.
- The plasma membrane of the axon is termed the *axolemma*, and the cytoplasm of the axon is termed the *axoplasm*. The axoplasm contains neurofilaments and microtubules but lacks Golgi apparatus and Nissl substance.
- The thicker axons have concentric wrappings of the enveloping Schwann cell in PNS and oligodendrocyte in CNS that forms the myelinated sheath. The nerve fibers wrapped with myelinated sheaths are called *myelinated fibers*.
- The myelin sheaths increase the velocity of conduction of an impulse. Myelin also forms an insulating sheath around the axons in the CNS and PNS.
- In myelinated axons the initial portion, between the axon hillock and the starting of the myelin sheath, is called the *initial segment*. Axons sometimes have right-angled branches the *axon collaterals*.
- Outside the myelin sheath in the PNS a thin layer of cytoplasm of Schwann cell and its cell membrane persists forming an additional sheath known as Schwann cell sheath or *neurilemmal sheath*.
- The neurilemmal sheath plays an important role in regeneration of a peripheral nerve after injury. Neurilemmal sheath is not found in CNS.

> **Clinical Importance**
> Hence, regeneration of an axon after injury is not possible in CNS due to the absence of neurilemmal sheath.

- Each unit of axon is myelinated by Schwann cell or oligodendrocyte. A gap occurs where axon is not covered by myelin. This gap is known as *node of Ranvier*.
- The segment of axon between two nodes of Ranvier is called *internode,* which is covered by a single Schwann cell whose nucleus is seen at the periphery.
- At the nodes of Ranvier a number of collaterals arise from the axon.
- Near the termination the axon divides into smaller branches called telodendria.
- The terminal parts of axon forms synapses with other neurons, muscle fibers and secretory units of exocrine glands.
- At the synapse the collaterals and terminals of axons form small bulbous expansions called boutons terminaux.

- Motor endplate is the specialized terminal of axon in a skeletal muscle.
- Bundles of axons form the peripheral nerve. In the CNS the axon forms the nerve fiber.
- An *endoneurial connective tissue sheath* surrounds each fiber.

Classification of Neurons

Anatomical:
- *According to polarity* (**Table 9.1** and **Figs. 9.3A to D**):
    - Unipolar
    - Bipolar
    - Pseudounipolar
    - Multipolar
- *According to length of processes*:
    - Golgi type I: A neuron with long process, e.g., pyramidal cells of cerebral cortex and Purkinje cells of cerebellar cortex
    - Golgi type II: A neuron with short process, e.g., cerebellar cortex neurons.
- *According to shape of cell bodies* (**Figs. 9.4 A to C**):
    - Stellate or star shaped, e.g., in spinal cord.
    - Triangular or pyramidal, e.g., in cerebral cortex.
    - Flask-shaped, e.g., Purkinje cells in cerebellar cortex.

Table 9.1: Description of different types of neurons (Figs. 9.3A to D).

Neurons—description	Structure (Figs. 9.3A to D)
Unipolar neuron: ❑ Have single process extending from cell body that is usually a dendrite ❑ *Example*: Mesencephalic nucleus of trigeminal nerve	A
Bipolar neurons: ❑ These have two processes, i.e., one dendrite and one axon extending from each end of the cell body ❑ *Examples*: Retina, olfactory epithelium, sensory ganglia of vestibular and cochlear nerves	B
Pseudounipolar neurons: ❑ Have a single, short process that extends from the cell body and bifurcates forming a T-shape. One of it is peripherally directed and receives information from the peripheral receptors. Other process enters the central nervous system and conveys the information ❑ *Example*: Sensory ganglia on dorsal roots of spinal nerves	C
Multipolar neurons: ❑ They possess single axon and several dendrites extending from the cell body ❑ *Example*: Most common type of neurons present in the spinal cord, cerebrum and cerebellum. They are also present in autonomic ganglia	D

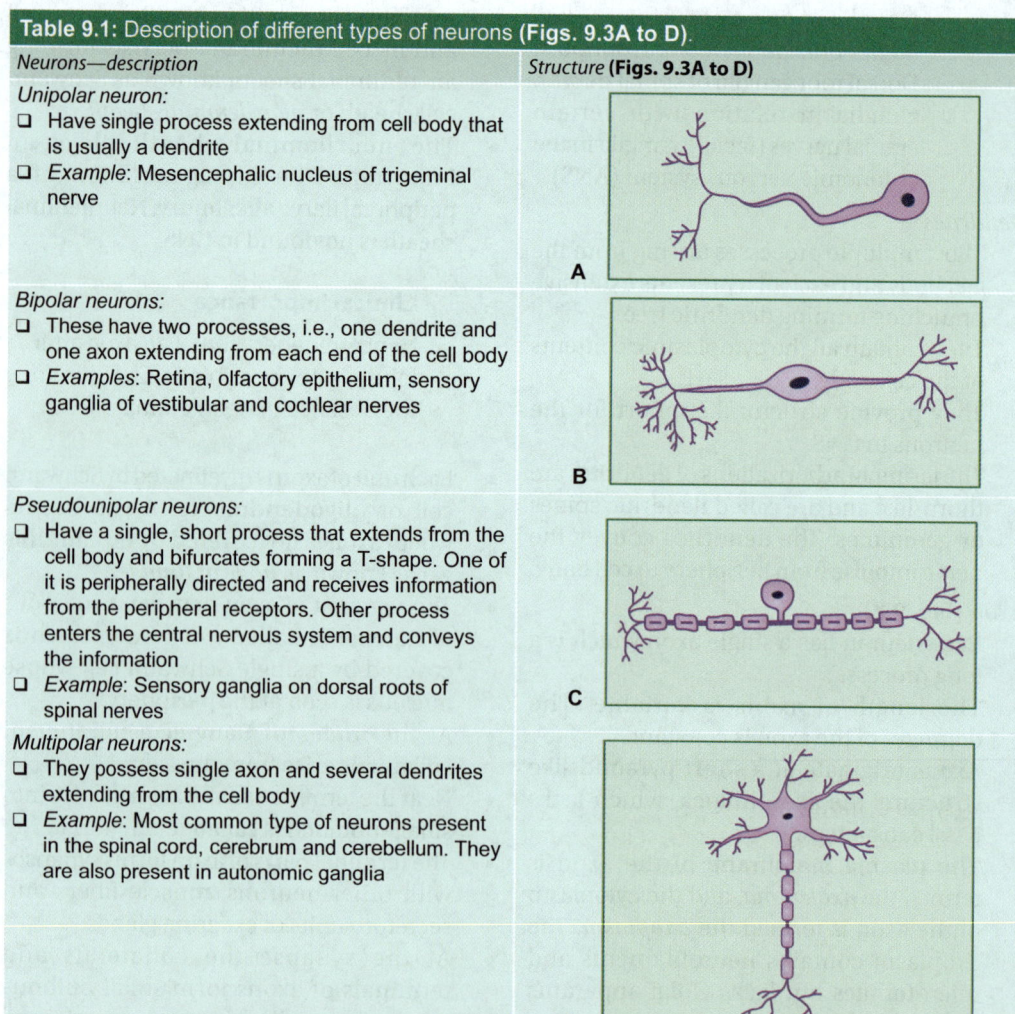

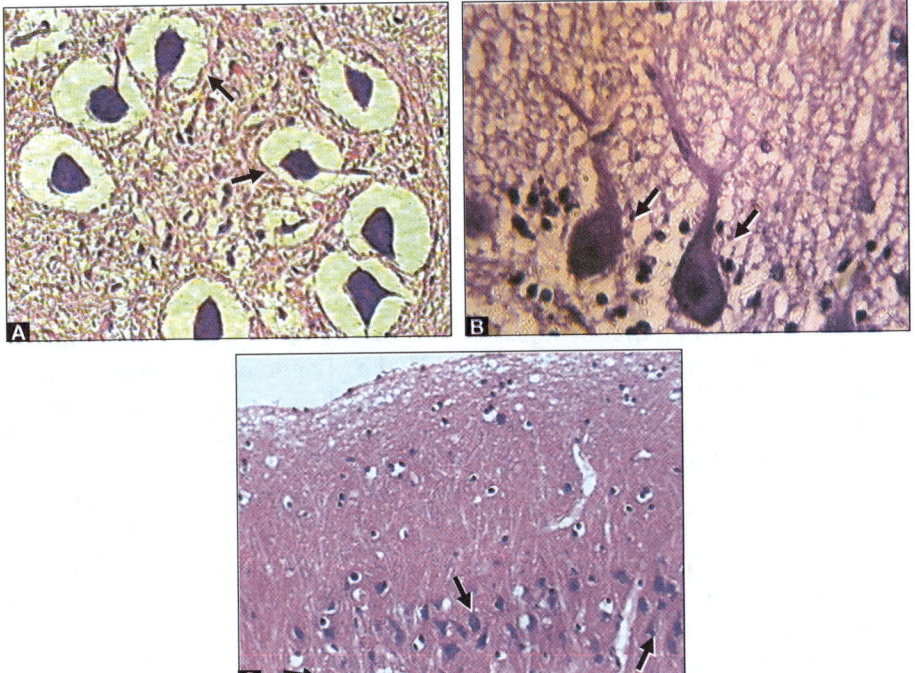

Figs. 9.4A to C: Classification of neurons—according to shape of cell body: (A) Stellate or star-shaped cell bodies in spinal cord; (B) Flask-shaped cell bodies (Purkinje cells) in cerebellar cortex; (C) Triangular-shaped cell bodies in cerebral cortex.

Functional:
- **Sensory neurons**: Receive sensory stimuli from the environment (from receptors) and from within the body. Example: Pseudounipolar neurons and bipolar neurons. The cell bodies of all sensory neurons lie outside the CNS except mesencephalic nucleus of trigeminal nerve.
    - **Motor neurons**: These control the effector organs (muscles, exocrine glands, and endocrine glands). They are located in CNS *except* postganglionic autonomic neurons. There are two types of motor neurons:
        1. *Upper motor neurons*: These are confined to cerebral cortex.
        2. *Lower motor neurons*: These are confined to anterior gray horn of spinal cord and brainstem.
    - *Autonomic neurons*: These are arranged in two sets **(Fig. 9.5)**:

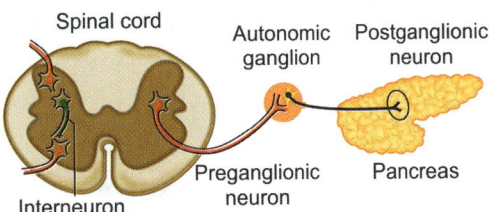

Fig. 9.5: Autonomic neurons.

1. Preganglionic neurons—located in CNS and are arranged as:
    - *Craniosacral (parasympathetic) outflow*—the preganglionic neurons are located in the brainstem (for cranial part) and sacral segments of spinal cord (for sacral part).
    - *Thoracolumbar (sympathetic) outflow*—the preganglionic neurons are located in the thoracic and lumbar segments of spinal cord.

2. *Postganglionic neurons*—situated outside CNS.
- *Interneurons (intermediate neurons)*: These are typically found in the CNS and connect other neurons (often between sensory and motor neurons). They are multipolar neurons, e.g., majority of ascending and descending tracts are axons of interneurons.
- *Neurosecretory neurons*: These are specialized neurons that synthesize and secrete hormones. These are present in the hypothalamus and produce the hormones antidiuretic hormone (ADH) and oxytocin.

AN7.7: Describe various type of synapse.

Synapse: Synapse is the site of contact between two neurons for easy transmission of information. It is a specialized junction. It contains three parts **(Fig. 9.6)**:
1. Presynaptic membrane of terminal bouton of one presynaptic neuron. It contains synaptic vesicles filled with neurotransmitter.
2. *Synaptic cleft*: It is an extracellular space between pre- and postsynaptic neurons. The neurotransmitter is released into this space.
3. Postsynaptic membrane of one postsynaptic neuron. Once the neurotransmitter comes in contact with this membrane action potential is generated.

Classification of synapses—based on the nerve cell components that are coming into contact they are classified as **(Fig. 9.7)**:
- *Axodendritic*: These are the *most common* type of synapses. In this type axon of presynaptic neuron makes contact with dendrites of postsynaptic neuron.
- *Axosomatic*: These are *less common*. In this type the axon terminal of presynaptic neuron comes into contact with the cell body or soma of postsynaptic neuron.
- *Axoaxonal*: The axon of presynaptic neuron makes contact with axon of postsynaptic neuron. These are *least common* type of synapses.

Neuroglia

- In Greek the term "Glia" means *glue*. These are the connective tissue cells in the nervous system.
- These are nonexcitable cells.

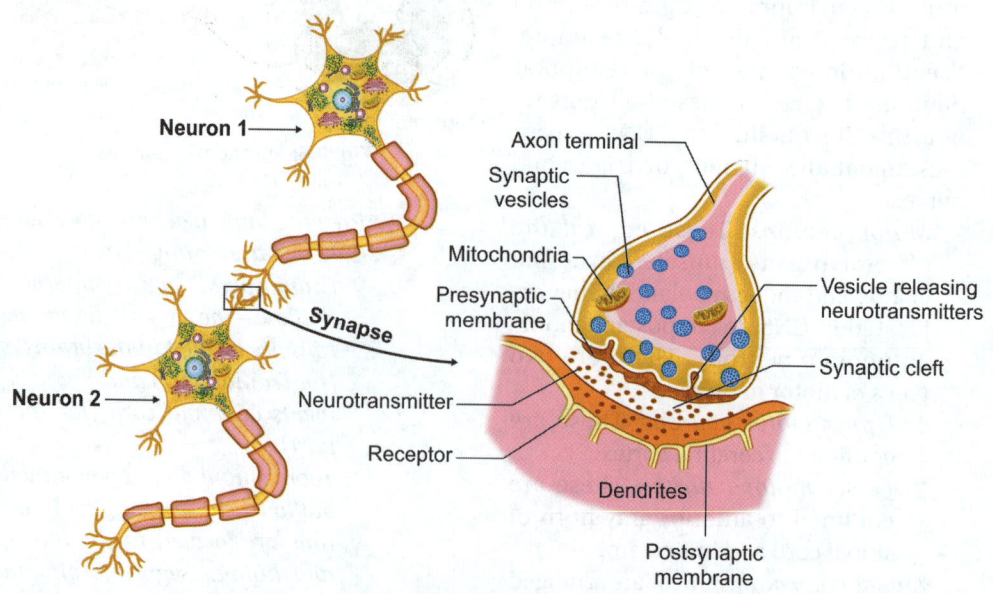

Fig. 9.6: Structure of synapse.

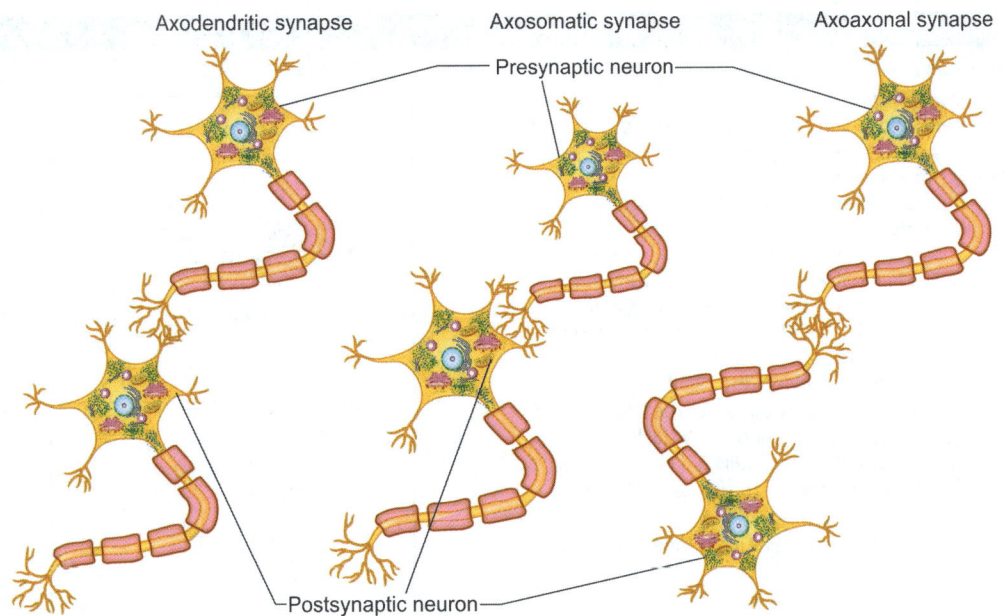

Fig. 9.7: Classification of synapse.

- They provide structural support for the neurons in CNS.
- In the PNS they form myelin sheath for the axons and are nutritional.
- They are capable of mitotic division throughout life.
- Tumors of brain can arise from neuroglia, meninges or blood vessels.
- The neuroglia are ten times more in number than the neurons.

Neuroglia in CNS: These are four types (**Table 9.2** and **Figs. 9.8A to E**):
1. *Astrocytes (astroglia)*
2. *Oligodendrocytes (oligodendroglia)*
3. *Microglia*
4. *Ependymal cells.*

The astrocytes, oligodendrocytes, and ependymal layer together are called *macroglia* and are derived from *neurectoderm*. Microglia is derived from *mesoderm*.

Neuroglia in PNS: Two types (**Table 9.2** and **Fig. 9.8F**):
1. *Schwann cells*
2. *Satellite cell.*

Nerve Ganglia

Ganglia are groups of nerve cell bodies (perikarya) outside the CNS. Two types of nerve ganglia can be distinguished based on their morphology and function.
1. Spinal ganglia (dorsal root ganglia)
2. Autonomic ganglia.

AN7.8: Describe differences between sympathetic and spinal ganglia.

Spinal ganglia (**Fig. 9.9A**):
- Found in the dorsal roots of spinal nerves and carry afferent sensory impulses from the periphery to CNS.
- The ganglion cells are grouped together at the periphery.
- Fascicles of nerve fibers course through the middle of the spinal ganglion.
- These ganglia contain *pseudounipolar neurons* with centrally located nuclei. The perikaryon is surrounded by two layers of capsule, an inner layer of glial cells known as satellite cells (capsule cells) with round or oval nuclei and an outer layer of fibroblasts.

Table 9.2: Description of different types of neuroglia.

Neuroglia	Structure (Figs. 9.8A to F)

Astrocytes (astroglia):
❏ Present only in the central nervous system (CNS)
❏ They are the largest of the neuroglia
❏ They are star shaped
❏ They have many long processes extending in all directions
❏ *Functions*: They provide structural and nutritional support to the neurons in CNS. Participation in the blood–brain barrier. They take part in repair processes following damage or injury to nerves
There are two types of astrocytes:
1. *Protoplasmic astrocytes* **(Fig. 9.8A)**:
  ➢ Present in the gray matter of the CNS
  ➢ Their processes are short and thick
2. *Fibrous astrocytes* **(Fig. 9.8B)**:
  ➢ These are present in the white matter of the CNS
  ➢ Their processes are much thinner and longer
	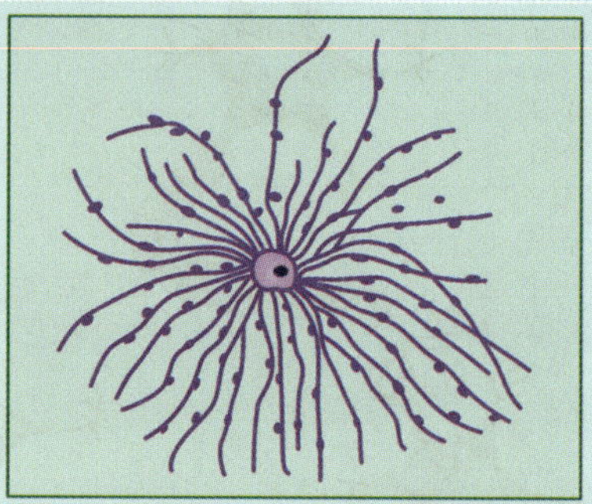 A 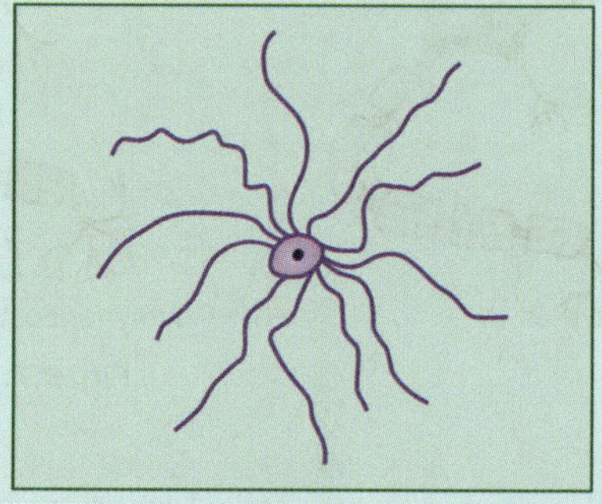
	
	B

Oligodendrocytes **(Fig. 9.8C)**: ❏ These are smaller than the astrocytes, with fewer and shorter processes ❏ They are found in both the gray- and white matter of the CNS ❏ *Function*: They are responsible for the formation of the myelin sheath surrounding axons in CNS	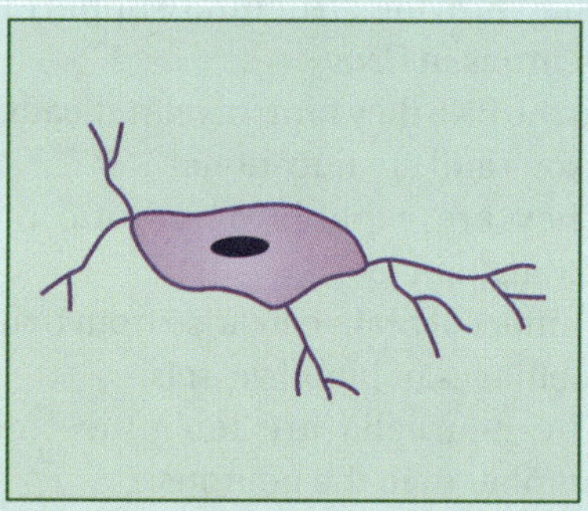 C
Microglia **(Fig. 9.8D)**: ❏ These are small cells, with elongated bodies, and relatively few processes ❏ They are found in both the gray- and white matter of the CNS ❏ *Function*: Perform phagocytic function like macrophages	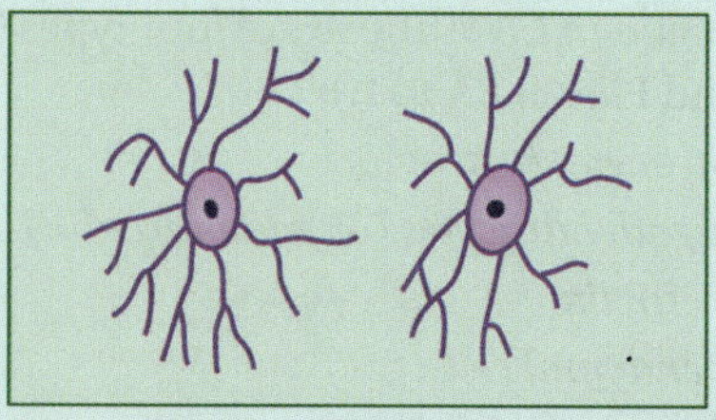 D
Ependymal cells **(Fig. 9.8E)**: ❏ These cells line the internal cavities (ventricles) of the brain and spinal cord (central canal) ❏ They are arranged as single layer of ciliated cuboidal or columnar cells ❏ *Function*: Formation and circulation of cerebrospinal fluid (CSF)	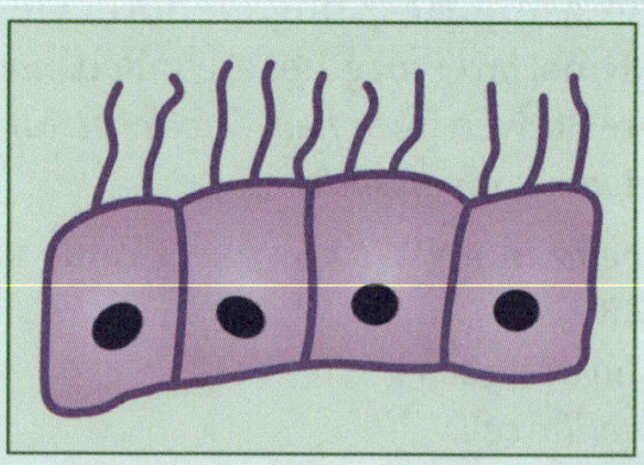 E

Contd...

Contd...

Neuroglia	Structure (Figs. 9.8A to F)
Schwann cells **(Fig. 9.8F)**: ❑ Schwann cells of the peripheral nervous system (PNS) are similar to the oligodendrocytes of CNS ❑ *Function*: They form the myelin sheath around peripheral axons *Satellite cells* **(Fig. 9.8F)**: ❑ These cells surround the cells of ganglia (spinal and autonomic) in the PNS. These are flattened cells with prominent nuclei ❑ *Function*: They provide nutritive support as they are the pathway for metabolic exchange. They also provide structural support in PNS	

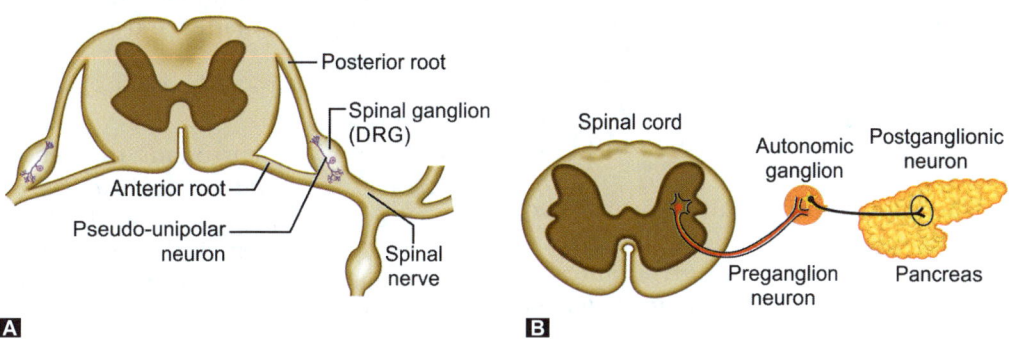

Figs. 9.9A and B: (A) Spinal ganglia; (B) Autonomic ganglia.

- Thick connective tissue capsule surrounds the ganglia.

Autonomic ganglia **(Fig. 9.9B)**:
- These are associated with nerves of the ANS.
- They are found as dilatations of autonomic nerves and may be encapsulated.
- In many cases the ganglia are seen in the walls of organs (intramural) and lack a capsule. They differ from spinal ganglia in that the neurons are multipolar.
- The perikarya are smaller, have fewer satellite cells and are more evenly distributed.

Blood–brain barrier:
- It is a selective semipermeable membrane at capillary level that separates the circulating blood form the brain, allowing passage of selective contents of blood to the nervous system thus preventing entry of toxic and harmful substances.
- It is formed by endothelial cells lining the cerebral capillaries that have tight junctions.
- Constituents of blood–brain barrier (BBB) are: (a) Capillary endothelial cell, (b) Basement membrane of the endothelium, and (c) End feet of astrocytes covering the capillary walls.

- It plays an important role in protecting the brain from fluctuations in blood plasma composition, from circulating chemicals that can disturb neuronal function. It protects the brain from a number of pathogens.

SPINAL CORD AND SPINAL SEGMENTS

Spinal Cord (Figs. 9.1 and 9.10)

- Spinal cord is the thin, elongated caudal part of CNS. It is 45 cm in length.
- It lies in the upper two-thirds of vertebral canal. It extends from the foramen magnum, to the level of 1st or 2nd lumbar vertebra.
- Above the level of foramen magnum it is continuous with medulla oblongata and below the level of L1/L2 vertebra it continues as filum terminale.
- It is cylindrical in shape and flattened anteroposteriorly. It is divided into cervical, thoracic, lumbar, and sacral regions.
- The spinal cord is divided into two symmetrical halves (right and left) by an *anterior median fissure* on anterior surface and a *posterior median septum* on posterior surface in the midline.
- Each half is further subdivided into anterior, lateral, and posterior areas by *anterolateral* and *posterolateral sulci*.
- Along the anterolateral sulcus the ventral/motor roots of spinal nerves exit from spinal cord. Along the posterolateral sulcus the dorsal/sensory root fibers enter the spinal cord.

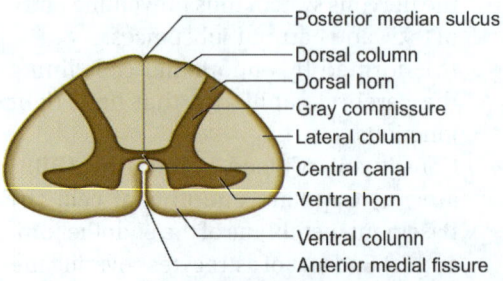

Fig. 9.10: Spinal cord.

- Between the posterolateral sulcus and posterior median septum *posterior intermediate sulcus* is present in cervical part of spinal cord.

Spinal Segment

- The *spinal* cord (**Figs. 9.11A and B**) is made up of 31 *segments*. They are:
  - Cervical: 8
  - Thoracic: 12
  - Lumbar: 5
  - Sacral: 5
  - Coccygeal: 1
- A pair of *spinal* nerves leaves each *segment* of the *spinal* cord. A total of 31 pairs of spinal nerves emerge from the spinal cord.
- *Cross-section of spinal cord*: Transverse section (TS) of spinal cord is circular or oval in shape and shows the following features:
  - Central gray matter and peripheral white matter.
  - Central canal is located in the center of gray matter.
  - Gray matter surrounds the central canal and is *butterfly* or *H-shaped*.
  - Gray matter presents a pair of anterior and a pair of posterior horns and a pair of intermediate horns if it is at thoracic level.
  - A cross-section of spinal cord at different levels differs in the proportion of gray matter and white matter and in the location of central canal. At lower levels, the amount of white matter is less. As it ascends up, the bulk of white matter increases.
  - Gray matter contains nerve cell bodies of multipolar neurons, neuroglia, initial parts of nerve fibers, and blood vessels. Multipolar neurons of spinal cord are star-shaped.
  - The gray matter presents collections of cell bodies of neurons called nuclei. Each nucleus has got specific function.
  - White matter is divided into anterior, posterior, and lateral columns. White matter contains myelinated nerve fibers and neuroglia.

Chapter 9: Introduction to Nervous System

Course of Typical Spinal Nerve (Figs. 9.11A and B)

AN7.4: Describe structure of a typical spinal nerve.

- Each spinal nerve is connected with the spinal cord by two roots, (1) a ventral root which is motor and (2) a dorsal root which is sensory. On the dorsal root lies the dorsal root ganglion nearer to the spinal cord in the intervertebral foramen.

- The dorsal and ventral roots unite in the intervertebral foramen to form the mixed spinal nerve. The mixed spinal nerve after emerging out from the intervertebral foramen gives off recurrent meningeal branches, and then divides into a *dorsal* and a *ventral ramus*.

- The dorsal ramus passes backward and supplies the intrinsic muscles of the back,

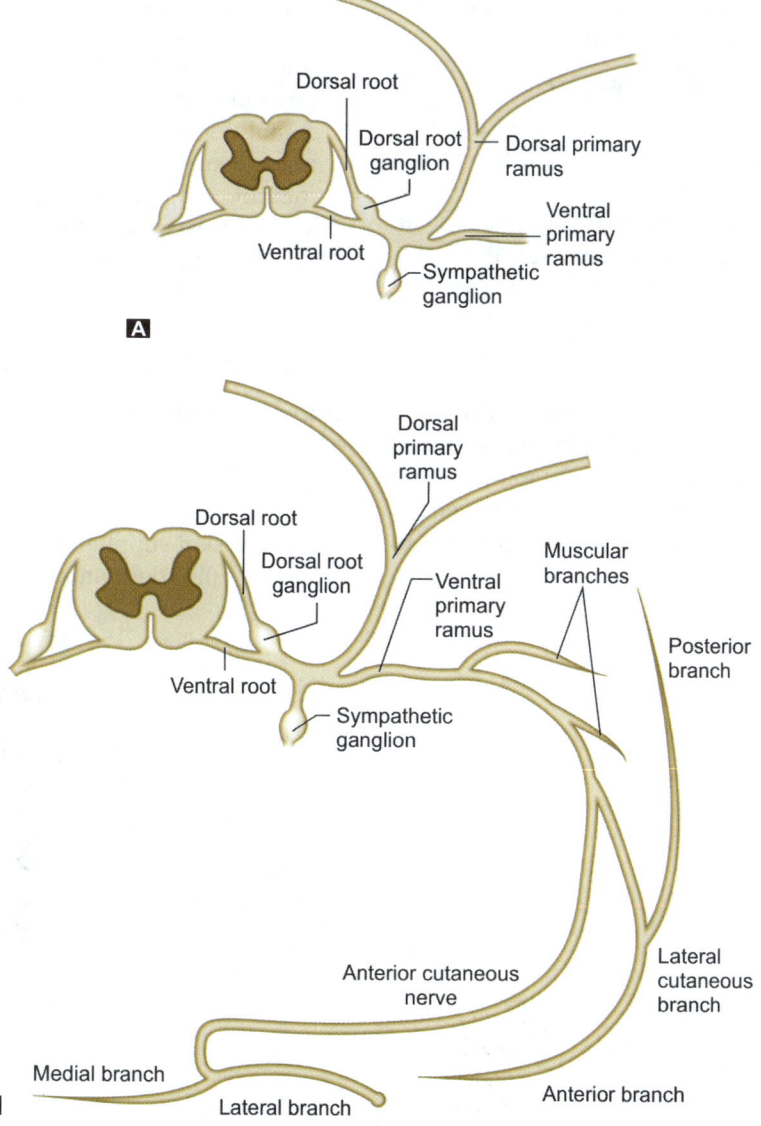

Figs. 9.11A and B: Spinal segment showing. (A) Course of typical spinal nerve; (B) Typical thoracic spinal nerve.

and the skin covering them. The ventral ramus is connected with the sympathetic ganglion, and is distributed to the limb or the anterolateral body wall.
- The ventral rami of all spinal nerves except thoracic join with neighboring ventral rami to form the nerve plexuses, i.e., brachial plexus, lumbar plexus for the supply of limbs.
- The *typical thoracic spinal nerve* gives off several muscular branches to intercostal muscles, a lateral cutaneous branch, and an anterior cutaneous branch.

Formation of Nerve Plexuses **(Fig. 9.12)**

- A nerve plexus is a branching network of intersecting nerves. It contains both motor and sensory fibers.
- All nerve plexuses are formed only by the ventral rami only. These supply the limbs.
- The spinal cord shows enlargements at the regions that contribute for the plexuses, e.g., "cervical enlargement" for the brachial plexus and "lumbar enlargement" for the lumbosacral plexus.
- Each ventral ramus divides into a ventral and a dorsal division. Each ventral division joins with neighboring ventral division in different ways to give rise to the branches.
- The branches of ventral division supply the flexor compartment, and that of the dorsal division, the extensor compartment, of the limb.
- Each division and in turn their branches supply specific muscles (motor) and an area of dermis of skin (sensory).
- The flexor compartments of limbs are richly innervated than the extensor compartments.
- Because of mixing of spinal nerves originating from different segments of spinal cords in plexus formation there is overlapping of dermatomes (area of dermis of skin supplied by one spinal nerve) and myotomes (a part of muscle supplied by one spinal nerve) that are supplied by segmental nerves. This suggests the composite origin of a muscle from adjacent segments and their migration into the trunk and limbs.

DERMATOMES

AN4.1: Describe different types of skin and dermatomes in body.

Definition

The area of skin supplied by a single spinal segment is called dermatome.

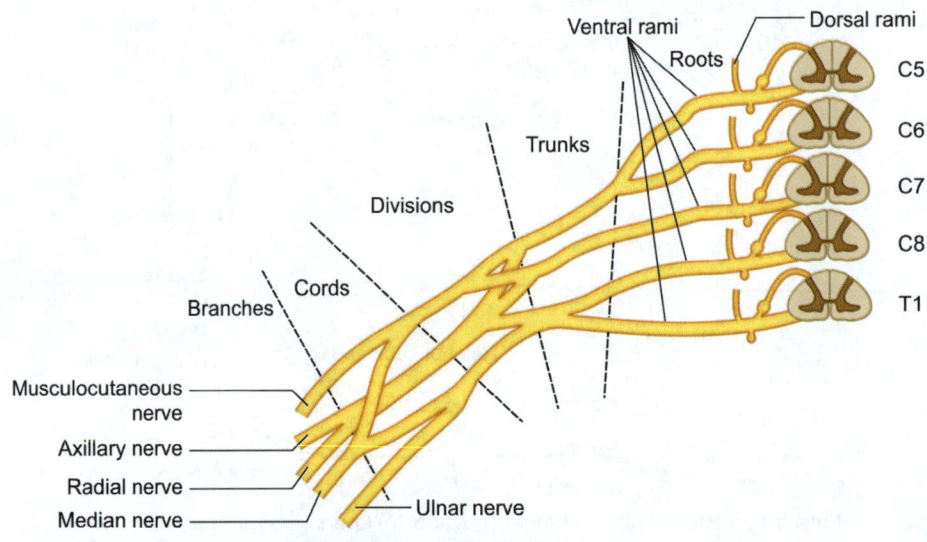

Fig. 9.12: Formation of nerve plexus.

- The cell bodies of sensory neurons are located in the dorsal root ganglion in relation to the afferent/sensory nerve.
- The spinal nerve roots supply the structures assigned to them according to their association with the spinal segment.
- There is overlap of spinal segments supplying adjacent/contiguous dermatomes. These overlapping dermatomes are called signature zones for identifying the spinal cord segment. This overlap of dermatomes is observed in T2-L1 segments.
- Dermatomes are represented as narrow bands of skin running horizontally in the trunk. Due to the growth and rotation of limb buds during development the dermatomes are arranged longitudinally along the long axis of the limb.
- There are 31 pairs of spinal nerves. But, the number of dermatomes are only 30. The reason being the dorsal ramus of C1 spinal nerve has no sensory root.
- The sensory innervation of scalp and face is by trigeminal nerve. Hence the first dermatome to begin with is C2 which overlaps with trigeminal nerve on the front of head and neck.
- The dorsal rami of C5-T1 are not involved in the supply of trunk due to the development of upper limb buds at these spinal segment levels. Hence, these segments are involved in the cutaneous innervation of upper limb. Because of this C4 dermatome is continuous with T2 dermatome.
- The dermatomal distribution of upper limb is C4-C6 segments along the lateral aspect of limb and C8-T1 along the medial aspect of limb with C7 in the middle.
- Due to the medial rotation of the developing lower limb along its long axis the dermatomal distribution is oblique in orientation. L1 and L2 dermatomes are placed adjacent to S2 and S3 as the intervening segments (L2-S1) moved into more distal parts of the limb. The dermatomes of lower limb are arranged in a downward sequence on the front and in an upward sequence on the back.

Clinical Application
- Knowledge of dermatomes is important in neurological examination to identify the involvement of a spinal segment or localization of injured spinal segment by testing for the loss of sensation in a conscious patient.
- Sectioning of single dorsal nerve root results in hypoesthesia (diminished sensation).
- Damage of at least three adjacent dorsal roots results in dermatomal anesthesia (total loss of sensation).
- Sharp radiating pain along the distribution of a dermatome suggests herniated intervertebral disc putting pressure on the segmental nerve.
- Pain or rash along the distribution of a dermatome indicates disease of the related nerve root. Most common cause is viral infection (varicella zoster that causes chickenpox and herpes zoster that causes shingles).

RECEPTORS

These are specialized cells that can detect changes in the environment (stimuli) either from the external or the internal (viscera) and convert them into electrical impulses. Most of them are located in the sensory organs like skin, eye, and ear and in the viscera and are called sensory receptors. The information they receive from different sources is relayed to the CNS via sensory neurons. In the CNS the information is integrated with the other sensory information and is analyzed for conscious perception of the stimulus. This will lead to making a decision about the appropriate motor response and its initiation by CNS. The receptors respond to four types of stimuli, i.e., chemical, mechanical, thermal, nociceptive, and photosensitive.

Classification of Receptors (Fig. 9.13 and Table 9.3)

Structural Classification

- *Free nerve endings*: Pain and temperature receptors located in the dermis.
- *Encapsulated nerve endings*: Lamellar corpuscles in dermis.
- *Specialized receptor cells*: Photoreceptor cells in the retina that receive light stimuli.

Classification based on location:

- Exteroceptors—receive information from outside the body. These include receptors for taste, smell, vision, hearing, equilibrium apart from pain, temperature, etc., Their function is to convey the information about the environment to the CNS.
- Interoceptors—receive information from the viscera like the hunger, thirst, fullness of bladder, stretching of viscera, blood pressure, and blood volume changes, etc. These are involved in maintaining homeostasis.
- Proprioceptors—present in the muscle, tendon and joint, and perceive the sensation of position, movement of the

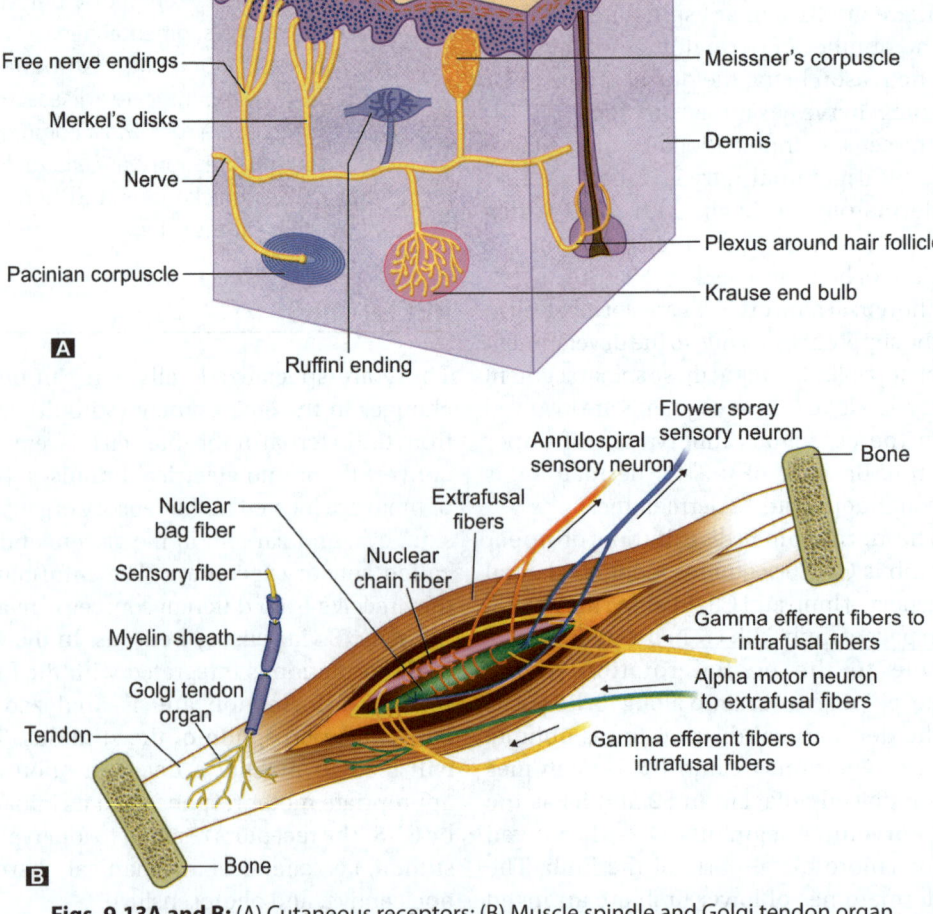

Figs. 9.13A and B: (A) Cutaneous receptors; (B) Muscle spindle and Golgi tendon organ.

Table 9.3: Various types of sensory receptors.

Receptor	Type	Location	Sensation
Free nerve endings	Nociceptor Thermoreceptor	Dermis	Pain, temperature (heat and cold), touch
Merkel disks	Mechanoreceptor	Epidermis-dermis junction	Vibration
Krause end bulb	Mechanoreceptor	Dermis, mucosa of oral cavity, conjunctiva	Touch and pressure
Ruffini endings	Mechanoreceptor	Dermis, subcutaneous tissue	Stretch
Meissner's corpuscles	Mechanoreceptor	Dermis especially finger tips	Light touch, vibration
Pacinian corpuscles	Mechanoreceptor	Dermis, subcutaneous tissue	Deep touch
Plexus around hair follicle	Mechanoreceptor	Wrapped around hair follicle	Movement of hair
Muscle spindle	Mechanoreceptor	Muscle fibers	Contraction and stretch of muscle
Golgi tendon organ	Mechanoreceptor	Tendon	Stretch of tendon
Rods and cones of retina	Photoreceptor	Eye	Vision
Hair cells in organ of Corti	Mechanoreceptor	Ear	Hearing
Hair cells in semicircular canals	Mechanoreceptor	Ear	Movement
Hair cells in vestibule	Mechanoreceptor	Ear	Gravity
Olfactory cells	Chemoreceptors	Nose	Smell
Taste cells	Chemoreceptors	Taste buds	Taste

limb, fingers, etc., These are responsible for touching your nose with the fingers with eyes closed.

Functional classification:
- Chemoreceptors—respond to chemical stimuli like smell, taste, and blood pH.
- Nociceptors—perceive the sensation of pain.
- Mechanoreceptors—respond to pressure, vibration, hearing, etc.
- Thermoreceptors—respond to changes in the temperature. They are located in skin and hypothalamus.
- Photoreceptors—respond to electromagnetic wave length, i.e., light for perceiving the colors.

REFLEX ARC (FIG. 9.14)

- This is the basic functional unit of nervous system. It is the path taken by a nerve impulse in response to a stimulus.
- This constitutes the various elements involved in the activities of nervous system.
- The functional components of a reflex arc are:
  - *Receptor*: Stimulation of the receptor in skin or skeletal muscle spindle initiates impulse.
  - *Afferent sensory neuron (pseudounipolar neuron)*: Propagation of an impulse via afferent sensory nerve (process of unipolar neuron), which enters the gray matter of the spinal cord.

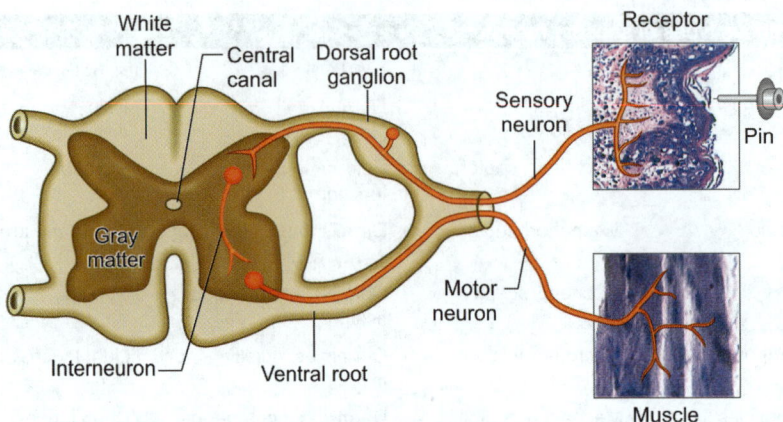

Fig. 9.14: Reflex arc.

- *Interneuron*: Connect sensory neuron with cell body of motor neuron in the ventral horn of spinal cord.
- *Efferent motor neuron*: Transmits the efferent impulse to an effector. It is present in ventral gray horn of spinal cord or in the brainstem.
- *Effector*—one that responds to the impulse, e.g., motor end plate of skeletal muscle or the gland.

♦ It defines the pathway by which the reflex (stimulus) travels from the source of stimulus (receptor) to sensory neuron, to motor neuron, to a reflex muscle movement or gland secretion (effector).

♦ Reflexes are involuntary and almost instantaneous.

♦ *Types of reflexes*: There are two types of reflexes depending on the number of neurons and the type of effector.

♦ *Depending on the number of neurons*:
  1. *Monosynaptic reflex*—contains only two neurons, (1) a sensory and (2) a motor. *Examples:*
     - *Knee jerk/patellar reflex*—sudden kicking movement of leg in response to a sharp tap on the patellar tendon located below the knee cap.
     - *Ankle jerk/Achilles reflex*—plantar extension or dorsiflexion of foot observed on tapping the tendon at the back of ankle.

     A brief stimulus of muscle spindle results in the contraction of the agonist (effector) muscle.
  2. *Polysynaptic reflex*—multiple interneurons are present in the interface between sensory and motor neurons. Majority of the reflexes in the body are polysynaptic. *Example:*
     - *Withdrawal reflex*—when a person touches a burning candle he/she withdraws the hand from the hot object without thinking about it. The heat of the object stimulates the temperature receptors in the skin, initiating sensory impulse that travels to the CNS. The impulse travels through sensory neuron, interneuron to the motor neuron and to the effector muscles of limb for withdrawal from the harmful stimulus.

♦ *Depending on the effector*:
  1. Somatic reflex arc—affecting the skeletal muscle.
  2. Autonomic reflex arc—affecting the inner organ or cardiac muscle.

Neurovascular bundle consists of a connective tissue sheath wrapped nerve, artery, and vein **(Fig. 9.15)**.

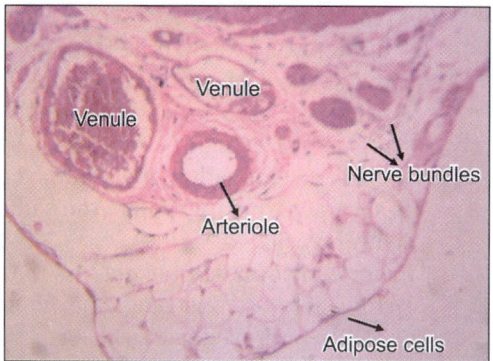

Fig. 9.15: Neurovascular bundle.

NERVE FIBERS AND THEIR MYELI-NATION (FIGS. 9.16 AND 9.17)

- Axon of a neuron is called the nerve fiber.
- Nerve fibers in brain and spinal cord receive support from neuroglial cells.
- The nerve fibers, leave the CNS to become constituents of peripheral nerves. They acquire a special sheath called neurilemmal sheath that is derived from the *Schwann cells*.
- At a later stage of development, a large number of nerve fibers, both inside and outside the CNS, develop another sheath between the neurilemma and the axon. This is called the *myelin sheath*.
- *Myelination* is the process of formation of a fatty covering on the axon that protects the neuron and facilitates effective conduction of nerve impulses. Myelin sheath increases the velocity of conduction of nerve impulse and reduces the energy expenditure in the conduction of impulse. The white matter in the brain and spinal cord looks white because of the presence of large number of myelinated fibers.

Process of Myelination in Peripheral Nervous System

- Single axon comes in contact with single Schwann cell.
- Axon invaginates into the cytoplasm of a Schwann cell.

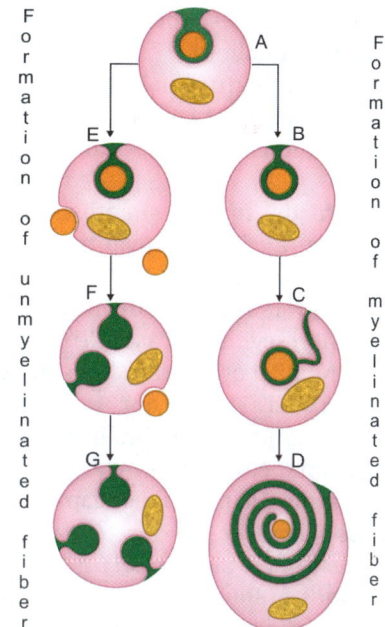

Fig. 9.16: Process of myelination in peripheral nervous system.

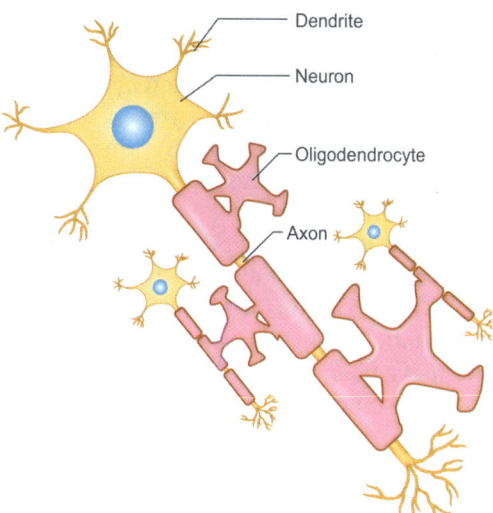

Fig. 9.17: Process of myelination in central nervous system.

- Along the line of invagination, the cell membrane of the Schwann cell becomes drawn into form a double layered mesentery called *mesaxon*.
- Mesaxon elongates and becomes spirally wound around the axon as several layers

- with one on the outside of the other (outward spiraling).
- Some fatty substances are deposited between adjacent layers of the mesaxon and, together with it, form the *myelin sheath*.
- Outside the myelin sheath is the cell membrane of the Schwann cell called *neurilemmal sheath*.
- Each Schwann cell provides myelin sheath for a short segment of axon. This suggests that a number of Schwann cells come into contact with a single axon. At the junction of two segments there is a gap where the axon is not covered by myelin sheath or neurilemmal sheath. These gaps are called *nodes of Ranvier*.
- Because of the absence of myelin sheath at nodes of Ranvier the nerve impulse jumps at the nodes, hence it is conducted faster along the whole length of the axon.

Process of Myelination in Central Nervous System

- In the CNS, there are no Schwann cells and the myelin sheath is formed by neuroglial cells called *oligodendrocytes*.
- In the CNS single oligodendrocyte provides myelin sheath for several nearby nerve fibers.
- Since a single oligodendrocyte cannot wind round several axons the newer layers of myelin are pushed under the older ones resulting in an inward spiraling toward the nerve fiber.
- Nerve fibers of CNS have no neurilemmal.

Types of fibers based on myelination:
- *Myelinated fibers*:
  - The axons of myelinated fibers are wrapped in a sheath of myelin that gives glistening white color to the nerve.
  - Myelinated fibers are found in the peripheral nerves and in the white matter of the CNS where they are arranged in the form of well-defined tracts.
  - Process of myelination in PNS and CNS are different.
- *Unmyelinated fibers*:
  - A number of axons come in contact with a single Schwann cell.
  - The axons invaginate into the cytoplasm of a single Schwann cell.
  - There is no elongation of the mesaxon as several axons invaginate the same Schwann cell.
  - *Examples*: Somatic fibers of less than 1µ thickness and postganglionic fibers of ANS are unmyelinated.
  - These fibers are present in gray matter of spinal cord and brain along with cell bodies of neurons.
  - These fibers are gray in color.

Composition of myelin: It contains 27% cholesterol, 43% phospholipids, and 30% proteins. Dietary fat is important for the formation of myelin sheath. Hence the infants should be encouraged to take more fat in their diet.

Regional and functional differentiation in myelination: Nerve fibers in different parts of the brain and spinal cord become myelinated at different stages of development. The process begins during the 4 months (16 weeks gestation) of intrauterine life. It begins in the brainstem and cerebellum before birth. The process of myelination is rapid in infancy and major part is completed when the child is 2-3 years old. But myelination of frontal lobe of brain that is concerned with cognitive functioning is completed during adolescent age. Nerve fibers become fully functional only after they have acquired their myelin sheaths.

Clinical Importance of Myelination
- Diseases that cause inflammation of nerves can cause damage to the myelin sheath. Such diseases are called demyelinating diseases.
- Damage to the myelin sheath causes slowing of conduction or even stoppage of nerve impulse leading to neurological problems.

- The severity depends on the type of disease, the part of NS affected and varies from physical disability (paralysis in severe cases) to impairment of speech, vision, etc.
- Examples are multiple sclerosis, Guillain-Barré syndrome, and certain types of encephalitis. People with these conditions suffer pain, muscle weakness, numbness, sensory loss, etc.,

Peripheral Nerve (Fig. 9.18)

- Axons of nerve cells form the nerve fibers. A nerve is one or more bundles of nerve fibers (axons) enclosed by connective tissue sheaths.
- The nerves emerge from the CNS through various foramina of skull (cranial nerves) and intervertebral foramina of vertebral column (spinal nerves). These carry information to and from the various organs of the body.
- The connective tissue covering in peripheral nerves is arranged in three layers.
  - *Endoneurium*: Each individual nerve fiber (with its enveloping Schwann cell) is surrounded by a loose vascular connective tissue called the *endoneurium*.
  - *Perineurium*: A large collection of nerve fibers is called a nerve fascicle or bundle and this structure is invested by a dense connective tissue called the *perineurium*.
  - *Epineurium*: If the peripheral nerve has more than one fascicle, all the fascicles are enclosed by a condensed, strong connective sheath the *epineurium*.
- Peripheral nerves are supplied by blood vessels that travel longitudinally within these three layers of connective tissue.
- *Classification of peripheral nerves based on conduction velocity and thickness*:
  - Group A fibers—conduct at a velocity of 5—20 m/s. They are 1–20 µ (microns) in diameter, e.g., myelinated afferent and efferent somatic fibers. These are further subdivided into four types based on the information they carry and the tissues they innervate.
    - A-alpha fibers: They innervate extrafusal muscle fibers.
    - A-beta fibers: These contribute for cutaneous mechanoreceptors.
    - A-delta fibers are free nerve endings that conduct the sensations of pain and temperature. These carry the sensation of sharp pain.
    - A-gamma fibers are motor to intrafusal muscle fibers.
  - Group B fibers—conduct at a velocity of 3–15 m/s. They are 1–3 µ in diameter, e.g., myelinated preganglionic autonomic fibers.
  - Group C fibers—conduct at a velocity of 0.5–2.0 m/s. They are 0.5–2 µ in diameter, e.g., nonmyelinated fibers. These carry slow, long lasting pain sensations (dull and aching pain).
- *Classification of peripheral nerves based on function*: Nerves can be categorized into two groups based on function:
  1. Sensory nerves constitute 40% of peripheral nerve and conduct sensory information from their receptors to the CNS, for processing the information. They are also called "afferent nerves".
  2. Motor nerves constitute 60% of peripheral nerve and conduct signals

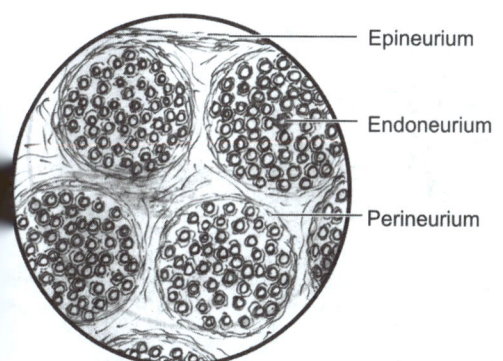

Fig. 9.18: Peripheral nerve—coverings.

from the CNS to muscles. They are also called efferent nerves. Motor fibers contain large myelinated alpha efferents that supply extrafusal muscle fibers, small myelinated gamma efferents that supply intrafusal muscle fibers and fine unmyelinated autonomic efferents that supply smooth muscle fibers in blood vessels.

- *Classification of peripheral nerves according to their connection with the CNS*: They are classified into those connected with the brain and those with the spinal cord.
- Those connected with the brain innervate the head and are known as *cranial nerves*. Those innervating the body are connected with the spinal cord through *spinal nerves*.
- *Functional components of cranial and spinal nerves* (**Figs. 9.19A to C**):
  - *Cranial nerves* have seven functional components (**Figs. 9.19A and B**)
    - General somatic efferent (GSE) that supply segmental somite derived skeletal muscles, e.g., that supplying eye ball muscles (III, IV, and VI CNs) and tongue muscles (XII CN).
    - Special visceral/branchial efferent (SVE) that supply skeletal muscles that are derived from pharyngeal arches, e.g., 1st to 5th arches that give rise to muscles of face, scalp, pharynx, larynx, and mastication (V, VII, and IX, X, XI CNs).
    - General visceral efferent (GVE) that supply smooth muscles and glands, e.g., lacrimal, salivary, etc., (III, VII, IX, and X CNs).
    - General visceral afferent (GVA) that carry visceral sensations from various viscera, e.g., X CN.
    - Special visceral afferent (SVA) that carry the sensation of taste, e.g., VII, IX, and X CNs.
    - General somatic afferent (GSA) that carry exteroceptive and proprioceptive from head and neck, e.g., V CN.

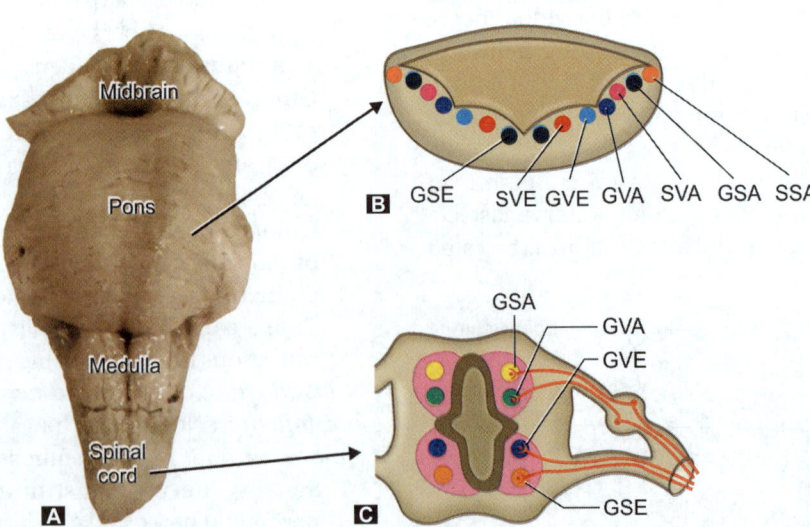

Figs. 9.19A to C: Functional components of cranial and spinal nerves. (A) Brainstem [origin of cranial nerves 3–12); (B) Cranial nerve functional components at the level of pons (see text for details)]; (C) Spinal nerve functional components (see text for details).
(GSE, general somatic efferent; SVE, special visceral efferent; GVE, general visceral efferent; GVA, general visceral afferent; SVA, special visceral afferent; GSA, general somatic afferent; SSA, special somatic afferent.

- Special somatic afferent (SSA) that carry the special sensations, e.g., smell (I CN) vision (II CN) hearing and equilibrium (VIII CN).
- Spinal nerves have four functional components **(Fig. 9.19C)**:
  - General somatic afferent (GSA)—carry the sensations from the specific dermatome and myotomic segments
  - General visceral afferent—carry the sensations from the internal organs, blood vessels and glands.
  - General somatic efferent—provides motor nerves to the skeletal muscles.
  - General visceral efferent—provides motor nerves to the smooth muscle, cardiac muscle and glands.

Neuronal Injury and its Degeneration and Regeneration

- *Causes for injury to a nerve*: Injury to nerve fiber, obstruction to blood supply and degenerative diseases can damage the cell bodies, synapses, and axons that form peripheral nerve.
- *Degenerative changes after injury*: When a nerve fiber is injured, various changes occur in the nerve fiber and nerve cell body. All these changes are together called the degenerative changes. The degenerative changes are of two types, i.e., (1) retrograde and (2) anterograde.

Retrograde Degeneration

- Chromatolysis within 48 hours of injury. This causes disintegration and disappearance of Nissl bodies.
- Swelling of the cell and eccentric migration of nucleus.
- Regrowth of axon in proximal segment.

Anterograde (Wallerian) Degeneration

- Degeneration distal to the site of injury.
- It starts within 24 hours of injury.
- Swelling and breakdown of axons forming myelin sheath fragments and neuronal debris.
- Neurilemmal sheath is unaffected.
- But the Schwann cells multiply rapidly. Macrophages invade from outside and remove the debris of axis cylinder and fat droplets of disintegrated myelin sheath. All these changes take place for about 2 months from the day of injury.

Regeneration

- It is the process of regrowth of lost part of a neuron.
- The injured and degenerated nerve fiber can regenerate.
- The neuronal debris and myelin sheath fragments are phagocytosed by microglia.
- Proliferation of neighboring astrocytes replaces the damaged neuron and form scar tissue.
- Regeneration from injury in a peripheral nerve is possible because of the presence of neurilemmal sheath and endoneural tubes.
- It starts as early as 4th day after injury and reaches the peak by 30th day and is completed in 80 days.
- The gap between the cut ends of the nerve should not be more than 3 mm for regeneration to take place. The neurilemma and nucleus should be intact and the cut ends should be in the same line.

AUTONOMIC NERVOUS SYSTEM

- It is the part of nervous system that controls the involuntary activities of internal organs, i.e., stomach, liver, intestines, kidneys, urinary bladder, lungs, heart, sweat, and salivary glands, etc., The activities include salivation, sweating, blood pressure, heart rate, water and electrolyte balance, respiration, body temperature, intestinal peristalsis, digestion, urination, defecation, etc., It stimulates cardiac muscle, smooth muscle and many glands.
- The two subdivisions of the ANS are sympathetic and parasympathetic.

Clinical Importance of Peripheral Nerve

AN7.5: Describe principle of sensory and motor innervation of muscles.
AN 7.6: Describe concept of loss of innervation of a muscle.

- *Nerve irritation:*
  - Irritation of motor nerve—causes muscle spasm.
  - Irritation of sensory nerve—mild irritation of a sensory nerve causes tingling and numbness. If severe it causes pain along the distribution of the nerve.
- *Damage to a nerve:*
  - Damage to motor nerve—causes paralysis of muscles.
  - Damage to a sensory nerve—causes localized anesthesia and analgesia.
  - Damage to a mixed nerve—results in both the sensory and motor losses.
- *Nerve injury*—different types and terms used **(Figs. 9.20A to D):**
  - Neuropraxia (demyelination)—minimal lesion with temporary functional loss (motor and sensory) without nerve degeneration. Here nerve sheath (Schwann cell and endoneurium) and axon are intact. Recovery is spontaneous and complete, e.g., compression of radial nerve due to faulty posture resulting in wrist drop; sudden stretching of nerves in fractures/dislocations. This type of lesion is more common in athletes.
  - Axonotmesis (demyelination + axon loss)—is a more significant lesion where axon and myelin sheath are damaged. But nerve sheath (Schwann cell and endoneurium) is intact. Although continuity is preserved, true Wallerian degeneration occurs. Regeneration takes place in due course, e.g., traction and crush injuries.
  - Neurotmesis (demyelination + axon loss + endoneurium loss)—is the complete division of a nerve. It is a more severe injury. Complete crushing of nerve with disruption of axon, Schwann cell and endoneurial sheath. For regeneration to occur the cut ends must be sutured.
- *Nerve pain (neuralgia):* Pain along the distribution of a nerve is called *neuralgia*. e.g. *intercostal neuralgia* (pain along the distribution of an intercostal nerve), *trigeminal neuralgia* (pain along the distribution of trigeminal nerve).
- *Nerve inflammation (neuritis):* Inflammation of a nerve is called *neuritis*. The symptoms may include pain, weakness (paresis), sensation of pins and needles (paresthesia), anesthesia, paralysis, etc.
  - Neurological examination—neurologists diagnose nerve disorders by testing the reflexes, muscle weakness, cutaneous sensations followed by nerve conduction study, electromyography and CT scan, and MRI.

Both sympathetic and parasympathetic systems innervate the organs. They act as antagonists. For example, sympathetic stimulation increases the heart rate, while parasympathetic stimulation reduces it.
- To maintain equilibrium for optimal functioning of the organs the two systems are to be complimentary to each other and work in coordinated fashion. The sympathetic activities are for fighting the emergency situations and are widespread/diffuse. The parasympathetic activities are for providing comfortable environment and are isolated/discrete.

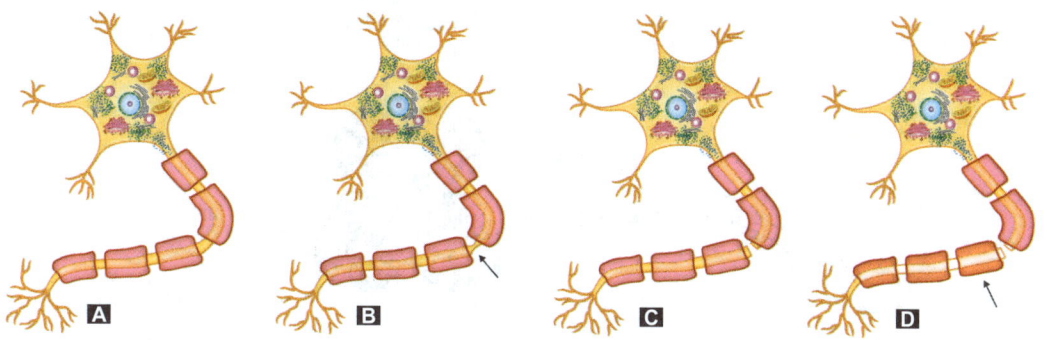

Figs. 9.20A to D: Types of nerve injury. (A) Normal; (B) Neuropraxia; (C) Axanotmesis; (D) Neurotmesis.

- The components of the autonomic pathway are:
  - Preganglionic neuron in CNS (brainstem or spinal cord).
  - Preganglionic fibers: These are usually myelinated.
  - Ganglia (collections of nerve cell bodies) for relay of preganglionic fibers. These are located outside CNS. Majority of the ganglia of sympathetic system are on either side of spinal cord. The ganglia of parasympathetic system are near or in the organs with which they connect.
  - Postganglionic fibers connect with internal organs (smooth muscle, glands, etc.). These are unmyelinated fibers.
- The difference between somatic and autonomic system is that the somatic system has the somatic nerves reaching the site of distribution without intermediary ganglia.

Sympathetic Nervous System (Fig. 9.21)

It extends from T1 to L2/3 segments of spinal cord. Hence, it is also called *thoracolumbar outflow*. Myelinated preganglionic fibers arise from the lateral horn of spinal cord present in the T1 to L2/3 regions of spinal cord. These travel through the ventral roots of spinal nerves and relay in the lateral ganglia of sympathetic chain located on either side of spinal cord in paravertebral region or in the collateral ganglia that located near the organs (e.g. celiac or renal ganglia). The unmyelinated postganglionic fibers arising from either the lateral or collateral ganglia run for some distance to reach the target organ.

The preganglionic fibers innervating sweat glands, hair and smooth muscle of cutaneous blood vessels traveling in the ventral root of spinal nerve enter the sympathetic trunk through white ramus communicantes and relays in the sympathetic ganglion. From the ganglion starts the unmyelinated postganglionic fibers and join the mixed spinal nerve by way of gray ramus communicans to reach the effector organ through branches of the peripheral nerve.

Parasympathetic Nervous System (Figs. 9.22A and B)

It is also known as craniosacral outflow as it has a cranial and a sacral part. The cranial part arises from the brainstem (III, VII, IX, and X cranial nerve nuclei) and the sacral part arises from the 2nd to 4th sacral segments of the spinal cord.

The preganglionic fibers travel a longer distance to reach the target viscera. The ganglia are located in the viscera and are called terminal ganglia. The postganglionic fibers are very short.

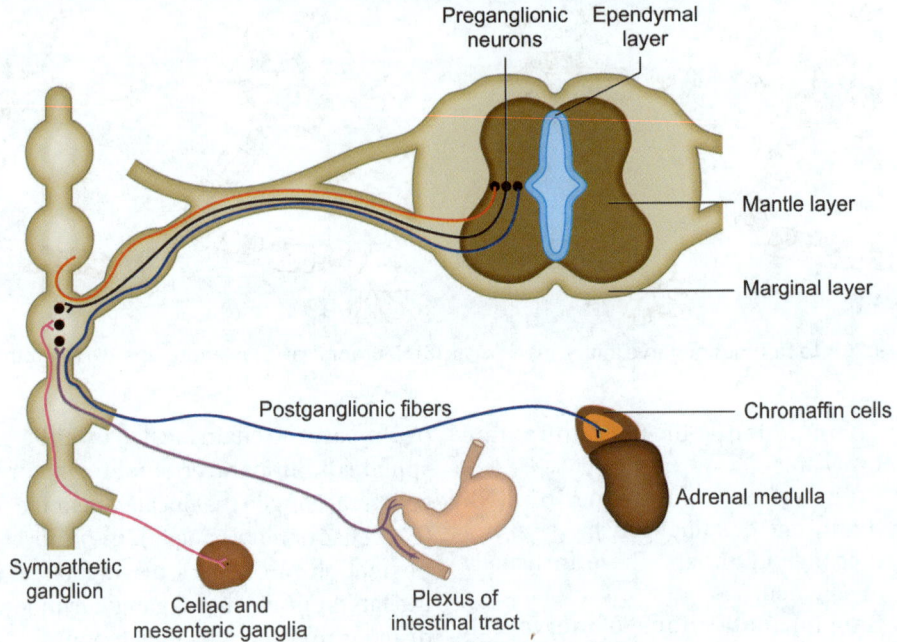

Fig. 9.21: Sympathetic nervous system.

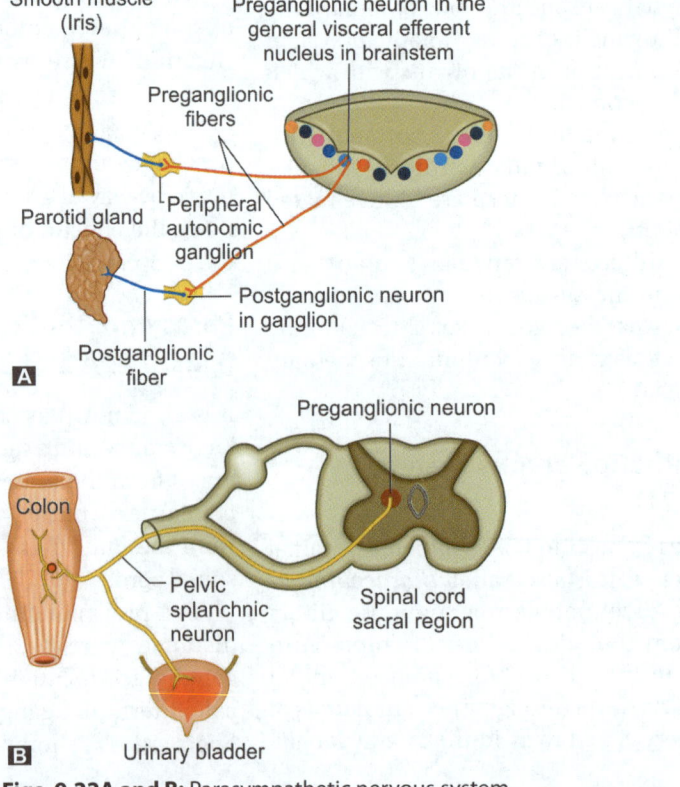

Figs. 9.22A and B: Parasympathetic nervous system.

Chapter 9: Introduction to Nervous System

Anatomical Basis for Clinical Condition

Case Scenario

Problem: A 30-year-old person complaints of frequent episodes of the following symptoms with normal health in between for the past 5 years:
- Tingling and numbness of face and fingers
- Fatigue and weakness
- Muscle stiffness
- Frequent urination and inability to control the bladder movements
- Blurring of vision
- Slurred speech.

Questions:

1. What could be the probable diagnosis?
2. What investigations will be ordered by the attending physician to confirm the diagnosis?
3. What could be the probable anatomical explanation for this condition?

Anatomical explanation:

1. The probable diagnosis is relapsing and remitting multiple sclerosis.
2. The investigations that are to be advised are:
    - Blood tests to rule out other causes for the condition.
    - Spinal tap to find out abnormal antibodies in cerebrospinal fluid.
    - Magnetic resonance imaging (MRI) of brain and spinal cord to find out areas with lesions.
    - Evoked potential tests to record the electrical signals produced by brain in response to stimuli.
3. It is an autoimmune disease with a cause unknown. The disease is caused by inflammation of nerves resulting in damage to the myelin sheath which plays an important role in the conduction of nerve impulse for appropriate response to a stimulus. Damage to the myelin sheath causes slowing of impulse conduction or even stoppage of nerve impulse leading to neurological problems. The severity of neurological problems depends on the severity of the disease, part of nervous system affected. It varies from mild to severe physical disability, impaired speech, vision, etc.

☞ Key Concept

Take Home Message—Nervous System

- The nervous system is broadly divided into central nervous system (CNS) and peripheral nervous system (PNS).
- The CNS is broadly divided into brain and spinal cord. The PNS consists of 12 pairs of cranial nerves, 31 pairs of spinal nerves that are connected to brain and spinal cord.
- The nervous tissue is classified into excitable neuron and nonexcitable neuroglia.

Contd...

Contd...

- The parts of a neuron are cell body, a single long process the axon and the short, multiple processes the dendrites.
- Collections of nerve cell bodies with in CNS are called nuclei whereas the same outside the CNS are called ganglia.
- The neurons are classified based on their function into motor and sensory. Based on number of processes they are classified into unipolar, bipolar, and multipolar. Majority of the neurons are multipolar.
- The axons of neurons unite to form tracts in CNS and peripheral nerves in PNS.
- Peripheral nerves contain various functional components that will differ in cranial and spinal nerves.
- Basic sensations from external and internal environment are received by specialized cells called receptors. Majority of receptors are located in the dermis.
- Reflex arc is the basic functional unit of nervous system and consists of a receptor, sensory neuron, interneuron, motor neuron, and an effector.
- Myelination of axon in CNS is by oligodendrocytes and in the PNS by Schwann cells.
- Myelination of the nerve fibers facilitates conduction of nerve impulse.

QUESTIONS

1. Structure of neuron.
2. Classification of neurons.
3. Neuroglia.
4. Myelin sheath.
5. Process of myelination.
6. Peripheral nerve.
7. Formation of a nerve plexus.
8. Reflex arc.

MULTIPLE CHOICE QUESTIONS

1. Myelination of nerves in central nervous system is by:
   A. Schwann cells
   B. Microglia
   C. Oligodendrocytes
   D. Protoplasmic astrocytes

2. Bipolar neurons are seen in:
   A. Sympathetic ganglia
   B. Dorsal root ganglion
   C. Retina
   D. Spinal cord

3. Nissl granules are absent in:
   A. Cell body
   B. Axon
   C. Dendrites
   D. Axon hillock

4. Central nervous system contains all the following types of neuroglia, *except:*
   A. Astrocytes
   B. Oligodendrocytes
   C. Satellite cells
   D. Microglia

ANSWERS

1. C   2. C   3. D   4. C

CHAPTER 10

Introduction to Splanchnology

Competencies:
This chapter is a preliminary introduction to various organ systems that will be studied in the gross anatomy under various relevant system-wise competencies.

LEARNING OBJECTIVES

- Definition of splanchnology
- Introduction to respiratory system—subdivisions
- Introduction to digestive system
- Introduction to urinary system
- Introduction to male genital system
- Introduction to female genital system
- Introduction to endocrine system

INTRODUCTION

The term *splanchno* is derived from Greek, meaning "viscera". *Splanchnology* is the study of visceral organs, i.e., respiratory, digestive, urogenital, nervous, circulatory, and endocrine system.

The various cavities of the body are **(Fig. 10.1)**:
- *Dorsal cavities*: Cranial and vertebral cavities where the brain and spinal cord are located and they are organs of nervous system.
- *Ventral cavities*: The thoracic cavity containing the heart with surrounding

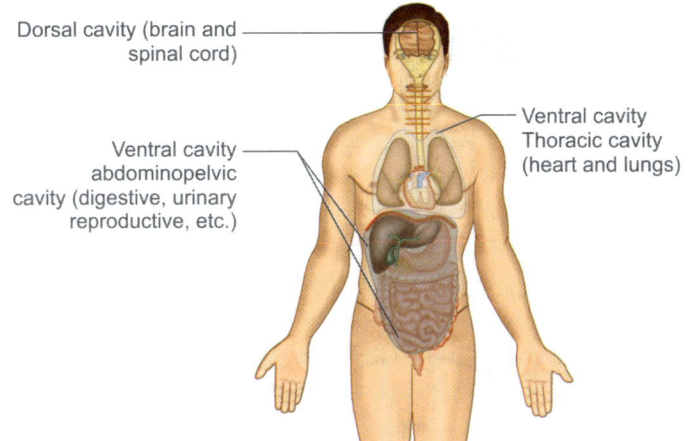

Fig. 10.1: Cavities of the body.

pericardium in the mediastinum and the two lungs enclosed by the serous membrane, the pleura. The abdominopelvic cavity contains the organs of various systems, i.e., digestive, urinary, reproductive, and endocrine systems. Some of them are enclosed by the serous membrane the peritoneum on all sides (e.g., stomach). Those not enclosed by the peritoneum on all sides are called retroperitoneal organs (e.g., kidney). To understand the location of the organs of the abdominopelvic cavity it is divided into nine quadrants [*detailed description in Surface Anatomy (Chapter 12)*].

To provide a comprehensive view of the whole body this chapter was included giving basic details. In-depth understanding of these organs will be provided in the textbooks of regional anatomy.

In this chapter the viscera are organized system wise.

- Respiratory system
- Digestive system
- Urinary system
- Genital system
- Endocrines.

RESPIRATORY SYSTEM (FIG. 10.2)

- The respiratory system works along with the circulatory system to provide oxygen and to remove the waste products of metabolism from the tissues. It also regulates pH (acid-base balance) of the blood.
- Parts of respiratory system are used for sensing the smell, for the production of sound (speech), for staining during coughing, defecation and child birth.
- It consists of pair of lungs and a series of air passages that extend to and from the lungs.
- *Subdivisions of respiratory system*:
  - *Upper respiratory tract*:
    - Nose
    - Nasal cavity
    - Paranasal air sinuses
    - Pharynx
    - Larynx
  - *Lower respiratory tract*:
    - Trachea
    - Bronchi
    - Terminal bronchioles
    - Respiratory bronchioles In lungs
    - Alveolar ducts
    - Alveoli.

The line of demarcation between the two is the vocal cord.

Nose: It is the beginning of respiratory system/passage. It is an organ for sense of smell as olfactory receptors are located in the upper part of nasal cavity. Upper part is lined by olfactory mucosa and the rest of nasal cavity by respiratory mucosa. Nose is divided into two main parts—*external nose* and *nasal*

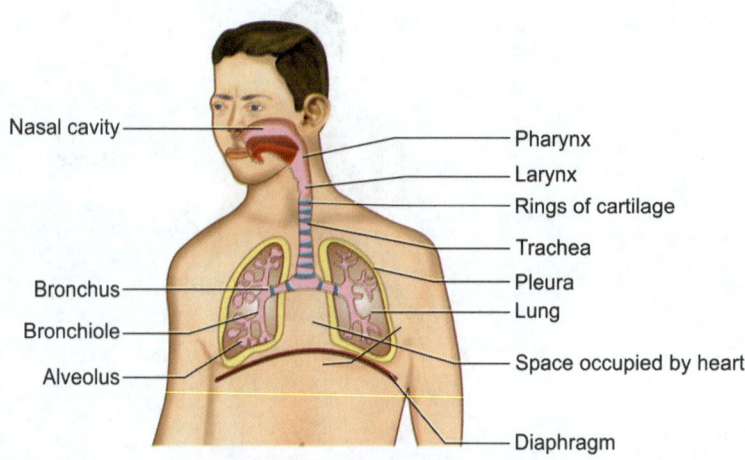

Fig. 10.2: Respiratory system—parts.

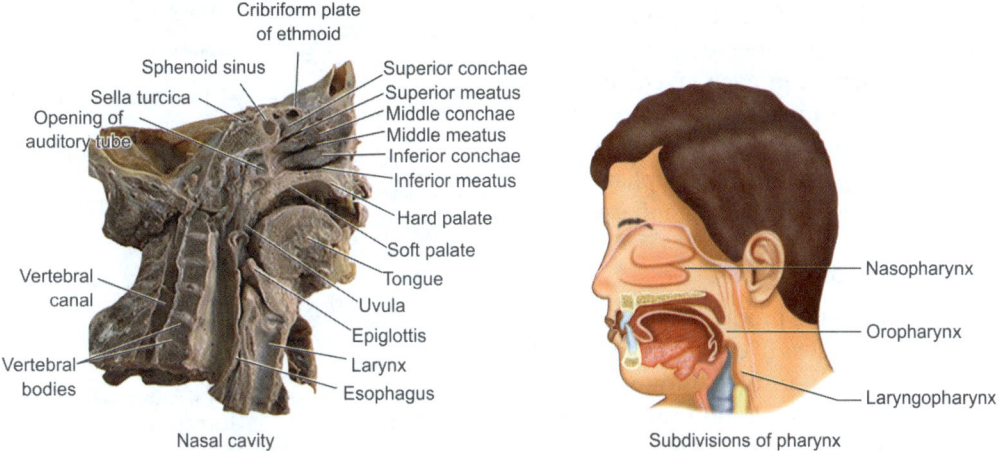

Fig. 10.3: Pharynx—subdivisions.

cavity. External nose is partly bony and partly cartilaginous.

Nasal cavity (**Fig. 10.3**): It is a pear-shaped irregular space and is divided into right and left halves by nasal septum. The nasal cavity has *a roof, floor, medial, and lateral walls.* Each half of nasal cavity is separated from the other by a partition called nasal septum (medial wall). The nasal septum is cartilaginous anteriorly and osseous posteriorly. The middle part of roof is separated from the cranial cavity by a thin bone (cribriform plate of ethmoid). Floor of nasal cavity is formed by hard palate (osseous) and separates it from the oral cavity. Lateral wall is irregular due to the presence of three curved bony projections called conchae (superior, middle, and inferior). Meatuses are the passages beneath concha which communicates with nasal cavity proper. Meatuses are three in number—(1) superior, (2) middle and (3) inferior. The paranasal sinuses and nasolacrimal duct open into these meatuses.

Paranasal air sinuses (**Fig. 10.4**): The paranasal air sinuses are *the* air filled spaces present with in the frontal, ethmoid, sphenoid and maxilla bones. These are of different sizes and communicate with nasal cavity through lateral wall of nose. Mucous membrane lining the paranasal air sinuses is respiratory epithelium. Anatomy of paranasal sinuses is

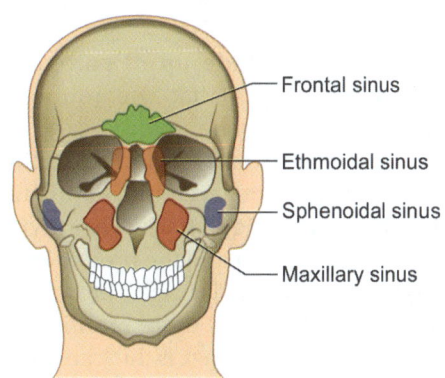

Fig. 10.4: Paranasal air sinuses.

important as they lighten the bones of face and add resonance to the voice.

Pharynx: It is a common muscular tube for digestive and respiratory systems. It is situated behind nose, mouth, and larynx. It is divided into three parts from cranial to caudal (**Fig. 10.3**).

They are:
1. Nasopharynx—transmits only air. It is the continuation of nasal cavity. The auditory tubes open into this part.
2. Oropharynx—transmits both food and air. The paired palatine tonsils are located in its lateral wall.
3. Laryngopharynx: It is inferior to oropharynx and behind the larynx. It directs the air and ingested food into respiratory and digestive passages respectively.

The musculature of the pharynx is arranged as outer circular and inner longitudinal layers with three muscles in each layer. The outer circular layer of muscles are the superior, middle, and inferior constrictors. The inner longitudinal muscles are the stylopharyngeus, palatopharyngeus, and salpingopharyngeus.

Larynx (or) Voice Box

It is an organ for the production of voice (or) phonation. It consists of cartilages and elastic membranes. It is part of respiratory system and acts as sphincter at the inlet of lower respiratory passage. It lies in anterior midline of neck and extends from root of tongue to trachea. It shows sex differences in position and size.

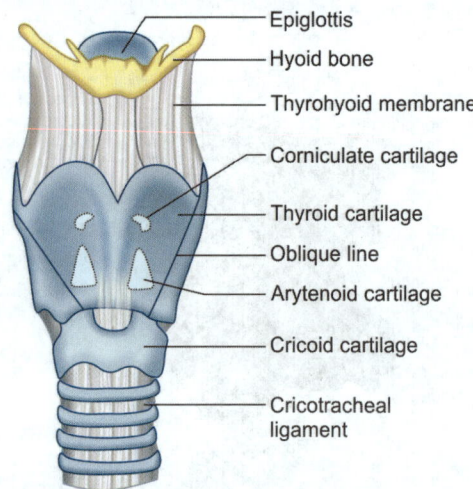

Fig. 10.5: Larynx—cartilages.

The larynx is made up of paired and unpaired cartilages that are joined by membranes. The three unpaired cartilages are thyroid, cricoid, and epiglottis. The three paired cartilages are arytenoid, corniculate and cuneiform **(Fig. 10.5)**. The thyroid cartilage is the largest and the prominence it makes in males is called laryngeal prominence or *Adam's apple*. This is more prominent in males. The cricoid cartilage is thick and forms a ring. The three smaller, paired cartilages—the arytenoids, corniculates, and cuneiforms attach to the epiglottis and the vocal cords. The muscles of larynx are divided into extrinsic and intrinsic muscles that facilitate movement of the mucosal folds of larynx, and cartilages of larynx in producing sounds and in the passage of air. The interior of larynx is lined by mucosa.

The cavity of larynx extends from inlet to lower border of cricoid cartilage. The inlet of the larynx is bound by epiglottis, arytenoid cartilages and aryepiglottic folds. The cavity is divided by two folds of mucous membrane (cranial vestibular and caudal vocal folds). The space between the vestibular (false vocal cords) is called rima vestibuli. The space between the vocal folds (true vocal cords) is the narrowest part of larynx and is called rima glottides **(Fig. 10.6)**.

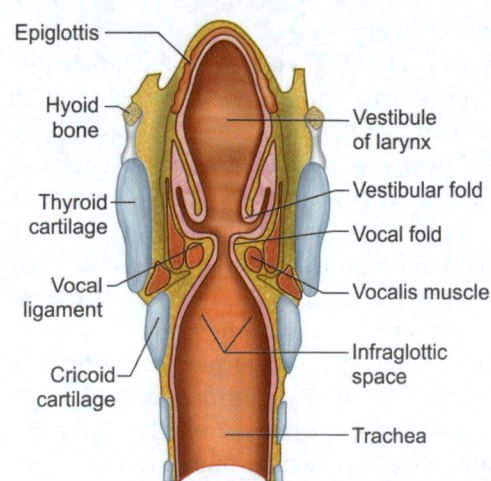

Fig. 10.6: Larynx—cavity.

Trachea (Wind Pipe) (Figs. 10.7A and B)

It is a wide noncollapsible tube that serves to conduct air to and from the lungs for respiration. It begins at the lower border of cricoid cartilage opposite to C6 vertebra. It passes downwards in the midline into the superior mediastinum of thorax. At the level of T5 vertebra it divides into right and left principal bronchi. Wall of trachea is made up of fibromuscular tissue and is supported by 16–20 "C"-shaped cartilaginous rings that are deficient posteriorly to allow distension of esophagus during swallowing.

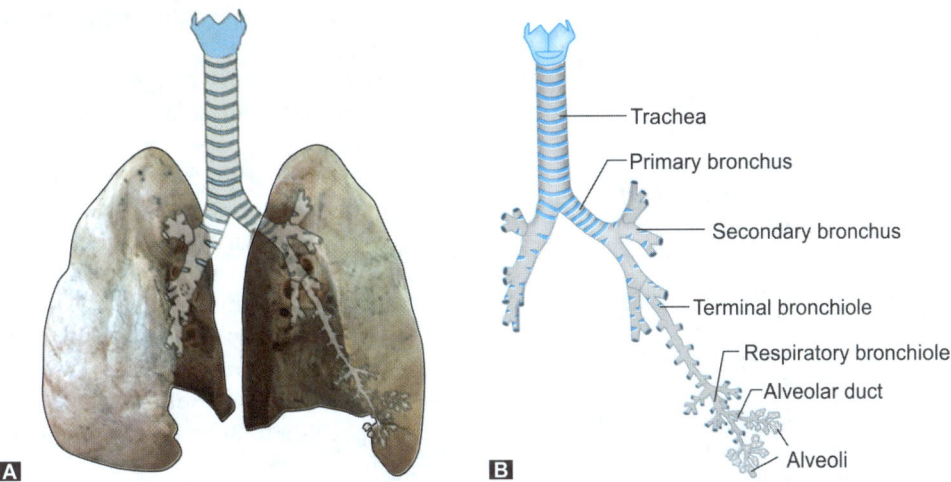

Figs. 10.7A and B: Respiratory system—trachea, bronchial tree, and lungs.

Bronchi, Bronchioles, Alveolar Ducts, Alveolar Sacs and Alveoli (Figs. 10.7A and B)

- After a short course each bronchus enters the hilum of respective lung and divides into *lobar bronchi* for three lobes in right lung and two lobes in left lung.
- Each lobar bronchus divides into segmental or *tertiary bronchi*.
- The subdivisions of tertiary bronchus are called *bronchioles* that divide and give rise to *terminal bronchioles*.
- Terminal bronchioles branch to form *respiratory bronchioles*.
- Each respiratory bronchiole gives rise to *alveolar ducts* which in turn lead to *alveolar sacs*.
- Each alveolar sac shows the sacculated alveoli in its walls. The alveoli are the site where actual gaseous exchange takes place and are the functional units of lung.

Lungs (Figs. 10.7A and B)

- The lungs are a pair of spongy, air-filled respiratory organs located on either side of the chest (thorax). The lungs are covered by a thin tissue layer called the pleura. There are two layers of pleura called parietal and visceral with a potential space in between the two called the pleural cavity.
- Right and left lung are separated by the mediastinum. In young age they are brown in color and in adults they are mottled black due to the deposition of inhaled carbon particles.
- *Parts*: Each lung is conical in shape having an apex, base, three borders (anterior, posterior and inferior) and two surfaces (costal and medial).
- Hilum of lung is a large depressed area that lies near the center of the medial surface. Various structures enter and leave the lung via its root.
- *Fissures and lobes of lungs*: The right lung is divided by two fissures (oblique and horizontal) into three lobes. The left lung is divided by a single oblique fissure into two lobes. Each lobe is divided into bronchopulmonary segments. There are 10 bronchopulmonary segments in each lung.

Clinical Importance of Respiratory System

- *Rhinitis* is inflammation of nasal mucosa.
- *Rhinorrhea* is a condition where the nasal cavity is filled with a significant amount of mucus fluid.
- *Sinusitis* is inflammation of paranasal air sinuses.

- *Pharyngitis* is inflammation of pharynx.
- *Laryngitis* is inflammation of larynx. It causes hoarseness of voice.
- *Tracheostomy* is a surgical procedure to create an opening in the neck for direct access to the trachea. It is performed in cases of airway obstruction.
- *CSF leak through nose*: Fracture of cribriform plate of ethmoid bone that forms the roof of nasal cavity causes leakage of cerebrospinal fluid into the nasal cavity. Spread of nasal infection into the cranial cavity occurs through the apertures in the roof.
- *Surgical approach to pituitary gland* is through the posterior part of roof.

DIGESTIVE SYSTEM (FIG. 10.8)

- The digestive system includes all those structures that are concerned with swallowing, digestion, and absorption of food. The system consists of an alimentary canal which starts at the mouth and ends at the anus.
- Each of the organs of digestive system has specific location, shape, structure, and function.
- The organs of digestive system can be broadly categorized into those of tubular gastrointestinal tract and the glands associated with the gastrointestinal tract. These are classified into:
  - Organs of gastrointestinal tract or hollow organs—have a lumen and a wall made up of four layers with a specific structural arrangement to suite to the function.
  - Organs associated with gastrointestinal tract or parenchymal organs.

Parts of Gastrointestinal Tract

Mouth or Oral Cavity **(Fig. 10.9)**

- Digestive system begins with oral cavity.
- Ingestion of food and its fragmentation into small pieces (bolus) by teeth and

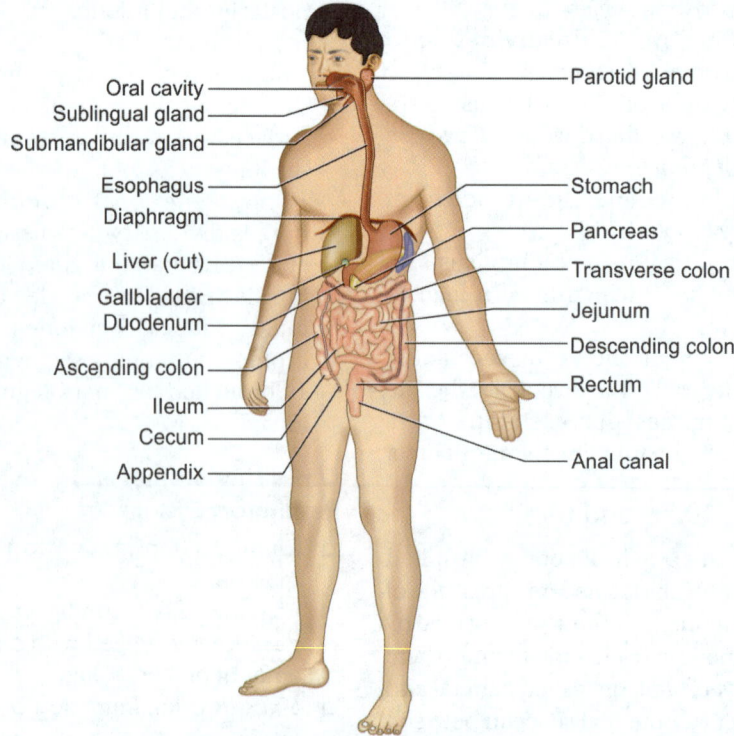

Fig. 10. 8: Digestive system—parts.

Chapter 10: Introduction to Splanchnology

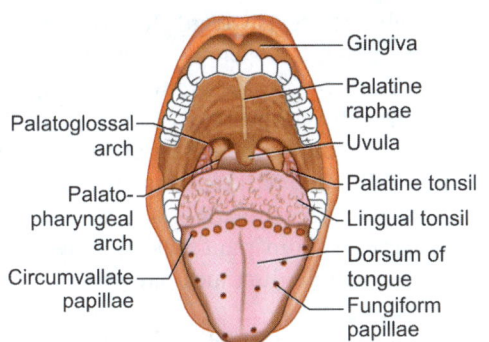

Fig. 10.9: Mouth—parts.

moistening by saliva secreted from major salivary glands takes place in the oral cavity.
- The mucous membrane lining the oral cavity (oral mucosa) is lined by stratified squamous nonkeratinized epithelium supported by lamina propria of loose connective tissue containing minor salivary glands.
- The external opening of the mouth is the *oral fissure* and is bounded by the upper and lower lips.
- Within the mouth cavity (or *oral cavity*) there are the *teeth* for chewing food; and the *tongue* which helps the processes of chewing and swallowing in addition to being an organ of taste.
- The roof of the mouth is formed by the *palate* (which separates the mouth from the nasal cavities).
- Posteriorly, the mouth opens into the *oral part of the pharynx* that is continuous, below, with the *esophagus*.

Wall of Gastrointestinal Tract (Fig. 10.10)

- The gastrointestinal tract is a muscular tube lined with mucosa.
- The structure of tube is similar from esophagus to anal canal with minor variations in the arrangement of muscular components and marked changes in the mucosa in different parts.
- Its wall consists of four main layers enclosing the lumen.
- From lumen to periphery they are: (1) mucosa, (2) submucosa, (3) muscularis externa, and (4) serosa or adventitia.

Esophagus

It is a muscular tube that passes through lower part of neck, thorax, and pierces the diaphragm to enter the abdomen. Hence, it has cervical, thoracic and abdominal parts.

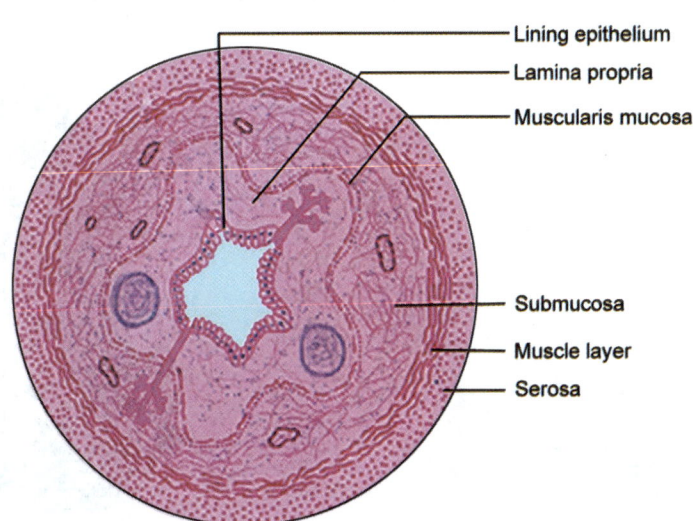

Fig. 10.10: Structure of wall of gastrointestinal tract.

The thoracic part is the longest and the abdominal part is the shortest that continues as the stomach.

Stomach **(Fig. 10.11)**

- The stomach is a large sac-like organ located in the left hypochondriac and epigastric regions.
- It is usually J-shaped. It presents two ends (esophageal and duodenal), two curvatures (lesser and greater), two surfaces (anterosuperior and posteroinferior) and has three parts (fundus, body, and pylorus).
- Its wall presents four layers. The duodenal end continues into duodenum of small intestine.
  - *Fundus*: It is dome-shaped and is filled with gas in the upright body position.
  - *Body*: It is the largest part of the stomach. It presents the lesser curvature and the greater curvature.
  - *Pyloric part*: It is the caudal part of stomach that is perpendicular to the long axis of the stomach. The pylorus sphincter marks the end of the stomach and is the entrance to the duodenum.

Small Intestine **(Fig. 10.12)**

- The three parts of small intestine are: (1) duodenum, (2) jejunum, and (3) ileum. It is about 20 feet in length. It is continuous with large intestine.
- Duodenum is 10 inches in length, C-shaped. Within the concavity of the C is the head of pancreas. It presents four parts. The 2nd part receives the bile from the liver and gallbladder and pancreatic secretions from pancreas by means of common bile duct and pancreatic duct respectively.
- The mesentery of small intestine suspends most of it from the posterior abdominal wall.
- Structurally the mucosa of small intestine is thrown into folds called the villi to increase the surface area for absorption. The protection from the toxins and microorganisms that were ingested with food is by the presence of lymphatic aggregations the *Peyer's patches* in ileum.

Large Intestine

The major parts of large intestine are cecum and appendix, colon (subdivided into ascending, transverse, descending, and sigmoid colon), rectum, and anal canal. The rectum is continuous with anal canal that opens to the exterior at the anal opening. The mucosa of large intestine is rich in mucus secreting goblet cells that protect the mucosa from the abrasion by rough particles of digestion.

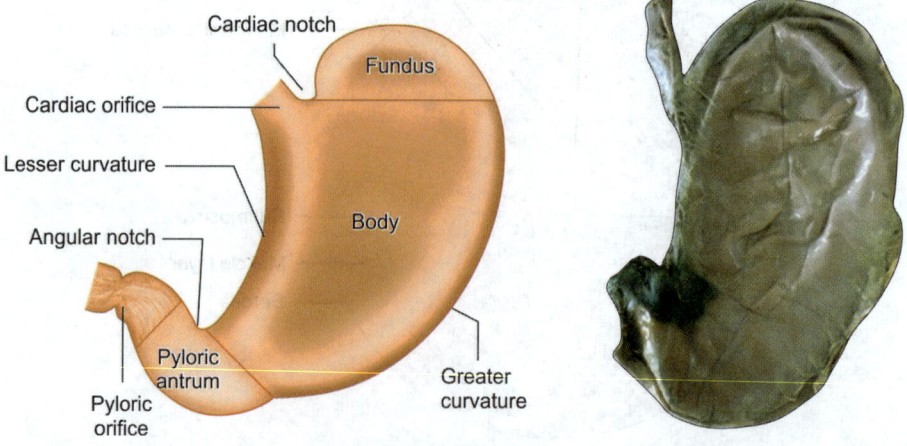

Fig. 10.11: Stomach—parts.

Chapter 10: Introduction to Splanchnology

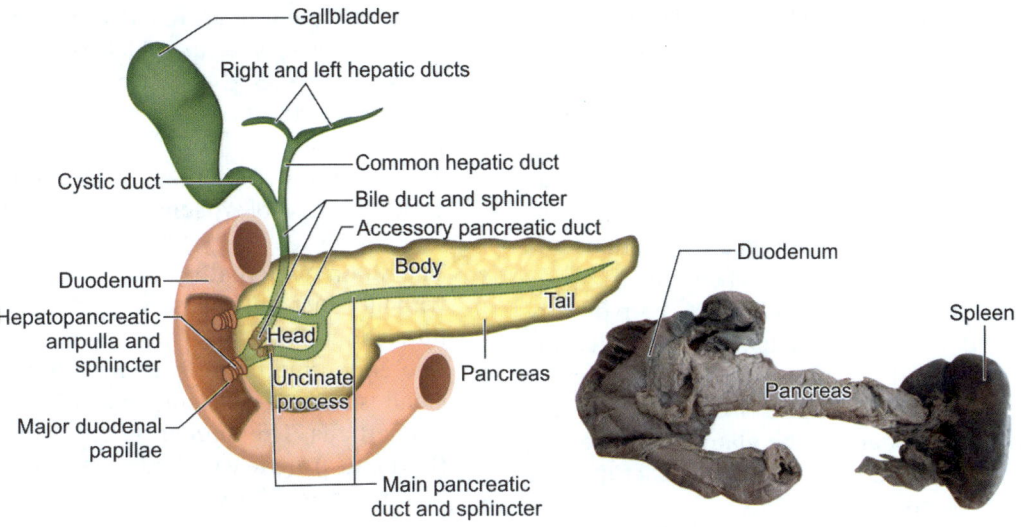

Fig. 10.12: Duodenum and pancreas.

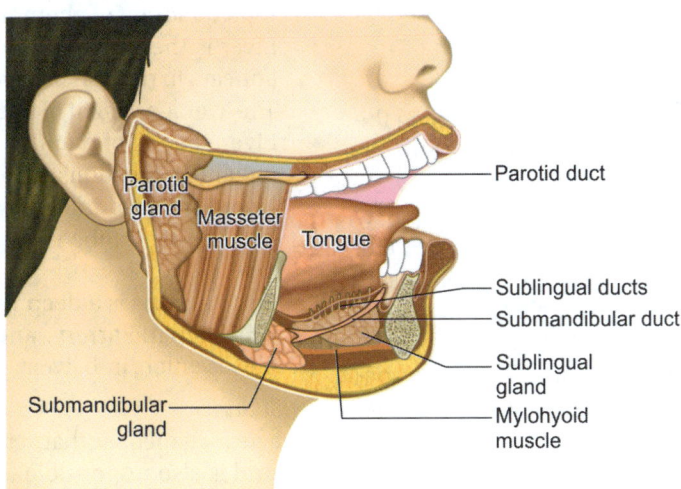

Fig. 10.13: Salivary glands.

Accessory Organs Associated with Alimentary Canal

Closely related to the alimentary canal there are several accessory organs. There are three accessory digestive glands in gastrointestinal tract (**Figs. 10.12 to 10.14**):
1. Salivary glands
2. Pancreas
3. Liver.

Salivary glands (**Fig. 10.13**): In the region of the mouth there are three pairs of *salivary glands*. Around the oral cavity there are three pairs of salivary glands which produce a fluid called *saliva* that helps to keep the oral cavity moist. They are:
1. Parotid glands
2. Submandibular glands
3. Sublingual glands.

In addition to these there are many small glands in tongue, palate, and lips. These glands maintain the oral cavity moisture.
- *Parotid gland*: These are largest salivary glands. It is situated below the external acoustic meatus. It appears like three-dimensional pyramid. The parotid duct carries the parotid gland secretions and opens into vestibule of mouth.
- *Submandibular gland*: A pair of sub-mandibular salivary glands which are located on either side just below the mandible. It appears like a size of wall nut and J-shaped. The glandular secretions are drained by Wharton's duct into the floor of the oral cavity.
- *Sublingual salivary glands*: These are the small glands. It consists of many ducts that will directly open into the floor of the mouth on the summit of the sublingual folds.

Pancreas (Fig. 10.12):
- It is a large glandular organ located in the abdominal cavity close to the stomach and duodenum.
- The pancreas is the gland that is partly endocrine and partly exocrine. The exocrine part produces pancreatic juices and endocrine glands produces hormones.
- It is soft elongated gland located trans-versely across the posterior abdominal wall.
- It is retort-shaped structure and presents head, neck, body, and tail.
- The enlarged right end called the *head*. Next to head is the short constricted *neck*. The neck is continuous with the *body* at the left extremity of which is the *tail*.
- The head of the pancreas is C-shaped and lies within the curve of duodenum.
- Neck of the pancreas is constricted part of the pancreas.
- The body of pancreas is elongated and extent in between neck and tail.
- The tail of the pancreas lies in between the folds of peritoneum along the splenic vessels.
- Exocrine tissue is arranged into small masses known as "acini" which produces digestive enzymes. The exocrine secretions are transported to duodenum through pancreatic ducts.
- The exocrine pancreas is drain by pancreatic duct of Wirsung and accessory ducts.
- The main pancreatic duct combines with bile duct and opens into 2nd part of duodenum.
- The endocrine tissue is in the form of small islands of cells known as islets of Langerhans. The endocrine secretions (hormones) are released into the adjcent blood vessels.

Liver (Fig. 10.14):
- Liver is the wedge-shaped large gland in the body and it is situated in the upper right quadrant of abdominal cavity.
- Liver is the soft and friable organ which appears in reddish brown in color.
- The average weight of liver is 1,500 g.
- Liver secrets bile and performs various metabolic functions.
- Liver is divided into two lobes; right and left. The right lobe is larger than the left lobe.
- Porta hepatis is a deep fissure, the portal vein, hepatic artery, and hepatic nerve plexus enters into liver.

Gallbladder:
It is a pear-shaped sac that acts as a reservoir of bile and is also responsible for concentration of bile. It is situated in the fossa on the inferior surface of right lobe of liver. It presents the parts fundus, body, and neck. Fundus is the lower expanded free end. The neck is continuous with cystic duct. The cystic duct joins with common hepatic duct to form bile duct.

> **Clinical Importance of Digestive System**
> - *Gastritis*: Inflammation of stomach
> - *Duodenal ulcers*: These are more common in the first part of duodenum as this part is more exposed to the acid secretions of the stomach.

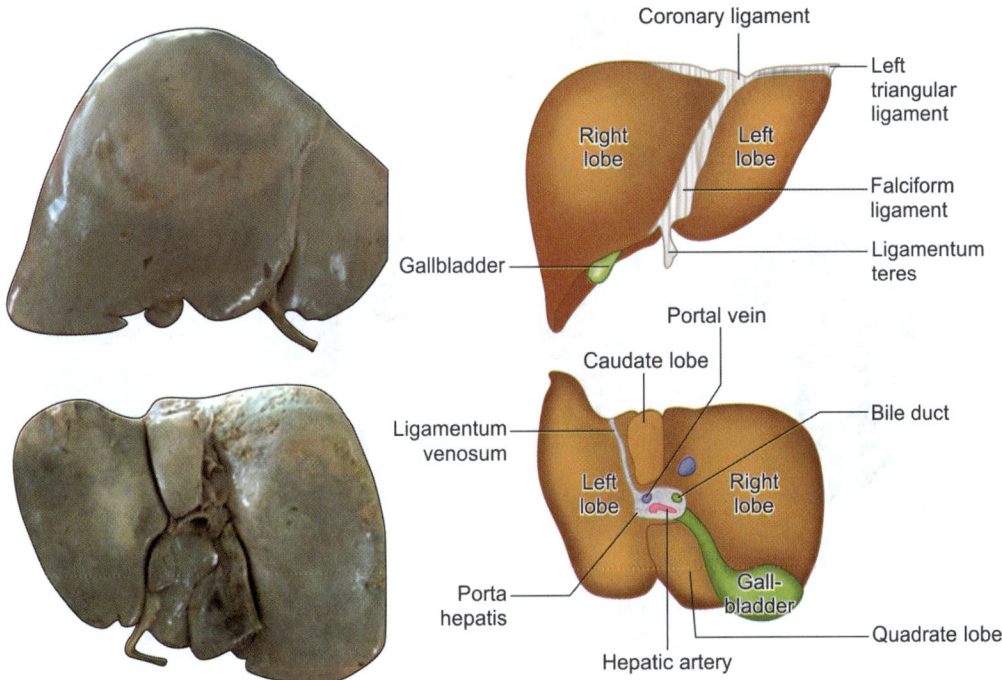

Fig. 10.14: Liver.

- *Enteritis*: Inflammation of small intestine.
- *Colitis*: Inflammation of colon.
- *Appendicitis*: Inflammation of vermiform appendix.
- *Hepatitis*: Inflammation of liver.
- *Cholecystitis*: Inflammation of gallbladder.
- *Cholelithiasis*: Stone formation in gallbladder.

URINARY SYSTEM

This system is concerned with the organs of the body that are concerned with formation of urine and its elimination from the body. Urine is formed in the right and left *kidneys* which lie on the posterior wall of the abdomen. This urine passes through narrow tubes, the right and left *ureters*, to reach a sac-like reservoir called the *urinary bladder*. The urinary bladder lies in the true pelvis. It is connected to the exterior by a tube called the *urethra* (Fig. 10.15).

Kidneys

- The kidneys lie obliquely on the posterior abdominal wall behind the peritoneum (retroperitoneal organs), on either side of vertebral column, under cover of the costal margin.
- Each kidney is bean-shaped having a convex border (lateral) and a concave border hilum (medial).
- Hilum transmits the renal vessels and nerves and the renal pelvis (beginning of ureter) anteroposteriorly.
- Hilum of the right kidney lies just below, and that of left kidney lies just above the transpyloric plane 5 cm (2 inches) from the midline.
- The kidneys extend from the level of last thoracic (T12) to the third lumbar (L3) vertebrae and the rib cage partially protects them.

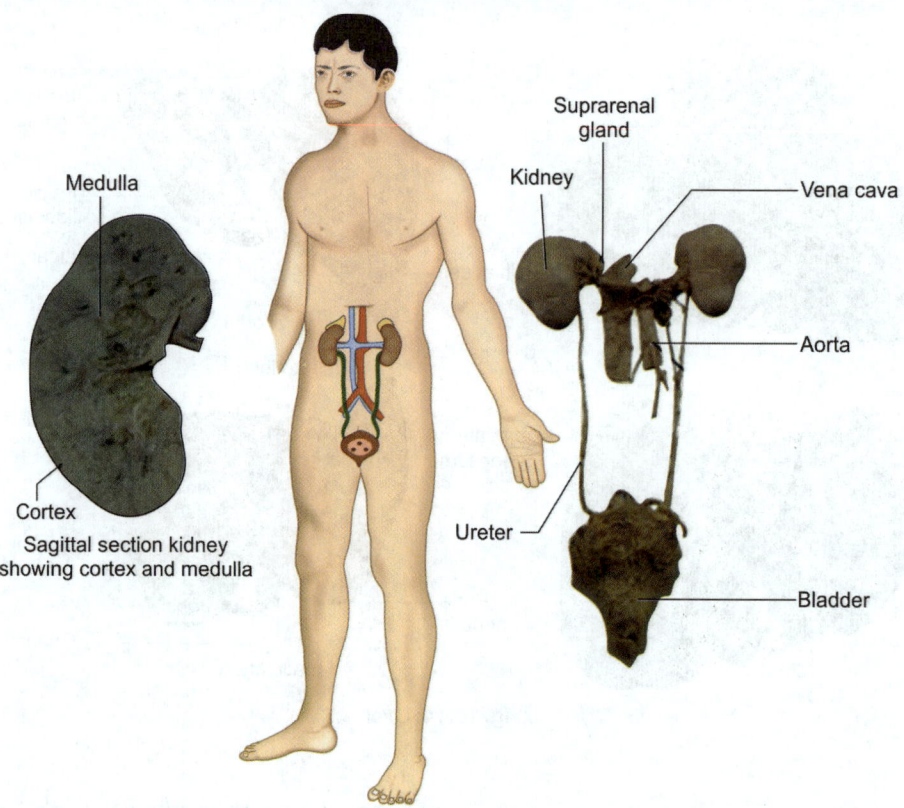

Fig. 10.15: Urinary system—parts.

Coverings of Kidney

Each kidney is covered by three layers of fascia from inside out. They are:
1. *Renal capsule/true capsule*, a layer of fibrous connective tissue, surrounding each kidney.
2. *Perirenal fat/perinephric fat*, a dense layer of adipose tissue, in turn, surrounds the renal capsule. It acts as a shock absorber, cushioning the kidneys against mechanical shock.
3. *Renal fascia/fascia of Gerota* is the thin outer most layer of connective tissue that surrounds the perirenal fat. It helps to anchor the kidneys and surrounding adipose tissue to the abdominal wall.

Ureter

- Ureter is a 25–30 cm long muscular tube. It transports urine from kidney to urinary bladder. It begins as a continuation of renal pelvis.
- It courses through abdomen, pelvis, and wall of urinary bladder and opens into the bladder cavity.
- Urinary bladder muscle contracts mechanically and closes off ureteral orifice which prevents a reverse flow of urine toward the kidney.

Urinary Bladder

- Urinary bladder is located immediately behind the pubic symphysis.
- Shape and relations of urinary bladder vary according to the amount of urine present in it.
- An empty bladder in adults is entirely a pelvic organ; as it fills, it rises up into the hypogastric region. In young children, it projects above the pelvic inlet.

Chapter 10: Introduction to Splanchnology

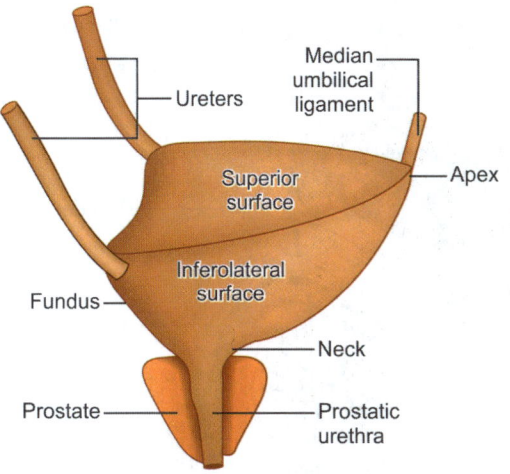

Fig. 10.16: Urinary bladder.

- An empty bladder is pyramidal in shape having (**Fig. 10.16**):
  - An apex
  - A base (posterior surface)
  - A superior surface
  - Two inferolateral surfaces
  - A neck.
- *Interior of the urinary bladder*: Mucous membrane is thrown into folds except in the triangular region in the base of bladder, between the openings of the two ureters and the urethra. This region is called the "trigone". Here, the mucous membrane is always smooth even when the bladder is empty.

Urethra

- In males it is about 8 inches (20 cm) long and extends from the neck of bladder to the external urethral orifice present at the tip of the glans penis. It is divided into three parts, i.e., prostatic, membranous and penile.
- In females it extends from neck of urinary bladder to open externally through the external urethral orifice (anterior to the vaginal opening).

REPRODUCTIVE SYSTEM

The term reproduction means formation of new living organism that closely resembles the parents. In higher animals it is accomplished by separate male and female sexual organs. Reproduction involves the process of production of gametes, sexual intercourse, fertilization, pregnancy, development of fetus, delivery of fetus, and lactation are complicated.

MALE REPRODUCTIVE SYSTEM

It consists of (**Fig. 10.17**):
- External genital organs which include:
  - Penis
  - Scrotum and its contents: Testis, epididymis, and part of spermatic cord.
- Internal genital organs:
  - Gonads
  - Epididymis
  - Vas deferens
  - Prostate
  - Seminal vesicle.

Penis

It consists of two parts, the *root* that is attached to the perineum and the free and movable *body*. The body contains three elongated masses of erectile tissue namely two corpora cavernosa and a corpus spongiosum. *Glans penis* is an elongated conical part at the distal end of penis and presents external urethral orifice at its summit.

Scrotum

It is an extension of layers of anterior abdominal wall from superficial to deep. It is seen as a pendulous sac of skin below and behind the penis and divided into right and left sacs by a median septum that extends to under surface of penis in front and to the anus behind. Each sac contains the gonad (testis), epididymis and initial part of spermatic cord.

Testis

It is the male gonad where the male gametes the spermatozoa are produced. It is suspended in the scrotal sac by spermatic cord. It is oblique in position. It is oval in shape. It has two poles (upper and lower), two surfaces

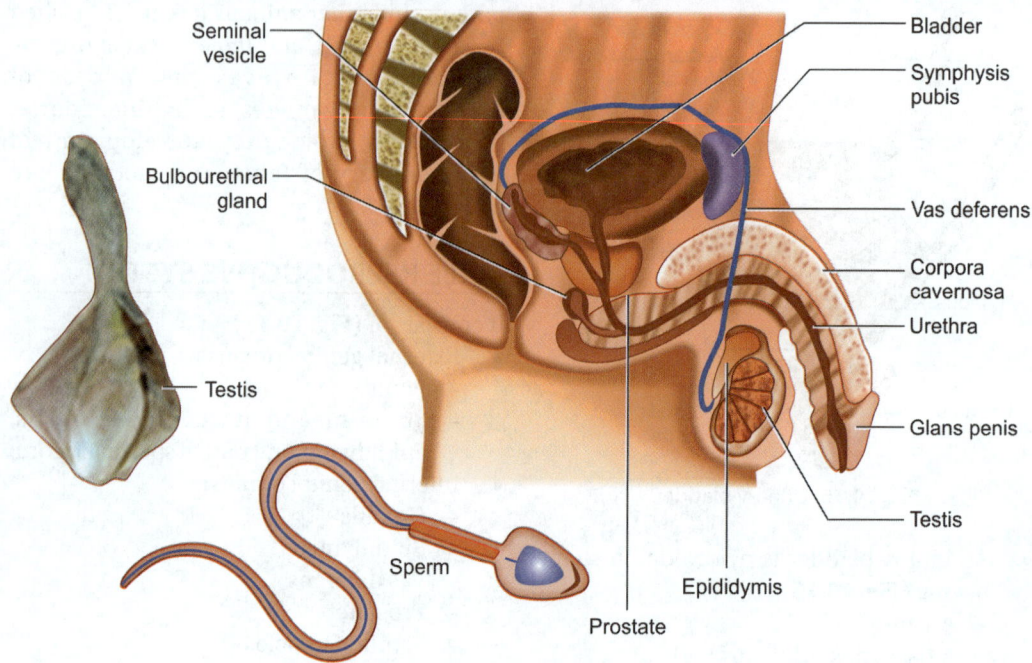

Fig. 10.17: Male reproductive system.

(lateral and medial) and two borders (anterior and posterior).

Epididymis

It is a comma-shaped structure along the posterolateral aspect of testis. It is made up of a single, highly coiled duct of epididymis through which passes the spermatozoa. The parts of epididymis are head, body and tail. Tail is continuous with vas deferens.

Prostate Gland

It is a fibromuscular and glandular organ that surrounds proximal part of male urethra.

Seminal Vesicles

A pair of convoluted, pouch like glands sandwiched between base of urinary bladder and rectum.

Ejaculatory Ducts

Ejaculatory duct is formed by union of ampulla of vas deferens and duct of seminal vesicle at the base of prostate and traverses through the prostate to terminate in the prostatic part of urethra.

Bulbourethral Glands or Cowper's Glands

A pair of small glands located in the deep perineal pouch, one on either side of membranous urethra.

Their ducts open into the penile urethra. The secretions protect the sperms and lubricate the tip of penis and urethra to prevent damage to spermatozoa during ejaculation.

Spermatic Cord

A group of structures that pass from inguinal canal to testis. It is a tubular sheath containing vas deferens, vessels and nerves of testis and epididymis. It receives three coverings from the anterior abdominal wall during descent of testis that become continuous with the corresponding layers of scrotum.

FEMALE REPRODUCTIVE SYSTEM

It consists of **(Figs. 10.18A to C):**
- External genital organs—vulva.

Chapter 10: Introduction to Splanchnology

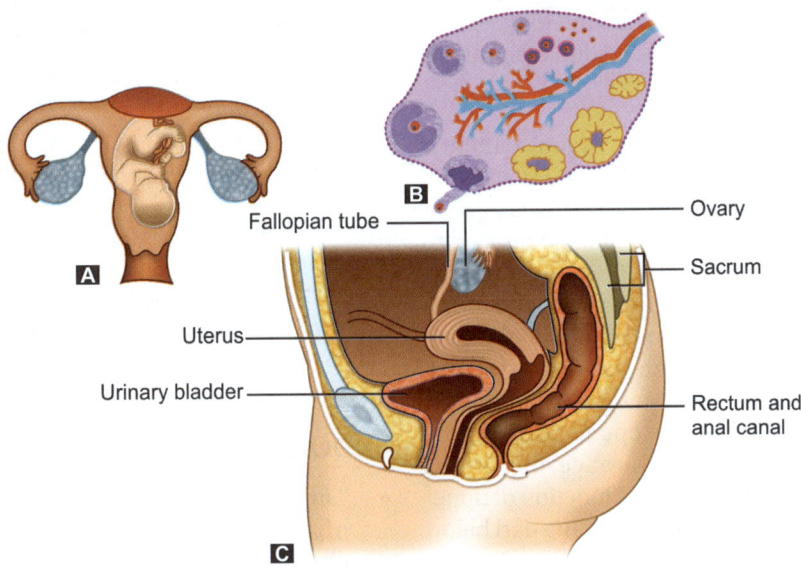

Figs. 10.18A to C: Female reproductive system. (A) Showing fetus in uterus; (B) Cut-section of ovary showing follicles in different stages of development; (C) Sagittal section of pelvis showing female reproductive organs.

- Internal genital organs—female gonads known as ovaries, uterine or fallopian tubes, uterus and vagina.
- Mammary glands.

Functions

- Ovaries—produce oocytes, female sex hormones (estrogen and progesterone).
- Uterine tubes—transport the oocyte to uterus and are the seat of fertilization.
- Uterus is the seat of implantation of fertilized ovum, growth of embryo and fetus during pregnancy and delivery of fetus at labor.
- Vagina—receives penis during copulation and is the site of release of sperms. It is the passage for child birth.
- Mammary glands—synthesize, secrete and eject milk for nourishing the newborn.

Ovaries

Ovaries are female gonads and are almond-shaped structures. They are located one on either side of uterus below and behind the corresponding uterine tube. They are attached to the posterior layer of broad ligament by a fold of peritoneum called mesovarium. It presents two ends (upper and lower), two surfaces (medial and lateral) and two borders (anterior and posterior). The substance of ovary is divided into cortex and medulla. Cortex contains the follicles in different stages of development. During the reproductive age of females the follicles mature from primordial follicle to Graafian follicle which is releases from the surface of ovary at monthly intervals (ovulation).

Uterine Tubes

These are a pair of ducts that transport sperms to reach an ovum, and transport ova from ovary to uterine tube for fertilization and fertilized ovum from uterine tube to uterine cavity. It presents two openings and four parts. The two openings are uterine ostium that communicates with the uterus and the pelvic ostium through which it communicates with the peritoneal cavity. The margins of pelvic ostium present finger-like processes called fimbriae. From medial to lateral it presents four parts—(1) intramural (1 cm), isthmus (3 cm), ampulla (5 cm), and infundibulum

(1 cm). Ampulla is the widest and longest part of uterine tube where fertilization takes place.

Uterus

It is a pear-shaped hollow organ, which is broad above and narrow below. It is located in the true pelvis. Long axis of uterus is at right angles to the long axis of vagina and is said to be in anteverted position. The angle it makes with itself because of forward bending of uterus is called anteflexion. The caudal part of cervix opens into the anterior wall of vagina. It presents fundus, body and cervix. Fundus is the broad part above the openings of uterine tubes. On the external surface the uterus presents a constriction at the junction of upper two-thirds and lower one-third. The part below the constriction is cervix. The two openings are uterine ostium by that communicates with the uterus and the pelvic ostium through which it communicates with the peritoneal cavity.

Clinical Importance of Urogenital System
- *Anomalous shape and position* of kidneys.
- *Hydronephrosis*: Dilatation of renal pelvis and kidney.
- *Hydroureter*: Dilatation of ureter due to obstruction.
- *Pyelonephritis*: Infection of lower urinary tract.
- *Cystitis*: Inflammation of urinary bladder.
- *Urethritis*: Inflammation of urethra.
- *Salpingitis*: Inflammation of uterine tubes.

ENDOCRINE SYSTEM (FIG. 10.19)

- The endocrine system is the collection of glands that produce hormones or chemical messengers that regulate the body's growth and development, sexual function, reproductive function, sleep, and mood.

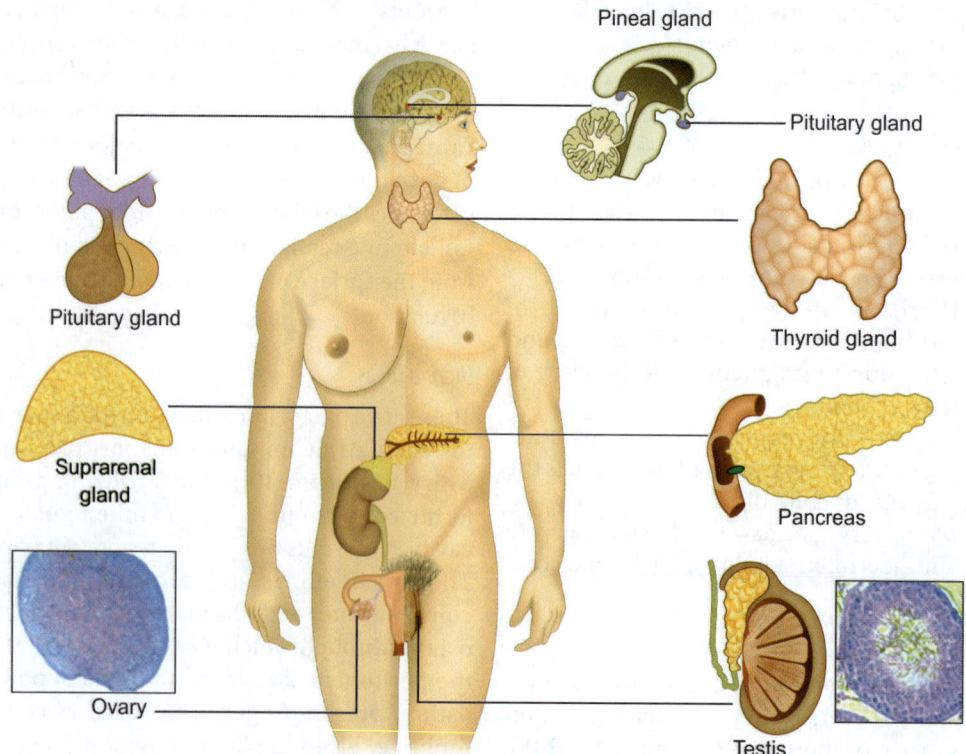

Fig. 10.19: Endocrine system.

- Hormones are chemical substances produced in the body. They are produced by one group of cells and act on cells at distant places. The hormones are released into the bloodstream and may bring out action of one or coordinated action of several organs throughout the body.

Mechanism of Action of Endocrine System

- The endocrine system is regulated by feedback mechanism to the hypothalamus. For the hormones that are regulated by the pituitary gland, the hypothalamus sends a signal to the pituitary gland in the form of a "releasing hormone", which stimulates the pituitary to secrete a "stimulating hormone" into the circulation.
- The stimulating hormone sends signals to the target gland for secretion of its hormone. When the level of this hormone secreted by the targeted gland rises in the circulation, the hypothalamus and the pituitary gland shut down the secretion of the releasing and stimulating hormones, which in turn, slows the secretion by the target gland. This results in stable blood concentration of the hormones that are regulated by the pituitary gland.
- All the endocrine glands pour their secretions into the circulation except the thyroid that stores the secretion and releases into the blood stream on demand.

Major glands of human endocrine system:
- Pituitary gland
- Thyroid gland
- Parathyroid glands
- Adrenal glands
- Pineal body
- Thymus
- Pancreas
- Gonads (ovaries and testes)
- Placenta.

Pituitary Gland

It is the master gland of endocrine system. It is a small pea-sized gland located in a small depression in the sella turcica of the sphenoid bone. It is situated below the hypothalamus of the diencephalon (base of brain) and connected to it by infundibular stalk.

It has two distinct lobes: (1) posterior and (2) anterior. Anterior lobe is called adenohypophysis. Posterior lobe is called neurohypophysis. These two are different in structure, function, and development.

Posterior Pituitary

It is a small extension of the hypothalamus. It consists of infundibulum and pars nervosa or pars posterior, through which axons of some of the neurosecretory cells of the hypothalamus extend. Neurosecretory cells of hypothalamus produce the following two hormones that are stored and released by the posterior pituitary.
- *Oxytocin*: It triggers uterine contractions during childbirth and the release of milk during breastfeeding.
- *Antidiuretic hormone (ADH)*: It prevents water loss in the body by increasing the re-uptake of water in the kidneys and decreases blood flow to sweat glands.

Anterior Pituitary

It is true glandular part of the pituitary gland. It consists of pars distalis or anterior, pars intermedia and pars tuberalis. It is controlled by the releasing and inhibiting hormones of the hypothalamus. Anterior pituitary secretes seven hormones:

1. Thyroid stimulating hormone (TSH) stimulates thyroid gland.
2. Adrenocorticotropic hormone (ACTH) stimulates adrenal cortex, external portion of adrenal gland to produce its hormones.
3. Follicle stimulating hormone (FSH) stimulates follicle cells of gonads to produce gametes (ova in females and sperm in males).
4. Luteinizing hormone (LH) stimulates gonads to produce sex hormones (estrogen in females and testosterone in males).
5. Human growth hormone (HGH) affects several target cells throughout the body by stimulating their growth, repair, and reproduction.

6. Prolactin (PRL) has several effects on the body, primary is that it stimulates mammary glands to produce milk.
7. Melanocyte stimulating hormone (MSH)—it controls the production of melanin granules that are responsible for color of skin and iris.

Thyroid Gland

- It is a butterfly-shaped gland located at the base of the neck and wrapped around the lateral sides of the trachea.
- It is the largest and highly vascular endocrine gland.
- It presents two conical lateral lobes and an isthmus connecting them. The isthmus is located on the anterior aspect of trachea over the 2nd to 4th tracheal rings. Each lobe extends laterally up to the oblique line of thyroid cartilage.
- The gland is enclosed by true and false capsules. True capsule is the condensation of connective tissue. The false capsule is provided by the pretracheal layer of deep fascia of neck.
- The gland is related to two tubes (esophagus and trachea), two nerves (recurrent laryngeal and external laryngeal).
- It produces three major hormones. They are calcitonin, triiodothyronine (T3), and thyroxine (T4).
  - Calcitonin is released when calcium ion levels in the blood rise above a certain set point. Its function is to reduce the concentration of calcium ions in the blood by aiding the absorption of calcium into the matrix of bones.
  - T3 and T4 hormones combined together regulate the body's metabolic rate. Increased levels of T3 and T4 lead to increased cellular activity and energy usage in the body.

Parathyroid Glands

- These are four small masses of glandular tissue found on the posterior aspect of the thyroid gland. There is a pair of superior parathyroid and a pair of inferior parathyroid glands.
- They are different in developmental origin. The position of superior parathyroid glands is constant whereas the position of inferior parathyroid is variable.
- They produce the parathyroid hormone (PTH) that is involved in calcium ion homeostasis. PTH is released from the parathyroid glands when calcium ion levels in the blood drop below a set point. PTH stimulates the osteoclasts to break down the calcium containing bone matrix to release free calcium ions into the bloodstream. PTH also triggers the kidneys to return calcium ions filtered out of the blood back into the bloodstream so that it is conserved.

Adrenal Glands

A pair of glands found superior to the kidneys in the posterior abdominal wall behind peritoneum. Right gland is triangular and left gland is semilunar in shape. It is made of two distinct parts: (1) the outer adrenal cortex and (2) inner adrenal medulla that are different in structure, function, and development.

- *Adrenal cortex*: Produces the following hormones:
  - *Glucocorticoids*: These have many diverse functions like breakdown of proteins and lipids to produce glucose. They reduce inflammation and immune response.
  - *Mineralocorticoids*: These regulate the concentration of mineral ions in the body.
  - *Androgens*: Testosterone produced at low levels in the adrenal cortex regulates growth and activity of cells that are receptive to male hormones.
- *Adrenal medulla*:
  - Produces hormones epinephrine and norepinephrine under stimulation by the sympathetic division of the autonomic nervous system.
  - These hormones help to increase the flow of blood to the brain and muscles to improve the "fight-or-flight" response to stress.

Pineal Gland/Body

- It is a small gland located near the posterior wall of third ventricle of brain, below the splenium of corpus callosum and above the superior colliculi of midbrain.
- It is also called *epiphysis cerebri*.
- It produces hormones that influence other endocrine glands. The important hormones are melatonin that is responsible for circadian rhythm.

Pancreas

- The pancreas is a heterocrine or mixed gland as it contains both endocrine and exocrine glandular tissue.
- The endocrine portion of the pancreas is made up of small bundles of cells called *islets of Langerhans*. Within these islets there are two types of cells—(1) alpha and (2) beta cells. Alpha cells produce the hormone glucagon that is responsible for raising blood glucose levels.
- Beta cells produce the hormone insulin, which is responsible for lowering blood glucose levels after a meal.

Gonads

The gonads are ovaries in females and testes in males. They are responsible for producing the sex hormones that regulate secondary sex characteristics of adult females and adult males.

Testes

- A pair of ellipsoid organs found in the scrotum of males.
- Produces male sex hormone testosterone at puberty.
- The effects of testosterone are on many parts of the body, including the muscles, bones, sex organs, and hair follicles.
- Growth and increase in strength of the bones and muscles, including the accelerated growth of long bones during adolescence.
- During puberty, testosterone controls the growth and development of the sex organs and body hair of males, including pubic, chest, and facial hair.

Ovaries

- A pair of almond-shaped glands located in the pelvic cavity lateral and superior to the uterus in females.
- Produces female sex hormones *progesterone* and *estrogen*.
- Progesterone is most active in females during ovulation and pregnancy and maintains suitable environment to support a developing fetus.
- Estrogen functions as the primary female sex hormone. The release of estrogen during puberty activates growth of female secondary sex features such as uterine development, breast development, and pubic hair. Estrogen triggers increased growth of bones during adolescence.

Thymus

- Soft, triangular-shaped, specialized primary lymphoid organ.
- It is made up of two lobes and is located in the superior mediastinum.
- This is the only lymphatic organ that is fully developed at the time of birth. Other lymphatic organs reach their full development in postnatal life.
- Thymus enlarges during childhood and atrophies at adolescence.
- Its function is to receive immature T-cells produced in red bone marrow and train them to protect the body from pathogens throughout a person's entire life.
- It produces the hormone thymosin that stimulates production of T cells that fight against infection.

Placenta

- In pregnant women, the placenta produces several hormones that help to maintain pregnancy.

- Progesterone is produced to relax the uterus, protect fetus from the mother's *immune system* and prevent premature delivery of the fetus.
- Human chorionic gonadotropin (hCG) assists progesterone by signaling the ovaries to maintain the production of estrogen and progesterone throughout pregnancy.

Clinical Importance of Endocrine System

- *Gigantism*: Excessive growth before fusion of epiphyses due to the excessive production of growth hormone.
- *Acromegaly*: Excessive growth of head, hands and feet after fusion of epiphyses.
- *Cushing's syndrome*: Abnormal deposition of fat in the face, neck, and trunk due to excessive secretion of adrenotropic hormones.
- *Goiter*: Benign enlargement of thyroid gland is called goiter.
- *Cretinism*: Hypothyroidism in infants is called cretinism.
- *Myxedema*: Hypothyroidism in adults.
- *Thyrotoxicosis*: Hyperthyroidism.
- *Thyroiditis*: Inflammation of thyroid.
- *Tumors of pineal gland*: It can press the colliculi of midbrain and the oculomotor nucleus causing paralysis of oculomotor nerve.
- *Myasthenia gravis*: It is an autoimmune disorder due to the abnormality of thymus.
- *Diabetes mellitus*: Deficiency in the production of insulin by beta cells of pancreas results in this condition.

Anatomical Basis for Clinical Condition

Problems and Questions:

1. A person had a fall from the motor bike on his face and was brought to the casualty with a complaint of clear watery fluid leaking through the nose, but without any external injuries. What could be the cause?
2. What do you call a condition when stones in the gallbladder are identified in an ultrasound and if the patient complaints of pain in the right upper abdomen? What do you call the investigation that is done in this case using contrast media?

Anatomical explanation:

1. Most probably it is a case of cerebrospinal fluid leaking through the nose due to the fracture of cribriform plate of ethmoid bone.
2. The process of stone formation in gallbladder is called cholelithiasis. Cholecystitis is inflammation of gallbladder that can produce pain in the right upper abdomen in the region of liver. By using contrast X-ray called cholecystography this condition can be diagnosed.

> **Key Concept**

Take Home Message—Splanchnology

- The important cavities of the body are the cranial and vertebral, thoracic and the abdominopelvic that contain the various organ systems, i.e., respiratory, urinary, reproductive, digestive, cardiovascular, nervous and endocrine.
- A brief introduction to each of the systems with clinical importance are provided in this chapter for overall understanding of the body. Details will be learnt while doing region-wise dissection and will be described in regional anatomy textbooks.

Autopsy or necropsy: It is postmortem examination of the dead body and dissection of its internal organs to determine the cause of death. An autopsy can diagnose

a. Disease not detected during life
b. Determine the extent of injuries or congenital defects(Congenital heart defects) or drugs effect and their contribution for the cause of death.
c. An autopsy is legally required in a criminal investigation, or to resolve legal disputes and for settling insurance benefits that depend on the cause of death.

QUESTIONS

1. Name the parts of respiratory system.
2. Name the parts of digestive system.
3. Name the parts of urinary system.
4. Name the parts of male reproductive system.
5. Name the parts of female reproductive system.
6. Name the endocrine glands.

CHAPTER 11

Introduction to Radiological Anatomy

LEARNING OBJECTIVES

- Radiology—definition and invention
- Different radiological procedures—classification
- Brief explanation of various procedures
- Clinical case with anatomical explanation

INTRODUCTION

- The term *radiology* meaning the science of radioactive substances and high-energy radiations, is a branch of medicine concerned with the use of radiant energy (such as X-rays) or radioactive material in the diagnosis and treatment of disease.
- This branch started with the discovery of X-rays by Wilhelm Roentgen in 1895.
- With the advent of X-rays that has the penetrating power, visibility of anatomy has increased and facilitated visualization of signs of pathology.
- It is also called *medical imaging* as it is the window to look into the internal details of the human body. By using the radiological techniques visual images of body can be created for clinical diagnosis, for undertaking medical interventions and for visual representation of function of some of the organs and tissues.
- Radiology is a complex and multifaceted science. There is explosive growth in radiology with the advent of newer imaging techniques that facilitate early diagnosis and treatment giving a greatest opportunity to cure the disease.
- Radiography is an investigation of choice as its findings are accurate in the detection of early stages of diseases as the procedure of radiographic method is a nondestructive testing of the living body.
- Interpretation of the radiological images requires a detailed knowledge of anatomy.
- A number of procedures fall under the preview of radiology. The earliest of these radiological techniques, utilized the interaction of ionizing radiation with the body, in order to create an image of the required part.

CLASSIFICATION OF RADIOLOGICAL PROCEDURES

AN 13.5: Identify the bones and joints of upper limb seen in anteroposterior and lateral view radiographs of shoulder region, arm, elbow, forearm and hand.
AN 20.6: Identify the bones and joints of lower limb seen in anteroposterior and lateral view radiographs of various regions of lower limb.
AN 43.7: Identify the anatomical structures in: (1) Plain X-ray of skull—anteroposterior view and lateral view; (2) Plain X-ray of cervical spine—anteroposterior and lateral views; (3) Plain X-ray of paranasal sinuses
AN 54.1: Describe and identify features of plain X-ray abdomen.
AN 54.2: Describe and identify the special radiographs of abdominopelvic region (contrast X-ray, barium swallow, barium meal, barium enema, cholecystography, intravenous pyelography and hysterosalpingography).
AN 54.3: Describe ERCP, CT abdomen, MRI, arteriography in radiodiagnosis of abdomen.

Chapter 11: Introduction to Radiological Anatomy

The various radiological procedures that are available for imaging the organs and tissues are:
- Diagnostic radiology
- Interventional radiology
- Computed tomography (CT scanning)
- Magnetic resonance imaging (MRI)
- Nuclear medicine and molecular imaging
- Positron emission tomography (PET)
- Single-photon emission computed tomography (SPECT)
- Ultrasonography/ultrasound
- Mammography.

All the procedures use ionizing radiation except ultrasound and MRI.

Diagnostic Radiology

Two types of radiographic images are used in medical imaging. They are:
1. Plain radiography
2. Fluoroscopy.

Plain Radiography **(Fig. 11.1)**

- These are often, called X-rays. These display the shadow of the body part on the film.
- It involves generating energy waves or X-rays by passing a stream of electrons (electrically generated cathode rays that come into contact with the metal plate) through X-ray tube that are directed at the particular part of the body that is to be examined.
- As these radiations can be harmful, procedures that restrict the area that is exposed and also that shield sensitive areas against the rays were developed.
- Various methods of detection of X-rays have been developed. The earliest of these relied on the direct interaction between photographic film and the X-rays. Subsequently, there was the development of methods for enhancement of images (using radiosensitive amplifying screens adjacent to X-ray film).
- During X-ray, a black and white image is recorded on a special film or computer. The image looks like a negative film of a black and white photograph. Each type of tissue allows a different amount of radiation to pass through and expose the X-ray sensitive film **(Fig. 11.1)**.
- The farther the body part is from the film, the more magnified it will appear, but also its borders will be less distinct.
- Additionally, since the image is a two-dimensional (2D) representation of a three-dimensional (3D) object, the

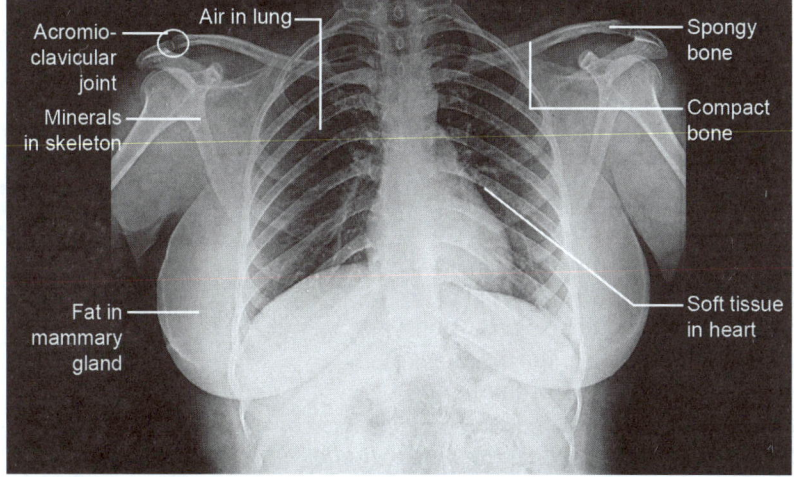

Fig. 11.1: X-ray chest [posteroanterior (PA) view].
Source: Saptagiri Scan Center, Tirupati.

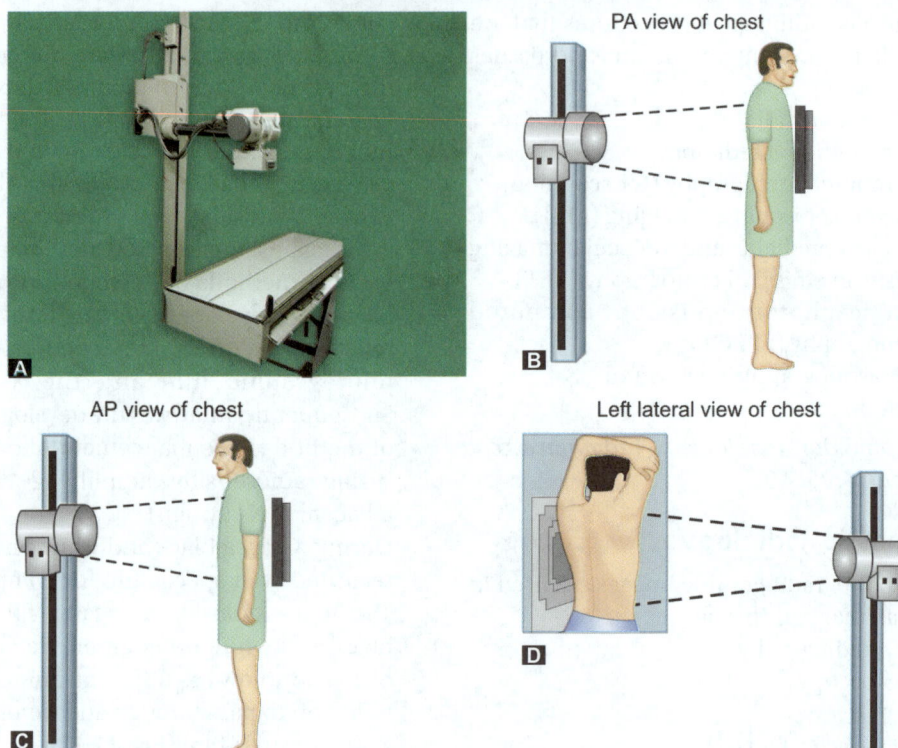

Figs. 11.2A to D: (A) X-ray machine; (B to D) Position of patient for X-ray. (PA, posteroanterior; AP, anteroposterior) *Source*: Saptagiri Scan Center, Tirupati.

anteroposterior location of structures must be inferred. Images taken from two perspectives may permit the skilled radiologist to interpret the anteroposterior location of objects by their displacement relative to one another in images taken from right angles. Plane film radiographs are still the most common method of viewing osseous structures or the chest **(Figs. 11.2A to D)**.

- X-ray images of the skeletal system and internal organs are used for a wide variety of diagnostic purposes. X-rays are especially useful in showing detailed images of skeletal structure **(Fig. 11.3)**.
- They are not of much use in the diagnosis of injuries or abnormalities of soft tissue, i.e. tendons, ligaments, etc.
- To understand the radiological imaging of structures the fundamental principles in *radio-opacity* and *positioning of the*

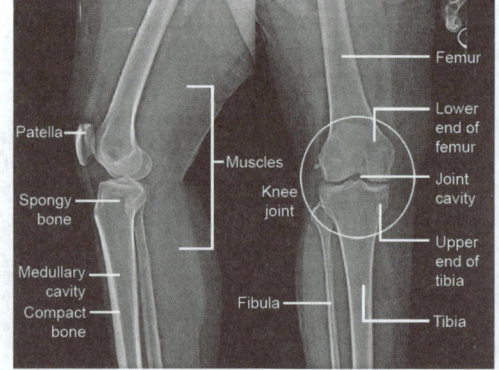

Fig. 11.3: General features of a long bone of adult. *Source:* Saptagiri Scan Center, Tirupati.

patient for radiographic imaging are to be known.

Radio-opacity:
- The fundamental principle of all radiographic tests that employ X-rays

Chapter 11: Introduction to Radiological Anatomy

is—different body tissues have a different capacity to block or absorb X-rays. For example, air and fat are black; bone, metal, and calcium are white and all other tissues are of varying shades of gray depending on the density of the structure.

- Contrast media are used if the density of structure to be observed is similar to that of the adjacent structures to make the structure in question to be more prominent. The contrast medial are of two types, i.e. (1) radiolucent and (2) radiopaque. The examples for radiolucent contrast media are air, nitrous oxide, and carbon dioxide. These are called negative contrast media because of their low density. The examples for radiopaque contrast media are barium sulfate, bromium (used for visualizing liver and spleen), and iodine. These are called positive contrast media because of their higher atomic number.
- The various tissues of the body exhibit different degrees of radio-opacity (whiteness/blackness) in the conventional radiography, in computerized tomography and in fluoroscopy. Radiographic image densities of various components can be compared as follows **(Figs. 11.1, 11.4, and 11.5)**.
  - Between air (e.g., in trachea and lungs), fat and soft tissues (e.g., heart and muscles) air is more radiolucent (black) than fat and soft tissues. In other words, soft tissues are more radiopaque (white) than air and fat.
  - Between bone and teeth the teeth are more radiopaque than bone because of presence of enamel in teeth.
  - Contrast media give more radiopaque (e.g., barium meal of stomach and intravenous pyelography of urinary system) appearance than plain X-ray.

Positioning of the patient for plain X-ray:
- Depending on the part of the body nearest to the film the views of the images of plain X-ray are named. Example: the position of film anterior, left lateral, and left anterior oblique.
- The alternate terms that are commonly used are depending on the direction of passage of X-rays through the object (part of the body) from the front or from the back. The term anteroposterior view (AP view) is used when X-rays are passed with the tube in front and the film behind the object. The term posteroanterior view (PA view) is used when X-rays are passed with

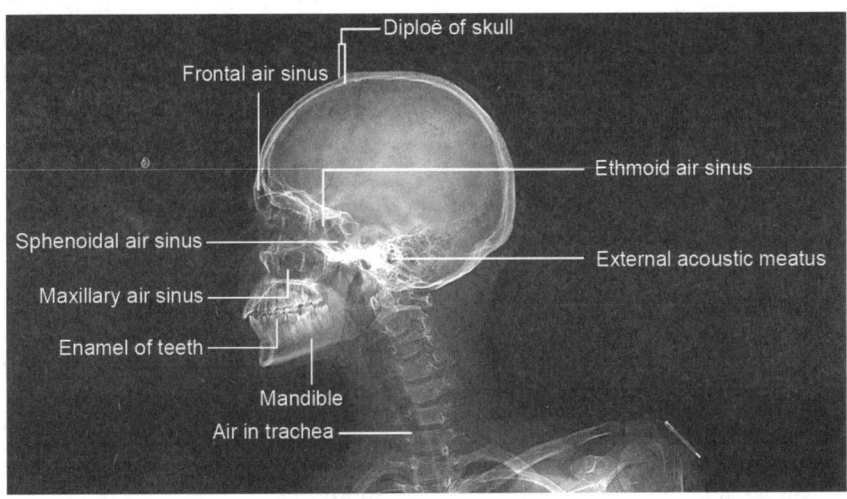

Fig. 11.4: X-ray—head and neck—lateral view.
Source: Saptagiri Scan Center, Tirupati.

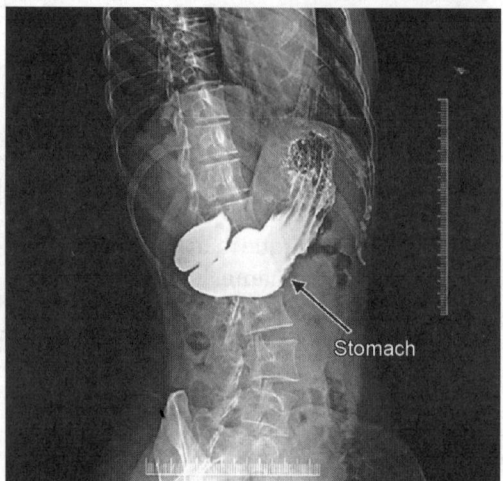

Fig. 11.5: Contrast X-ray—barium meal.
Source: Saptagiri Scan Center, Tirupati.

the tube behind and the film in front of the object. In lateral view, if the tube is on right side it is right lateral view, etc. **(Figs. 11.2A to D)**.

- Highly standardized radiographic positions facilitate appropriate interpretation of radiological findings, by highlighting the areas to be observed. For example, the heart is more anterior in position in thoracic cage and to get the well-defined shadow of the heart posteroanterior view is preferred. In the abdomen the kidneys and colon are posterior in location; hence an anteroposterior view is preferred.

Radiological anatomy of skeleton:
General features of a long bone in radiology **(Figs. 11.3 and 11.4)**:
- Compact bone is seen at the periphery as a thick, homogenous calcified-band.
- Nutrient canal is seen as an oblique radiolucent line passing through compact bone.
- Cancellous bone is seen as a network with spaces in between and is seen more clearly at the ends of shaft.
- Bone marrow and periosteum are not clearly distinguishable.
- In young bones uncalcified epiphyseal plate is seen as an irregular, radiolucent band and is known as epiphyseal line. Disappearance of epiphyseal line indicates fusion of epiphysis with diaphysis.
- Metaphysis is the calcified epiphyseal plate of cartilage and the newly formed bone near it.

Radiological appearance of a joint **(Figs. 11.3 and 11.6)**:
- The articular disc is not visible radiologically.
- The joint space is identified radiologically as the interval between epiphyseal areas of adjacent bones and is occupied by articular disc of cartilage (radiolucent) on the ends of bones that are taking part in the articulation. The space is 2–5 mm in width in the adult.
- The joint line is observed radiologically as the junction between radiopaque end of bone and the radiolucent articular cartilage.

Skeletal maturation:
- Maturation of bone differs with the time of appearance of ossification centers in the limbs.
- The accuracy in timing of appearance of ossification centers varies in sexes and also varies with the race, geographical location, and the nutritional status.
- The above points have to be considered while making a comment on maturation of bone by radiological appearance for estimation of age.

Fluoroscopy
- It is not used regularly.
- It is used for observing the moving body structures.
- The image is created and intensified electronically by striking X-rays on a fluorescent scene coated with a thin layer of phosphor is analyzed.
- *Advantage*: Observation of movement of moving components (e.g., blood) in a body part.
- *Disadvantage*: Higher radiation exposure and lesser resolution of image.

Chapter 11: Introduction to Radiological Anatomy

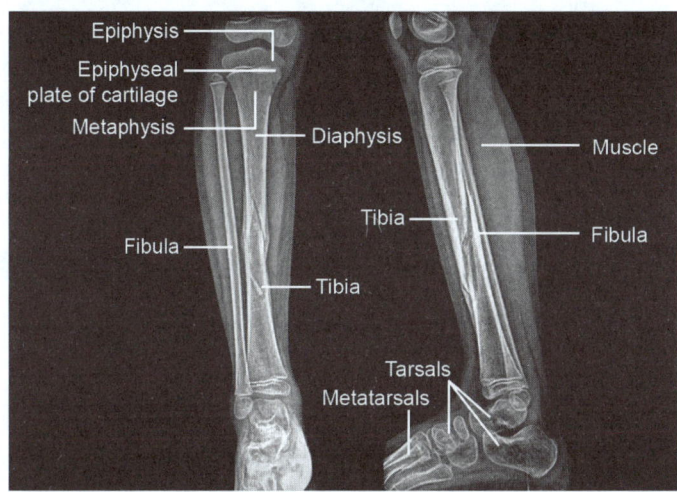

Fig. 11.6: Plain X-ray young bone—epiphyseal cartilage.
Source: Saptagiri Scan Center, Tirupati.

Use of contrast media in radiography (**Fig. 11.5**):

- To differentiate structures of same density contrast agents are used.
- For the diagnosis of abnormal constrictions and growths of gut tube.
- Iodinated contrast media are used for visualization of arteries (arteriogram) or veins (venogram) and to view spinal cord and nerve roots by injecting through spinal canal (intrathecal route).
- Digital subtraction angiograms are a type of fluoroscopy used to visualize blood vessels with minimal use of contrast media and with better clarity.
- Allergies to iodine and the renal problems as the dye is excreted by the kidney are the limitations for the use of contrast media.
- The various contrast radiographic procedures were represented in **Table 11.1**. For GIT are barium meal swallow and enema is used for visualization of esophagus, stomach, and large intestine, respectively.

Endoscopic Retrograde Cholangiopancreatography (ERCP)

A procedure with combined usage of X-ray and upper GI endoscopy to examine and treat the peoblems of biliary and pancreatic ducts, e.g., opening the narrowed ducts, removal of stones or for obtaining tissue for biopsy.

Cross-sectional imaging:

- Limitations in distinguishing objects of similar densities by plain X-rays because of limited resolution has brought revolutions in the field of medical imaging.
- Technological advances in electronic storage, modification and transmission of information has led to the evolution of CT scan, MRI, etc.

Table 11.1: Different contrast of radiographic procedures.

Organ system	Contrast radiography
Gastrointestinal tract (GIT)	Barium swallow—esophagus; barium meal—stomach; barium enema—colon
Salivary glands	Sialography
Trachea and bronchi	Bronchography
Biliary system	Cholecystography
Female reproductive system	Hysterosalpingography
Ventricles of brain	Ventriculography
Blood vessels	Angiography
Urinary system	Pyelography

Interventional Radiology

It refers to a range of procedures that use radiological images obtained by using fluoroscopy, ultrasound, CT and MRI to precisely target therapy.

These are safer alternatives to open and laparoscopic surgeries as these procedures are minimally invasive, minimal risk, low cost, greater comfort to the patient, quick recovery, and shorter hospital stay.

In these procedures needles/fine catheter tubes/wires are navigated into the body under image control. This procedure requires special skill and training. This procedure is used for the following conditions:

Vascular Diseases (Vascular Interventions)

- *Peripheral vascular diseases* where there will be reduced blood flow. These are treated by using balloons to stretch the vessels by a procedure called *balloon angioplasty*/percutaneous transluminal coronary angioplasty (PTCA) and sometimes by placing metal stents to keep the lumen patent.
- To prevent avascularity and subsequent limb amputation in cases of, rapid loss of blood supply to a limb because of a blood clot blocking the circulation in a vessel. The clot bursting drugs are pushed into the artery through catheter, to maintain blood supply to the limb.
- In cases of dilated arteries (aneurysms) that are at risk for rupture. In such cases a stent is placed for relining of the vessel.
- In cases of hemorrhage from gut or from injury, postpartum hemorrhage during cesarean delivery, etc. bleeding is stopped by blocking the vessel (embolization).
- Varicose veins and in cases of deep vein thrombosis (DVT), blood clot in lungs (pulmonary embolism) are treated by using the techniques of interventional radiology.

Nonvascular Interventions

This is also known as interventional oncology and is used for both benign and malignant conditions.

The examples are:
- Treatment of cancers—tumor ablation, etc.
- Drainage of fluid or pus in thorax or abdomen.
- To insert feeding tubes—gastrostomy, jejunostomy, etc.
- To relieve pressure effects of cancer on other systems—esophagus, kidney, liver, etc.
- Uterine fibroids—blocking blood vessels to stop heavy menstrual bleeding.
- Renal stones and gall stones—breaking the stone with special instruments and allowing drainage of the fragments.

Computerized Axial Tomography (CAT or CT Scan) (Fig. 11.7)

- *Principle*: To construct a cross-sectional image by passing X-ray beams in multiple directions along a 360° arc (tomography).
- *Technique*: A series of cross-sectional images (slices) are taken at 3 mm to 1 cm interval through the body parts to create 2D images. The 2D images can be reconstructed in 3D images for the organ or body part of clinical importance.
- The limitations for this technique are the patient is prevented from movement during the procedure and the hazard of ionizing radiation.
- *Uses*:
  - In trauma cases to detect fractures that are invisible by plain X-rays and if there is blood clot.
  - It enhances the visibility of structures when a contrast is used as in observing rupture of a blood vessel, e.g., in brain.

Magnetic Resonance Imaging (Figs. 11.8A and B)

- It is for creating cross-sectional images without using the ionizing radiation.

Chapter 11: Introduction to Radiological Anatomy

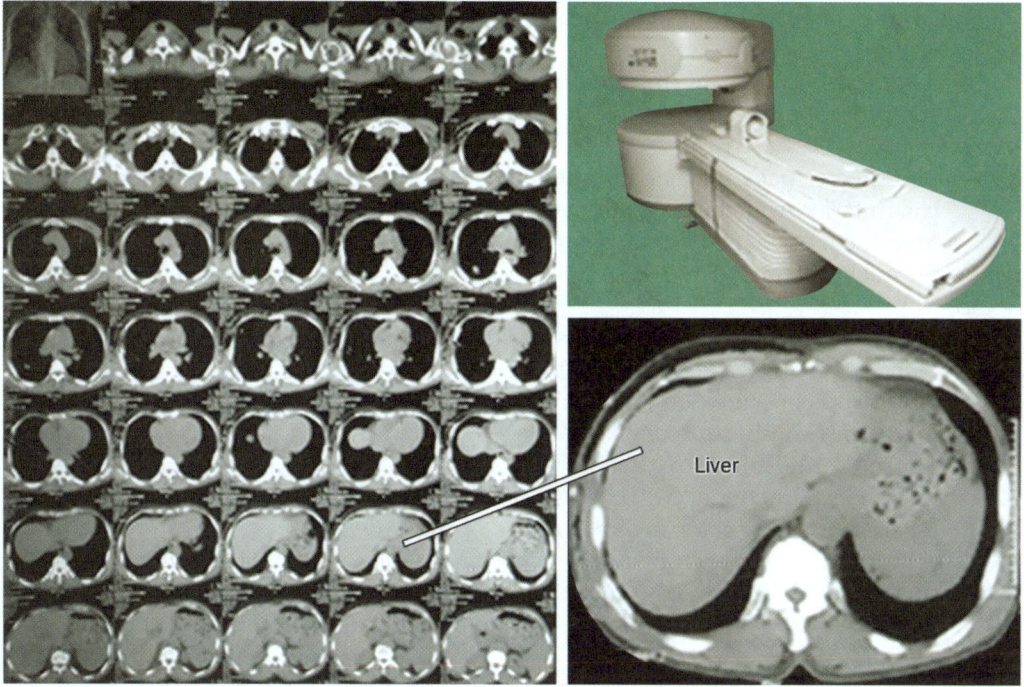

Fig. 11.7: Computed tomography (CT) scanner and image.
Source: Saptagiri Scan Center, Tirupati.

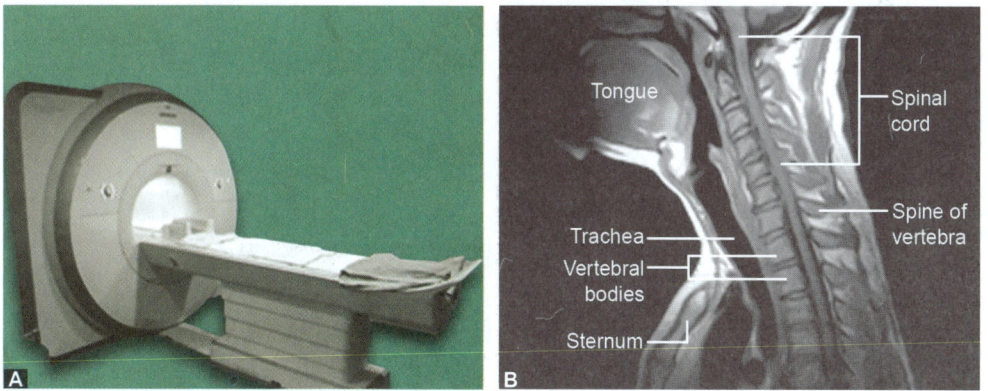

Figs. 11.8A and B: Magnetic resonance imaging (MRI) machine and image.
Source: Saptagiri Scan Center, Tirupati.

- *Principle*:
  - Alignment of polarized molecules in the body when placed in a strong magnetic field.
  - When subjected to radio waves the alignment of these molecules will be displaced.
  - When they are returning to aligned position the energy burst (echos) given up by them will be detected.
  - Depending on the chemical environment of the body the movement of polarized molecules varies, thus creating images characteristic for each

tissue depending on the pulse of radio waves.
- A series of images are collected by a computer application.

♦ *Limitations*:
- Presence of pace makers and metal clips interfere with the magnetic fields.
- Movement of the patient can degrade the quality of image.

♦ *Uses*:
- MRI is used for creating images of blood vessels (MR angiogram).
- To measure concentration of a chemical in a tissue (MR spectroscopy).
- To determine blood oxygen levels in tissues (functional MRI). This is especially useful for observing functional activity in certain areas of brain.

Nuclear Medicine Scans

♦ This facilitates understanding the anatomy and physiology in health and disease.
♦ *Technique*:
- By the use of radioactive contrast medium and observing the tracer radioactive element using SPECT.
- Specificity of the scan depends on the particular substance to which the radioactive tracer is bound, e.g., radioactive iodine is taken up by thyroid gland facilitating its visualization.
- In the case of fracture of bone and in tumors with bone metastasis it facilitates visualization as the radioactive tracer is taken up by osteoblasts.
- It facilitates visualization of blood flow and the progress of infection as the tracer is taken up by blood vessel and the white blood cells respectively.

Positron Emission Tomography (PET) Scan (Figs. 11.9A and B)

♦ *Technique*:
- It is a noninvasive, diagnostic technique used in nuclear medicine. In this procedure the radiation given off by a substance called radiotracer [e.g., fluorodeoxyglucose (FDG)] when it collects in different parts of the body is detected.

♦ *Uses*:
- The most common uses of the procedure are to:
  - Detect the malignant stage of tumor.

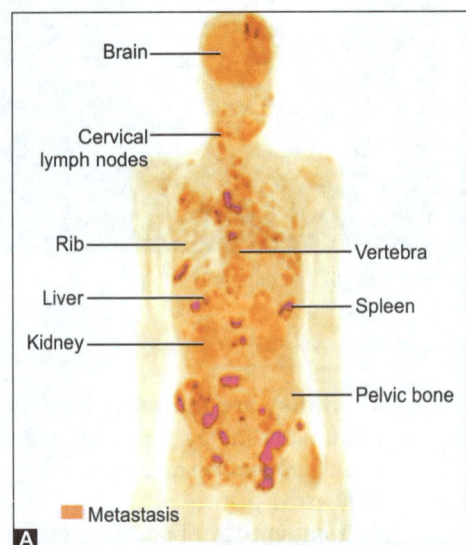
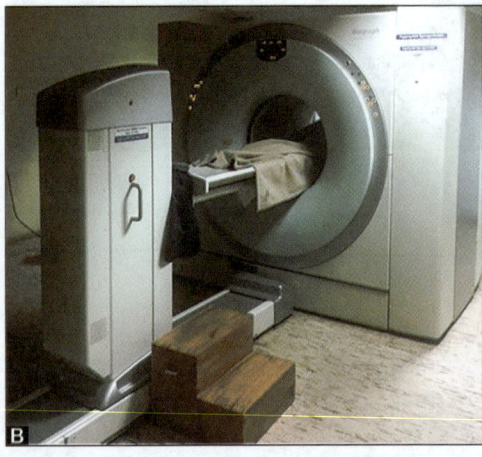

Figs. 11.9A and B: Positron emission tomography (PET) scan machine and image.
Source: Dr Ranadheer, Department of Nuclear Medicine, SVIMS, Tirupati.

Chapter 11: Introduction to Radiological Anatomy

- Evaluate brain function, e.g., Alzheimer's disease, and epilepsy.
- In pyrexia of unknown origin (PUO).
- To diagnose a condition or to track the progress of a disease to understand the response to medication.
- It can be combined with CT or MRI to show the exact localization, e.g., cancer imaging pinpointing its exact location, distinguishing between benign and malignant tumors, etc.

Single-photon Emission Computed Tomography

- It is imaging with radiotracers.
- *Principle and technique*:
  - Here radiopharmaceuticals (pharmaceuticals tagged with radioisotope) are injected and biodistribution studied. Different types of scans are taken and the images from each are merged.
  - It uses two technologies, i.e., (1) methylene diphosphonate (MDP) for osteoblastic activity and (2) sulfur colloid for reticuloendothelial function and a radioactive material (tracer) of natural element.
  - The tracer allows visualization of blood flow function, in a tissue or an organ. The tracer elements pass safely through the body.
  - It uses a special technique to create 3D images.
- *Uses*:
  - To detect spondylosis, disc infection, tumors of vertebra.
  - To find cancer progression and spread to the bone, hidden bone fractures.
  - For detection of inducible perfusion defects in myocardial ischemia, pulmonary thromboembolism.

Ultrasound (Figs. 11.10A and B)

- *Synonyms*: It is also called sonography or ultrasonography.

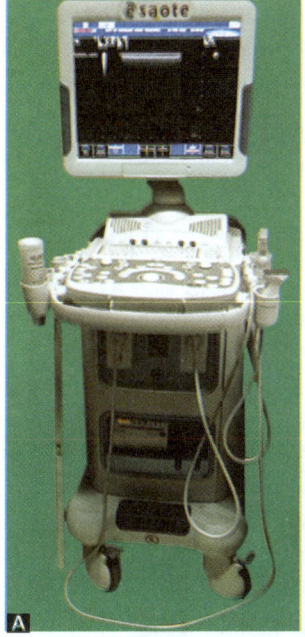
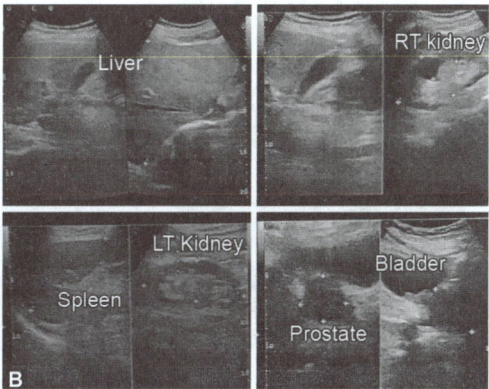

Figs. 11.10A and B: Ultrasound machine and image.
Source: Department of Radiology, SVIMS and Saptagiri Scan Center, Tirupati.

- Safe and effective procedure for observing internal organs.
- *Principle and technique*:
  - Short bursts of high frequency sound waves (1–10 MHz) are used to create images of internal organs. There is no risk of radiation exposure as it does not use ionizing radiation as in X-rays.
  - A small transducer (probe) and ultrasound gel are placed on the skin directly. High-frequency sound waves are transmitted from the probe through the gel into the body. The probe collects the sounds that bounce back and the computer converts the sound waves into an image.
  - Since the images are captured in real-time the movement of organs as well as blood flow can be observed.
- *Appearance*:
  - Solid tissues appear more homogeneous and white. Example: liver, spleen, kidney (not calyces).
  - Cystic structures—appear hypoechoic and black. Example: cysts (renal, liver, etc.), gallbladder, and bladder.
- *Uses*:
  - For evaluation of many organs like liver, kidneys, pancreas, gallbladder, bile ducts, heart, spleen, etc.
  - In women to examine breast, uterus, ovaries, tubes, and during pregnancy.
  - For fetal monitoring.
  - To diagnose heart condition and assess damage to the heart after a heart attack.
  - Certain procedures such as needle biopsies and draining the fluid are performed under the guidance of ultrasound.

Mammography (Figs. 11.11A and B)

- It is a specialized medical imaging of breast using low dose X-rays.
- It is also called mammogram.
- It aids in early detection of cancer of breast in women.

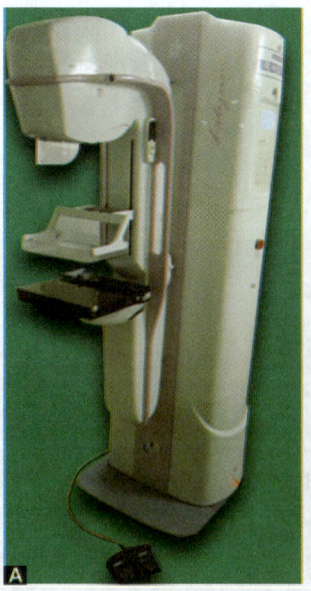
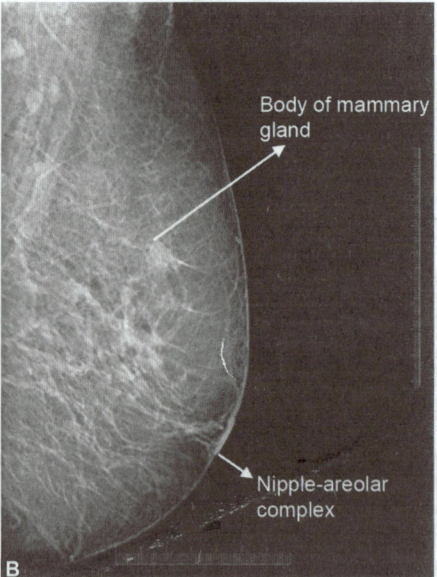

Figs. 11.11A and B: Mammogram machine and image.
Source: Department of Radiology, SVIMS and Saptagiri Scan Center, Tirupati.

Chapter 11: Introduction to Radiological Anatomy

Anatomical Basis for Clinical Condition

Case Scenario

Problem: What investigation can be suggested in the following conditions? Give your explanation for each with your anatomical knowledge.

Questions:

1. Estimation of age of a child of 10 years.
2. Ultrasound investigation in a case of sterility in a female of 35 years age.
3. Most common investigation suggested in a case of coronary artery disease.
4. The procedure for mass screening of breast cancers in a community.
5. Investigation for knowing the extent of spread of cancers in the bone.
6. Explanation for the image in **Figures 11.9A and B**.
7. Importance of single-photon emission computed tomography (SPECT) in brain tumors.
8. Investigation in a case of head injury.

Anatomical explanation:

1. Estimation of age of a child of 10 years. Plain X-ray of long bones should be advised for observing the presence of unfused epiphyses with diaphysis or epiphyseal plate of cartilage which will be seen as a translucent area.
2. Ultrasound investigation is advised in a case of sterility in a female of 35 years age. It is used for observing the normal appearance of reproductive organs and mainly for the study of maturity of ovarian follicles.
3. Most common investigation suggested in a case of coronary artery disease is the coronary angiogram for diagnosis of blockage or narrowing of coronary arteries to plan for angioplasty or stent, coronary artery bypass grafting (CABG) or medical line of management.
4. The procedure for mass screening of breast cancers in a community is by mammography to reduce the breast cancer mortality.
5. Investigation for knowing the extent of spread of cancers in the bone is by magnetic resonance imaging (MRI) for small metastases.
6. Positron emission tomography (PET) scan is advised for knowing the spread of cancers to other organs and bone metastases. It is a maximum intensity projection image showing physiological distribution of fluorodeoxyglucose (FDG) in the brain, liver, spleen, and bone and further excretion through kidney and bladder. Multiple areas of FDG concentration is noted in cervical and mediastinal lymph nodes. Increased FDG concentration was noted in the skull, vertebrae, ribs, and pelvic bones suggestive of metastases.
7. SPECT is used in brain tumors for differentiating high-grade from low-grade brain tumors.
8. Investigation advised in a case of head injury is CT scan to quickly visualize fracture, hemorrhage in the brain and blood clots in brain.

Chapter 11: Introduction to Radiological Anatomy

> ### ☞ Key Concept
>
> **Take Home Message—Radiological Anatomy**
> - Radiology is a complex and multifaceted science.
> - The advent of the newer imaging techniques facilitates early diagnosis and treatment giving a greatest opportunity to cure the disease.
> - Interpretation of the radiological images requires a detailed knowledge of anatomy.
> - Plain X-rays are useful in showing detailed images of skeletal structure and for viewing the chest.
> - Computed tomography (CT) scan is of particular utility in cases of trauma and in cases of traumatic hemorrhage in traffic accidents.
> - Magnetic resonance imaging (MRI) is particularly useful in the brain especially "functional MRI" is used to detect the areas of activity of the brain during certain tasks or activities.
> - Positron emission tomography (PET) and single-photon emission computed tomography (SPECT) are used in nuclear medicine.
> - Contrast media are used to enhance contours of structure. Contrast media are classified as radiolucent (e.g., air) and radiopaque (e.g., barium or iodinated contrast media).
> - Ultrasound is the procedure used for assessing fetal growth, for observing the ovarian follicular maturation and release in obstetrics.
> - Ultrasound-guided biopsies can be performed like chorionic villous biopsy, amniocentesis, etc.
> - Mammography procedure can be used for screening of breast cancers in females.

QUESTIONS

1. Importance of plain X-rays.
2. Ultrasonography.
3. Contrast X-rays.
4. Magnetic resonance imaging.
5. Interventional radiology.

MULTIPLE CHOICE QUESTIONS

1. Which one of the following is radiolucent contrast medium?
   A. Air
   B. Barium
   C. Iodine
   D. Bromine

2. Which one among the following is having highest radio-opacity?
   A. Air
   B. Heart
   C. Skeleton
   D. Barium

ANSWERS

1. A   2. D

CHAPTER 12
Introduction to Surface Anatomy

LEARNING OBJECTIVES

- ❖ Importance
- ❖ Techniques used
- ❖ Surface anatomy of important organs
- ❖ Imaginary lines and quadrants of abdomen
- ❖ Brief explanation of various procedures
- ❖ Important surgical incisions
- ❖ Clinical case with anatomical explanation

This is preliminary introduction required for understanding the competencies in gross anatomy

AN 4.5: Explain principles of skin incisions.
AN 13.6 and 13.7: Identification of important bony landmarks and palpation of important vessels and for testing important muscles of upper limb.
AN 20.7–20.9: Identification of important bony landmarks and palpation of important vessels and surface marking of important nerves of lower limb.
AN 55.1 and 55.2: Surface marking in abdominal and pelvic regions, structures and organs.

INTRODUCTION

Surface anatomy is a branch of gross anatomy that examines shapes and markings on the surface of the body of the structures that are deeply situated. An understanding of surface anatomy is essential for locating and identifying anatomic structures prior to studying internal gross anatomy.

IMPORTANCE

Healthcare personnel use surface anatomy to locate the anatomical structures by observation, palpation, percussion using landmarks. This helps in diagnosing medical conditions and to treat patients, as in taking arterial pulse, listening to heart beats, inserting a needle or tube for biopsy, or performing radiological investigation (CT, MRI, and ultrasound) or a surgical procedure or physical therapy.

TECHNIQUES USED

The techniques that are used in surface anatomy are visual inspection, palpation with hand, percussion using fingers and auscultation with stethoscope. *The readers are advised to go through the chapter of introduction to anatomy for the description of these methods.* The uses and examples of each of these techniques are described in **Table 12.1**.

Using *visual inspection*, one can directly observe the structure and mark for surface features through *palpation* (feeling with firm pressure or perceiving by the sense of touch), to precisely locate and identify the palpable anatomic features under the skin. Using *percussion* they tap firmly on specific body sites to detect resonating vibrations and through *auscultation* they listen to sounds produced from organs due to their physiological phenomenon.

Chapter 12: Introduction to Surface Anatomy

Table 12.1: Surface anatomy—techniques.

Method	Uses	Examples
Visual inspection	Direct observation of the structure with un-aided eye	Goiter (hyperthyroidism), kyphosis, scoliosis, lordosis, limping gait, hemiplegic hand, etc.
Palpation	Precisely locate and identify anatomical features under the skin with the palm of hands	Hepatomegaly, splenomegaly, subcutaneous lumps, body temperature, pulse, iliac crest, clavicle, spines of vertebrae, sternal angle, etc.
Percussion	Tap firmly with the middle fingers of both hands on specific body sites to detect resonating vibrations	Lungs (air/fluid-filled), abdominal bloating, etc.
Auscultation	Listen to sounds from various organs of the body using stethoscope	Heart sounds, breath sounds, etc.
Imaginary lines	Used to locate the particular organs of the body	Abdominal quadrants, McBurney's point in appendicitis, kidney marking, etc.

Surface anatomy of important organs in various regions of the body: There are certain important visible or palpable landmarks in the various regions of the body that serve as a guide for locating an organ or structure. As stated above in **Table 12.1** they can be identified by the techniques mentioned. To make the reader familiar certain examples are provided for each region in **Table 12.2**.

The palpable arteries that are used commonly for feeling and counting the pulse are shown in **Figure 12.1**.

Different types of percussion notes in health and disease were represented in **Table 12.3**.

Auscultation

Auscultation can be done with stethoscope to listen to the sounds inside the body. During auscultation, the stethoscope allows to hear what's happening inside the body. Abnormal sounds in these areas may indicate problems:
- Lungs
- Abdomen or bowels
- Heart
- Major blood vessels

Imaginary Anatomical Lines

These are the lines useful for the medical procedure and surface markings thus they are aids for localizing the underlying viscera or important events that takes place.

For example: Midclavicular line, midaxillary line (mammary line), midsternal line, parasternal line, midinguinal line, etc. These are described in **Table 12.4**. *Details of each of these will be dealt in the relevant regions in Textbooks of Gross Anatomy.*

Axillary Lines (Fig. 12.2)

- There are three axillary lines—(1) anterior, (2) mid, and (3) posterior.
- The anterior axillary line is used for placing the V5 lead of ECG.
- The midaxillary line is used as a guide for performing thoracocentesis procedure, V6 lead of 10 electrodes ECG.

Anatomical Lines of Thorax

The important lines are midsternal, lateral sternal and midclavicular lines. Important bony landmarks of thorax are the jugular (suprasternal) notch, manubriosternal angle (Louis angle) and xiphisternal angle.

Anatomical Regions of Abdomen

Division of abdomen into nine regions (**Fig. 12.3**): There are two horizontal and two vertical imaginary lines on the abdomen dividing into nine regions and the organs located in these regions are shown in **Table 12.5**.

Chapter 12: Introduction to Surface Anatomy

Table 12.2: Region-wise landmarks of importance.

Region	Landmarks of importance—examples of structures
Head region	☐ *Visible*: Ear, eyes, chin, and parts of nose ☐ *Palpable*: Inferior border and angle of mandible, external occipital protuberance, and facial artery pulsation at the lower border of mandible in relation with anterior border of masseter muscle
Neck region	☐ *Visible*: The sternocleidomastoid muscle can be made prominent by asking the person to turn the neck to the opposite side. This muscle subdivides each side of the neck into anterior and posterior triangles. The thyroid gland is visible on asking the person to swallow ☐ *Palpable*: Vertebra prominence or spine of C7 vertebra, hyoid bone
Trunk region	The trunk is divided into the thorax, abdominopelvic region, and back *Thorax:* ☐ *Visible*: Apex beat of heart, suprasternal notch ☐ *Palpable*: Sternal angle, ribs, and apex beat. ☐ *Percussion*: Borders of heart, position of heart valves, and lines of pleural reflection ☐ *Auscultation*: Breath sounds, heart beat *Abdominopelvic:* ☐ *Visible*: Umbilicus, costal margin ☐ *Palpable*: Linea alba, anterior superior iliac spine, inguinal ligament, and liver ☐ *Percussion*: For the limits of liver ☐ *Auscultation*: Bowel sounds *Back*: The triangle of auscultation is an area where breath sounds may be heard clearly with a stethoscope
Shoulder and upper limb region	☐ *Visible*: Clavicle, inferior angle of scapula ☐ *Palpable*: Radial and brachial artery pulse, styloid process of ulna and radius The surface anatomy of the shoulder and upper limb is used for drawing blood, providing nutrients and fluids, and for administering medicine The axilla, or armpit, is important clinically because of the blood vessels, nerves, and lymph nodes located there The thenar and hypothenar eminences are easily palpated on the anterior surface of the hand
Lower limb region	☐ *Visible*: The gluteal muscles form the prominences of the buttocks. Malleoli at ankle are visible ☐ *Palpable*: Femoral triangle and popliteal fossa are clinically important surface landmarks. Femoral artery pulsations and femoral artery ligations can be done at the femoral triangle (superior medial aspect of the thigh) The pulse of the dorsalis pedis artery may be palpated on the medial dorsal side of the foot above the navicular bone, or along the dorsal interspace between the first and second metatarsals

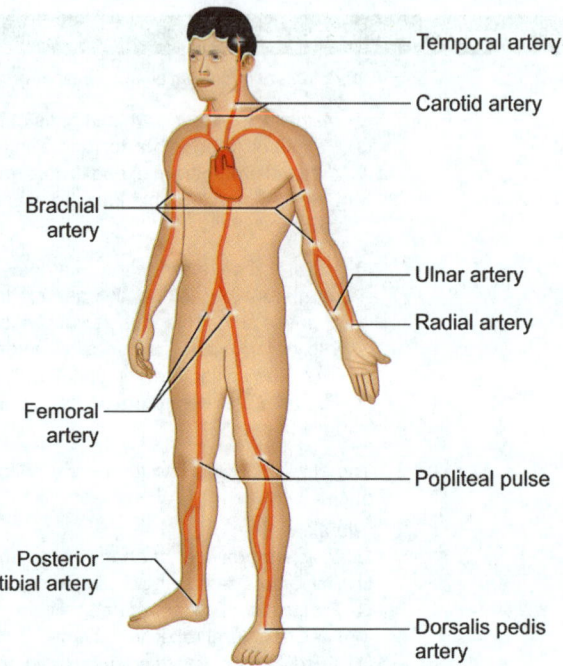

Fig. 12.1: Sites for recording arterial pulse.

Table 12.3: Different types of percussion notes.		
Normal percussion sounds	Organ or region heard	Abnormal percussion sounds
Resonance	Lung	❑ Dullness, which may be produced by pneumonia, tumor, infarction, or fluid collection ❑ Hyper-resonance or even tympanic, which may result from confluent air collection, as seen in pneumothorax or emphysema
Tympanic	Most portions of the abdominal cavity	❑ Dullness, which may be produced by intra-abdominal tumors or masses ❑ Shifting dullness may indicate presence of ascites
Dullness	Over solid organs (liver), heart and muscles	Heart: An expanded area of dullness may indicate cardiomegaly or pericardial effusion

Table 12.4: Anatomical landmarks of clinical significance.		
Region	Anatomical line	Bony/structural landmark
Head and neck and back	Planes used for measurements: ❑ Frankfurt plane ❑ Facial plane ❑ Mandibular plane	❑ *Vertebra prominence*— spine of C7 vertebra—junction of neck and back ❑ *Spine of scapula*—medial end to T3 vertebra ❑ *Inferior angle of scapula*—T7 vertebra ❑ Lower border of mandible ❑ Angle of mandible ❑ Tragus of ear ❑ Red margin of upper lip ❑ Ala of nose

Contd...

Contd...

Region	Anatomical line	Bony/structural landmark
Upper limb	Axillary folds	❑ Epicondyles of humerus ❑ Tuberosity of radius ❑ Radial styloid process ❑ Ulnar styloid process
Thorax	1. *Midsternal line*—tracing pleural reflection 2. *Parasternal line*—tracing the borders of heart, lines of pleural reflection 3. *Midclavicular line*—used as a reference point for locating the apex beat of heart; used along with extension into the abdomen for dividing the nine quadrants of abdomen	1. *Jugular notch*—corresponds to T2/T3 vertebra. Clinical significance in aortic aneurysm (suprasternal pulsations) in adult and coarctation of aorta in children 2. *Manubriosternal angle of Louis*—important events take place at this point. Corresponds to T4/T5 vertebra, e.g., termination of trachea, junction between superior and inferior mediastinum 3. *Xiphisternal angle*— corresponds to T9 Vertebra. 4. *Nipple*— position corresponds to 4th inter-costal space
Abdomen	1. *Subcostal plane*—it is a landmark—corresponds to L3 vertebra and 10th rib 2. *Transpyloric plane*—corresponds to L1 vertebra and position of certain structures, e.g., pylorus of stomach, hilum of kidney 3. *Intertubercular plane*—corresponds to L5 vertebra 4. *Intercristal plane*— corresponds to iliac crest L4 vertebra	1. *Umbilicus*—corresponds to junction of L3 and L4 vertebrae 2. *Anterior superior iliac spine*—inguinal ligament attachment—surgical landmark 3. *Pubic tubercle*—inguinal ligament attachment 4. *Pubic symphysis*—important in pelvimetry
Lower limb	1. *Midpoint of inguinal ligament* 2. *Mid-inguinal point*	1. *Ischial spine*—landmark for pudendal block in anesthesia 2. *Ischial tuberosity* 3. *Medial malleolus* 4. *Lateral malleolus*

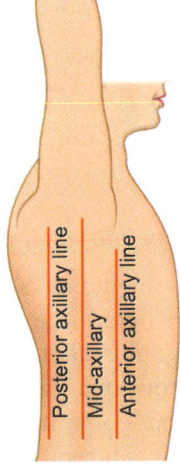

Fig. 12.2: Axillary lines.

Horizontal Planes

The following two horizontal planes are drawn by connecting easily palpable bony points:
1. *Subcostal plane*:
   - It corresponds to the line drawn connecting lower most projecting bony points on right and left parts of rib cage.
   - This corresponds to 10th costal cartilage anteriorly and body of L3 vertebra posteriorly.
   - This plane is the surface marking for certain structures, e.g., origin of inferior mesenteric artery, 3rd part of duodenum.

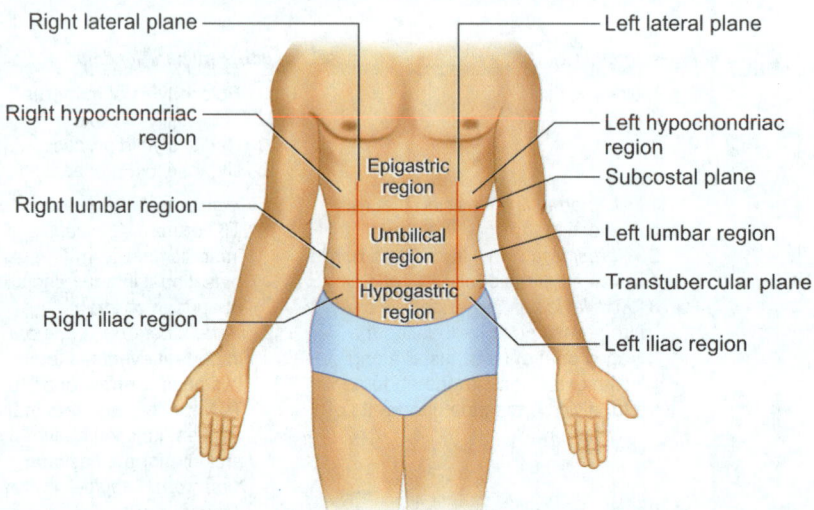

Fig. 12.3: Nine regions of abdomen.

Table 12.5: Location of organs in the various regions of abdomen.

Region	Organs
Right hypochondrium	Liver, gallbladder, right kidney, and small intestine
Left hypochondrium	Spleen, colon, left kidney, and pancreas
Epigastrium	Stomach, liver, pancreas, duodenum, spleen, and adrenal glands
Right lumbar region	Gallbladder, liver, and right colon
Left lumbar region	Descending colon and left kidney
Umbilical region	Umbilicus, jejunum, ileum, and duodenum
Right iliac fossa	Appendix and cecum
Left iliac fossa	Descending colon and sigmoid colon
Hypogastrium	Urinary bladder, sigmoid colon, and female reproductive organs

2. *Transtubercular plane*:
   - It corresponds to the line drawn connecting the two tubercles on iliac crest.
   - This line corresponds to upper border of L5 vertebra.

Vertical Planes
- These are two vertical lines connecting midpoint of clavicle to the mid-inguinal point.
- It passes just lateral to the tip of 9th costal cartilage which is a surface marking for gallbladder.
- This line can be used as a surface marking for the lateral border of rectus abdominis muscle.

Abdominal division into four quadrants:

Dividing the abdomen into various sections will help doctors determine what could be the cause of the illness. The abdomen can also be divided into four quadrants keeping the umbilicus as the midpoint. The importance of these four quadrants is represented in **Table 12.6** and **Figure 12.4.**

Chapter 12: Introduction to Surface Anatomy

Table 12.6: Importance of four quadrant of abdomen.

Abdomen quadrant	Clinical importance
Right upper quadrant (RUQ)	❑ To elicit the exact site of pain and tenderness by palpation ❑ This region contains the organs, e.g., liver, gallbladder, and duodenum ❑ Pain and tenderness of diseases of liver (hepatitis), gallbladder (cholecystitis) can be localized here
Right lower quadrant (RLQ)	❑ This quadrant contains the organs, e.g., appendix, right ureter and in women the right ovary and the uterine tube ❑ The pain and tenderness in this region gives a clue for the diagnosis of their origin form the viscera located in this region, e.g., appendicitis ❑ *McBurney's point*: This is the point of maximum tenderness felt on application of deep pressure along the line connecting umbilicus and right anterior superior iliac spine cases of acute appendicitis
Left upper quadrant (LUQ)	❑ The important organs located in this quadrant are the stomach, spleen, left lobe of liver, major part of pancreas, left kidney, and left suprarenal gland
Left lower quadrant (LLQ)	❑ The important organs located in this quadrant are the sigmoid colon, left ureter, left ovary, and left uterine tube ❑ Diseases originating from the viscera of this region can be diagnosed, e.g., colitis, ureteric colic, cysts and tumors of ovary, etc. ❑ The doctors will assess this area if there is abdominal pain in this region ❑ Abdominal pain in the LLQ may be a symptom of colitis, diverticulitis, or ureteric colic ❑ Pain in this region may also be caused by ovarian cysts or a pelvic inflammation ❑ Tumors found in this region can be serious determinants of colon or ovarian cancer

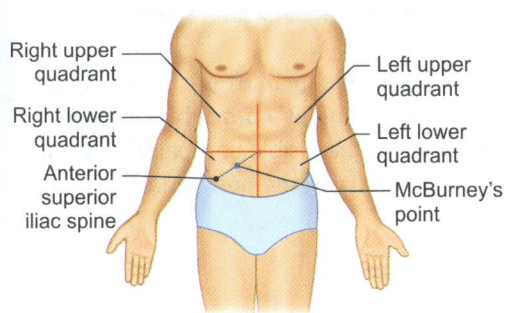

Fig. 12.4: Four quadrants of abdomen.

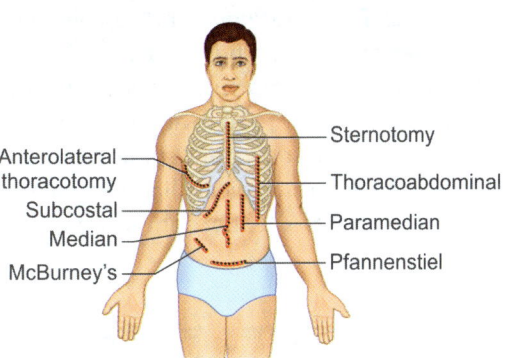

Fig. 12.5: Important skin incisions.

Skin Incisions (Fig. 12.5)

The skin incisions are used for approaching the body cavities. Each incision has got both advantages and disadvantages. The surgeon is the right person to choose the appropriate incision for the viscera or region in which he has to operate.

Thorax

- *Sternotomy*: Used for opening entire thoracic cavity.
- *Thoracotomy*: For surgeries on lung, esophagus, and for applying a clamp to abdominal aorta this is preferred.

Thoracoabdominal

- It is a single large incision involving both the thorax and abdomen.
- Because of the risk involved with such a wider incision it is rarely used.

Abdomen: In the abdomen, the vertical midline incision is the most frequently used.

- *Vertical midline*: Most commonly preferred because of:
  - Minimal blood loss
  - No risk of injuring the nerves
  - Ease of opening and closing
  - Wider exposure of most of the abdominal and pelvic viscera.
- *Pfannenstiel*:
  - It is a transverse incision above the pubis.
  - This is given for operations in pelvic region.
  - It has a good cosmetic advantage.
- *Subcostal*:
  - Rectus muscle is divided.
  - Used for surgeries on gallbladder on right side and spleen on left side.
  - Bilateral incision for upper abdominal surgeries.
- *Paramedian*:
  - It facilitates better exposure of structures that are placed laterally.
  - The chances of incisional hernia are less as the closure of abdomen is with multiple layers of fascia.
  - Extent of vertical incision is limited by costal margin.
  - Lower transverse incision is given just above the pubis.
  - Cosmetic advantage.
- *McBurney's*: This incision is given for surgery on appendix.

Clinical Application of Surface Anatomy
- Healthcare personnel use surface anatomy to locate the anatomical structures for diagnosis (e.g., biopsy and radiology) and for treatment (surgical procedures), physiotherapy.
- The techniques that are used in surface anatomy are visual inspection, palpation with hand, percussion using fingers and auscultation with stethoscope. These facilitate localization of organ of origin for the health problem.
- Division of a region into various subregions as in abdomen facilitates isolation of an area of health problem and its in-depth analysis for arriving at a probable diagnosis.
- Skin incisions for various surgical procedures is based on the visible and palpable bony points and the imaginary lines drawn on the body surface using the bony landmarks and the locational extent of normal organs in situ.

Anatomical Basis for Clinical Condition

Case Scenario

Problem: A male patient attends the emergency department with pain in the right lower abdomen of sudden onset, fever, and vomiting. The surgeon examined the patient and advised blood test for complete blood picture, X-ray abdomen, and ultrasound abdomen. Based on the clinical findings and investigation reports it was diagnosed as acute appendicitis. Surgeons plans for surgery of appendectomy.

Questions:
1. What was the relationship between the pain mentioned by the patient to right lower abdomen, right iliac fossa, and the diagnosis of appendicitis?
2. What clinical examination will diagnose the condition of acute appendicitis?

Contd...

Contd...

3. How the clinical examination does helps in ordering investigation of ultrasound abdomen?
4. How the knowledge of surface anatomy does helps in giving incisions at the appropriate area of organ?

Anatomical explanation:

1. The knowledge of surface anatomy facilitates localization of origin of pain to an area as in this case to the right lower abdomen, i.e., the right iliac fossa. As the appendix, the organ more commonly can get inflamed and the patient is male, it could be the organ of origin of the pain. In the case of female one should exclude the origin of pain from ovary/ uterine tube on right side.
2. The surgeon palpated, percussed and auscultated the right iliac fossa for tenderness and elicited the area of tenderness by asking the patient to confirm the pain area during examination. The surgeon confirmed that the area of maximum tenderness was at McBurney's point by marking it on the surface.
3. Based on history and physical examination investigation of ultrasound abdomen could be suggested for detailed radiological observation of right iliac fossa with special emphasis on appendix.
4. The knowledge of surface anatomy helps in giving appropriate, minimal surgical incision adequate for exposing the area for undertaking the surgery of an organ. In the present case it is at McBurney's point.

☞ Key Concept

Take Home Message—Surface Anatomy

- It is a branch of gross anatomy where based on the anatomical knowledge of internal organs their location can be mapped on the surface of the body.
- An understanding of surface anatomy is essential for locating and identifying anatomic boundaries of internal organs before opening the cavities or giving incisions for regions in surgical practice.
- The study of surface anatomy uses the basic techniques of visual inspection, palpation, percussion, and auscultation with the help of landmarks in health and disease.
- This helps in diagnosing medical conditions and to treat patients.
- Based on the surface bony points and landmarks different lines are drawn in different planes to divide the region into various areas for accurate localization of organ, its dimensions in health, in disease, for planning diagnostic and therapeutic methods.
- While giving skin incisions the type of incision depends on the extent of exposure required for surgical maneuvering, healing of scar, cosmetic aspect, etc.

QUESTIONS

1. What are the important arteries that are palpated for recording pulse?
2. What are the nine quadrants of abdomen? and What organs are located in each quadrant?
3. Importance of surgical incisions.

CHAPTER 13

Introduction to Dissection of Cadaver

LEARNING OBJECTIVES

- Definition of cadaver
- Definition of dissection
- Cadaver—respect, cadaveric oath and care
- Dissectors safety measures
- Dissection instruments
- Dissection procedure
- Clinical importance
- Clinical case with anatomical explanation

INTRODUCTION

Study of anatomy has to be carried out on the dead, preserved human body (cadaver) in which texture and appearance of structures and organs of the body has not been altered. The word cadaver is derived from the Latin word *cadre* means "to fall". The method used for understanding the organization of the various parts of the body is by dissection of cadaver. For carrying out the dissections it is important that the dissector should have basic knowledge of general structural plan of the body and the relationship of the layers, partitions and compartments one encounters when dissecting from superficial to deep in any particular region. Before *Vesalius* the descriptions in textbooks of anatomy were based on dissections conducted in animals. *Leonardo da Vinci* has painted descriptive pictures of human body though he is not an anatomist.

DISSECTION

- It is the process to separate and clean structures for proper visualization of their orientation.
- *Benefits*: Class and individual understanding of the subject will be enhanced.

It aids in identification of the part during clinical testing.

Before Proceeding for Dissection

- *Respect to laboratory partner*: Give respect to your laboratory partner (cadaver) and the structure or organ you are about to explore, observe and learn.
- *Personal care*: Take extra care with your dissection tools. Handle them carefully.
- *Check before cutting*: Double check before cutting a structure.

CADAVER RESPECT

AN 82.1 Demonstrate respect and follow the correct procedure when handling cadavers and other biological tissues.

- Every human cadaver that is subjected to anatomical dissection is enriching the knowledge of medical sciences. Hence, cadaver is the first teacher in the medical profession and has to be treated with utmost respect.
- Cadaver should be handled with due respect. As cadavers are obtained either as they are unclaimed or by voluntary donation. The anatomical donors are to

be treated with utmost respect at all times and in a professional manner.
- As persons donating their bodies are not receiving any financial compensation the cadavers are to be treated as gift.
- The dignity of cadaver/dead body is to be maintained by covering the body part that was not being dissected.
- Articulated skeletons, skulls, and isolated bones are to be afforded the same respect as cadavers.
- Take good care of the cadaver. Cover the cadaver with chemicals to prevent drying as once the part is dried softness cannot be restored.
- Disposable tissues should be put in the steel trash bins.
- Use of cameras, cell phones or other photographic or video equipment are not permitted in the dissection hall unless specifically authorized.
- Food and/or drinks should not be allowed at the cadaver.
- *Cadaveric oath*: The medical student should be made to take oath before starting cadaver dissection to sensitize them about the importance of cadaver as first teacher and first patient in enhancing their knowledge and for inculcating professional behavior.

CARE OF CADAVER

- The different chemical compounds and gases released from a dead body due to the action of microorganisms causes decomposition of the body and produce unpleasant odor.
- To protect the dead body from decomposition and to prevent the spread of infection to others and to the surroundings certain chemical substances are injected into the cadaver. The process is called *embalming* and the fluids that are injected are called *embalming fluids*.
- Before embalming, the dead bodies are subjected to pre-embalming treatment to remove blood clots.
- The bodies are preserved by injecting the embalming fluid containing a mixture of formalin, methanol, glycerin, water, etc. into the femoral artery or carotid artery. As the fluid is injected into an artery it is called arterial embalming. Some amount of embalming fluid is directly injected into the abdominal, pelvic, and thoracic cavities and into the cranial cavity through orbit.
- Embalming is done to temporarily preserve the body while waiting for the funeral. It is done permanently for long-term preservation for studying anatomy by dissection method. Embalmed cadavers are stored in tanks filled with formalin, water and some preservative salts.
- To prevent drying of the cadaver from varying temperatures it has to be appropriately draped at all times preferably by a cloth soaked in preservative fluid to prevent drying or the body can be painted with a chemical mixture to keep it moist.
- The well-preserved cadavers are used for anatomical dissection, research, and histological examination.
- The cadavers for dissection or research in anatomy department are obtained from the forensic department when they are declared as unclaimed bodies or by voluntary body donation of the deceased (expressed by a will during his lifetime) or by his close kith and kin. The human cadaver and its tissue for research, teaching, and training are governed by ethical issues.

Dissection Hall Maintenance

- Space for storing your books and dissection tools to be utilized for the personal safety and for the respect of the cadaver.
- Do not keep books/instruments on the cadaver.
- Do not lean or place hands/elbows on cadaver to support yourself.
- Keep the hall area grease-free and clean to avoid fall and getting injured.

DISSECTION SAFETY MEASURES

- *Remember*: Cadaver is your first patient and you usually do not know what your patient has when you first start interacting with him/her.
- Dress should not drag on the floor/cadaver. It is recommended to wear old clothes, tops with short sleeves or sleeves that can be rolled up if long sleeved. To protect the clothes from soiling use separate clothes for dissection hall. Wash them frequently with detergent and bleach.
- Apron should be worn compulsorily to avoid contact with the embalming fluid. Covered shoes to be used to protect from dropped sharp instruments like scalpel.
- Goggles to be used while cutting bones to protect the eyes from foreign bodies, using hammers and chisels.
- *Contact lenses*: Do not wear contact lenses in laboratory. Formaldehyde and other preservatives produce chemical vapors that can be absorbed by the contacts.
- Gloves to be used to prevent contact with preservatives and chemicals.
- Best is to use naked hand for palpation and for feeling of structures—nerves, arteries, veins, tendons, etc.
- Long hair to be secured in place with hair pins, hair bands, etc. before beginning dissection.
- Not to wear rings, bangles, etc. that comes in contact with cadaver.
- Wash your hands thoroughly before leaving the dissection hall.
- Not to wear flowers as a token of respect and to prevent carrying of any infective material from the dissection hall.

Know Anatomy before Beginning Dissection

Cadaver is the rare gift for you. Dissecting without preparation is never a good idea. It will result in the destruction of structures and loss of opportunity to learn from the cadaver.

- *Reading*: Thorough reading of dissection manual makes the dissector confident of structures to be exposed in the region of dissection.
- *Planning*: Procedure of dissection, i.e., incisions, tips for tracing the structures, etc., has to be planned in advance.
- *Check list*: A list of structures to be identified and the relations and the course to be traced, etc., facilitates learning anatomy with confidence.
- Dissection—prerequisites:
  - Dissection is an art. It requires:
    - *Skill*: It develops over time.
    - *Care, patience, and practice*: While doing dissection the dissector should show utmost care and patience while separating the various layers of tissue and should practice not to cut the important structures. This perfection with patience and practice improves their surgical skills during their subsequent clinical practice.
- *Techniques and tools*: To save time and to avoid the loss of details appropriate technique should be used for detailed exposure of the area of dissection under study. Use of appropriate tools reduces the time taken for completing the dissection in time.

Instruments Required for Dissection (Figs. 13.1A to L)

1. Surface marking pencil to mark on the skin surface
2. Probe
3. Scalpel with blade (fixed and removable)
4. Forceps (toothed and regular)
5. Scissors (small and medium sized)

- *Surface marking pencil*:
  - Surface marking of structures
  - Bony or other land marks on cadaver
  - Marking skin incisions
- *Probe* (**Fig. 13.1B**):
  - *Description*: One end is handle. Other end is angular with a rounded tip
  - *Uses*: Tearing tissues. Feeling structures like vessels and nerves

Chapter 13: Introduction to Dissection of Cadaver

- *Scalpel (Figs. 13.1C and D)*:
  - *Description*: One end is handle. Other end is the cutting edge.
  - *Uses*:
    - Used for sharp dissection
    - To cut and reflect skin
    - To cut tissues and dissection of tough connective tissue
    - To divide vessels, pedicles, and other structures
  - *Disadvantage*: It may cut or injure important structures during dissection
  - *Parts*:
    - Handle
    - Blade
  - *Types*:
    - Fixed handle and blade
    - Separated handle and blade.

  How to hold scalpel: It should be held with thumb, middle, and ring finger and the index finger should be placed on the upper edge to guide the **scalpel (Figs. 13.1C and D)**.

- *Forceps* **(Figs. 13.1E and F)**:
  - *Description*: Shaft is closed by thumb and fingers
  - *Uses:*
    - Blunt dissection—pulling or tearing (not for cutting)
    - To grasp, lift and hold tissues
    - To cut tissues and dissection of tough connective tissue
  - *Types*:
    - Plain: To hold delicate structures like vessels, nerves, and peritoneum
    - Toothed/tissue forceps: For others
  - *Uses*:
    - To hold tissues and for better grip
    - To insert blade over handle and to remove blade from handle
  - *Description*:
    - Two parts: Blade and tip
    - Outer surface: Serrations for better grip for holding
    - Inner surface: Plain forceps has ridges and grooves. Toothed forceps has tooth and socket to prevent slipping of tissue.

  How to hold forceps: It should be held between thumb and fingers with the middle finger playing a key role **(Figs. 13.1E and F)**.

- *Scissors* **(Figs. 13.1G and H)**:
  - *Uses*:
    - Cutting and sectioning of tissue
    - Cut tough structures like tendons, ligaments, etc.
  - *Types*:
    - Blunt dissection: Straight scissors
    - Delicate work: Curved scissors

- *Saw* **(Fig. 13.1I)**:
  - *Uses*:
    - Cutting bones
    - Electrical saw is available for reducing the time for cutting.

- *Bone cutting forceps* **(Fig. 13.1J)**:
  - *Uses*:
    - To cut small and large pieces of bone, edges of bones, spicules, spines, and processes of bones
    - Tearing away the remaining's of muscle, ligaments and pieces of periosteum of bones as it gives firm grip on the tissues without cutting them.

- *Chisel* **(Fig. 13.1K)**:
  - *Uses*:
    - To cut strong bones
  - *Description*: Handle and shaft
    - Handle: At one end is the head where hammer can be hit or stroked. At the other end is the shaft.
    - Shaft: Flat with one end continuous with handle and other end having cutting edge that is beveled on one side.

- *Hammer or mallet* **(Fig. 13.1L)**:
  - *Uses*:
    - To hit or stroke
    - Used along with chisel to cut the bones
  - *Description*: Handle and striking end
    - Striking end is heavier to increase the strength of stroke.

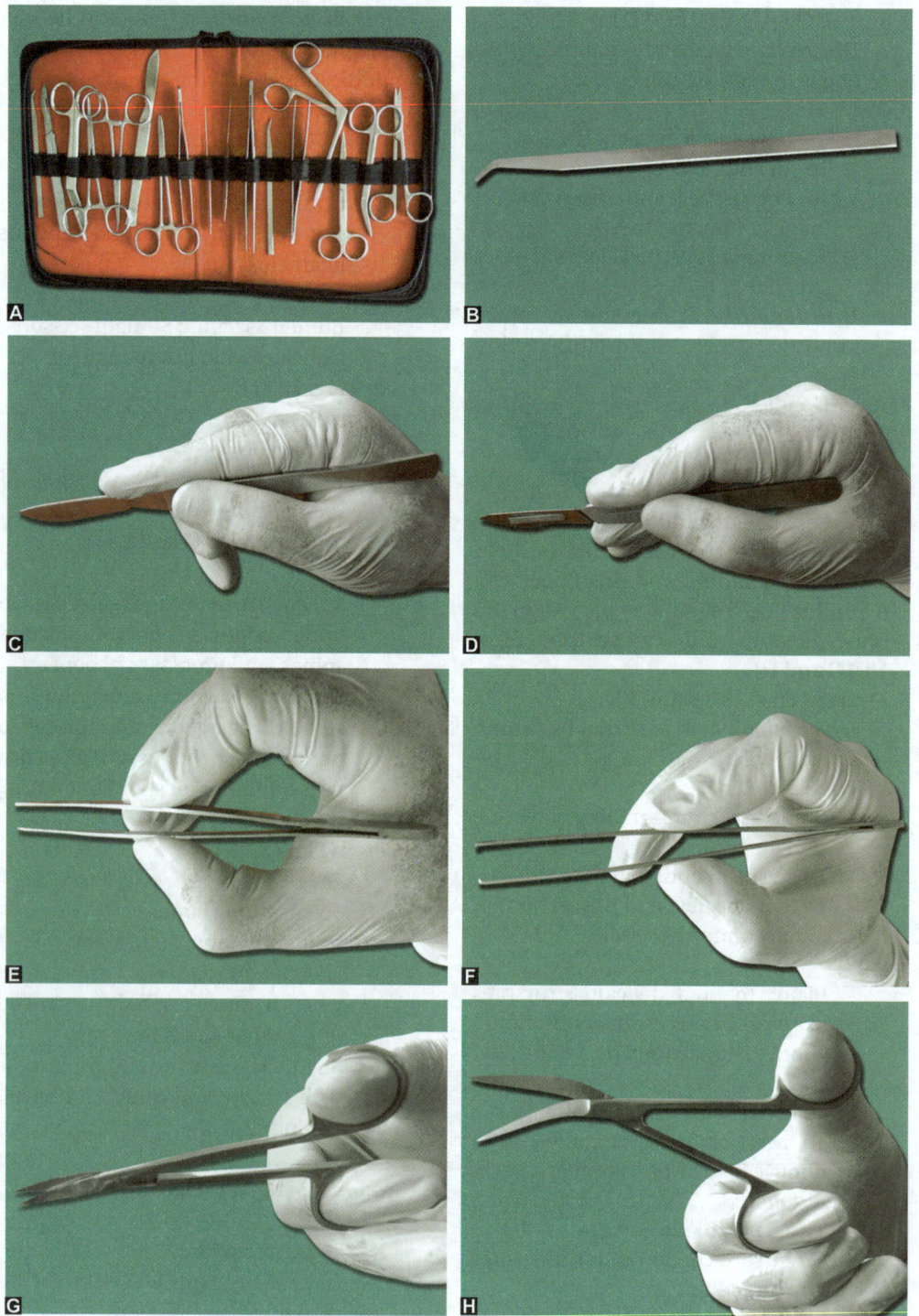

Figs. 13.1A to H: (A) Dissection kit showing instruments; (B) Probe; (C) Scalpel with fixed blade; (D) Scalpel with removable blade; (E) Forceps—untoothed; (F) Forceps—toothed; (G) Scissors—straight; (H) Scissors—curved.

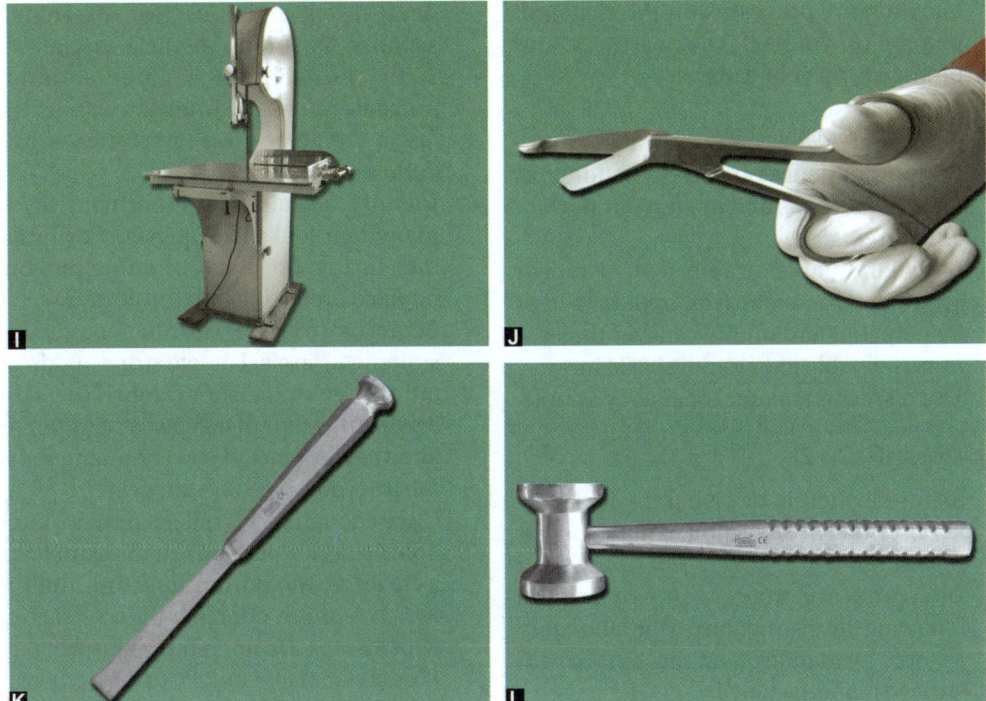

Figs. 13.1I to L: (I) Electrical bone and body cutting machine; (J) Bone cutting forceps; (K) Chisel; (L) Hammer.

Dissection Techniques

- Blunt dissection
- Sharp dissection

Blunt Dissection

- Pulling or tearing instead of cutting
- Done by:
  - Fingers—first and best
  - Probe—next best
  - Scissors—with its back edge—vessels and nerves
    - Scissor technique:
      - Insertion of closed pair of scissors into connective tissue or between two structures and then opening it
      - Scissors tears the connective tissue between two structures and cleans them

Sharp Dissection

Uses:

- Clean, precise cuts
- Incisions through skin
- Removal of fat and fascia.

Instruments:

- Done by scalpel and scissors
- To cut skin and reflect the skin flap scalpel is used
- Otherwise—no scalpel as it may cut wanted and important structures.

When dissecting rest the hand to reduce unsteady movements.

Orientation and Surface Anatomy

- Place cadaver in proper position.
- Observe and review surface anatomy of cadaver.
- Review bony anatomy.

- Locate bony processes on the skeleton, palpate on yourself, your partners, and ultimately on your cadaver.

Importance of Osteology

- Bony prominences are used as landmarks for skin incisions and to locate important structures.
- Bony landmarks on thin bodies appear as projections, on heavier bodies need to be palpated and on the cadaver they are more palpable after removal of skin.
  Use dissection manual or atlas as a guide.

Skin Incisions **(Fig. 13.2)**

- Skin reflection is by giving the incisions as described in dissection manual for that region.
- Incisions are made using a scalpel following the instructions in the laboratory manual by marking it on the surface with surface marking pencil.
- Incisions should pass through the skin and superficial fascia leaving the deep fascia and underlying muscle untouched.
- Depth of the incision varies depending on the amount of fat in the superficial fascia.
- Plane of deep fascia will most likely be seen during the next step.

Skin Reflection

- By grasping a corner of skin with a forceps, keep pulling up the skin while using a scalpel to cut or reflect the skin and superficial fascia from the underlying deep fascia and muscles. Alternately separate skin from superficial fascia.
- With the help of scalpel scraping movement of skin from the superficial fascia should be done rather than strictly cutting.
- Identify dermis and superficial fascia plane that looks like "pigskin" or pitted due to the presence of subcutaneous papillae projecting into the dermis.
- Remove skin leaving subcutaneous tissue/superficial fascia. For two strips of skin on either side of incision remove the skin, leaving the superficial fascia with nerves and vessels intact. If you are seeing red of muscle you have gone too deep.
- Once enough skin is reflected cut a button hole using scalpel through the skin. Place a finger in the button hole and pull up which is more effective than retracting with forceps. Do not remove the skin flap. Fix the skin flaps laterally to the body with hooks. Replace the flap over the dissected area when you have finished dissecting to prevent drying.

Superficial Fascia **(Fig. 13.3)**

- Superficial fascia is close to skin and contains fat, cutaneous vessels, and nerves. Removal of fat improves esthetics.
- Deep or investing fascia is a tough, but thin, layer of fibrous tissue, devoid of fat and is between superficial fascia and muscle. It can be readily demonstrated by making an incision in the superficial fascia, and raising a small portion of it.

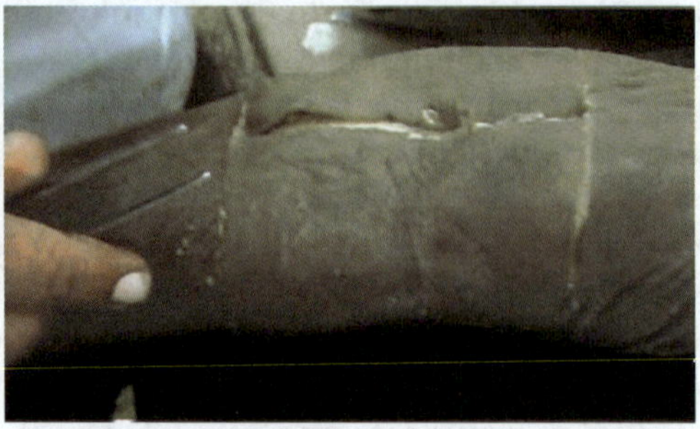

Fig. 13.2: Skin incisions for dissection of cubital fossa.

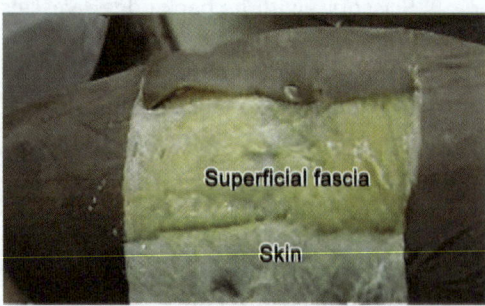

Fig. 13.3: Superficial fascia.

Nerves and Vessels in Superficial Fascia

- As you separate dermis and superficial fascia laterally, the nerves can be seen leaving the muscle and entering the superficial fascia.
- Use forceps to dissect and identify cutaneous nerves and vessels.
- Use blunt dissection and scraping to remove the fat.
- Blunt dissection (using probe and forceps) is necessary here as scalpel or sharp dissection generally severs most of the nerves before they are seen.
- Nerves always and almost accompanied by small artery and small vein.
- *Cutaneous nerves*—better to learn these structures by referring to diagrams except the larger branches that can be followed easily.
- *Small veins*—may be filled with blood, giving them a chocolate color, and are more obvious. These supply the skin and subcutaneous tissue and are not specifically named.
- *Larger veins*—run a solitary course to pierce the deep fascia and drain into the deep vein that contain valves to prevent reflux.

Deep Fascia (Fig. 13.4)

- After removal of subcutaneous tissue examine and remove deep fascia. But it is more difficult as it sends sheets between muscles enclosing each muscle. Deep or investing fascia covers the muscles and hides their details. Distinguish between investing fascia and muscular fascia.
- Superficial muscles are covered with an investing fascia that is relatively opaque and firmly adherent to the muscle. Removal of investing fascia and any other connective tissue or fat which may be obscuring the muscle has to be under taken. The fascia is elevated with toothed forceps and then cut away with the scalpel.
- The investing fascia is the denser connective tissue layer that "invests" the area like a stocking or sleeve, is usually named regionally (e.g. thoracolumbar fascia) (Latin word *septum* means "partition, wall").

Muscular fascia (**Fig. 13.5**):

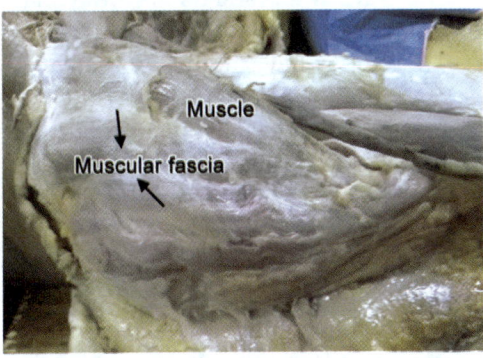

Fig. 13.5: Muscular fascia.

- Surrounds individual muscles directly
- The muscular fascia is removed by cutting it from the muscle at right angles to the muscle fascicles. Use fingers or forceps to separate one muscle from another. Use a scalpel or scissor to incise the deep fascia at the border of two adjoining muscles and then slide your fingers up and down the adjoining borders to free one muscle from another.
- It binds groups of muscles together as a unit and has partitions between the muscles called *intermuscular septa*.

Neurovascular plane and bundle (**Figs. 13.6A and B**):

- Veins, arteries, lymphatic vessels, and nerves often travel together in bundles.

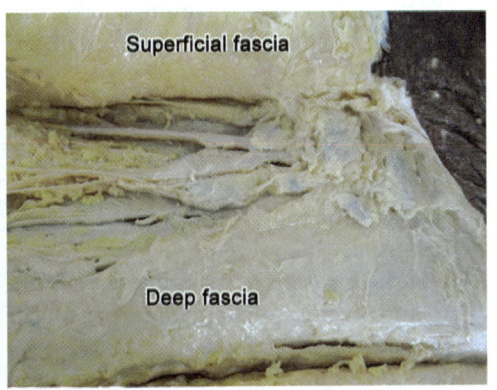

Fig. 13.4: Deep fascia.

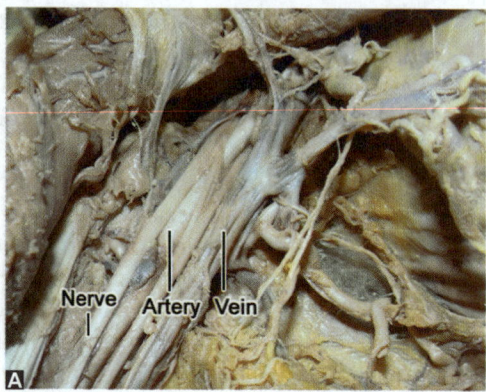
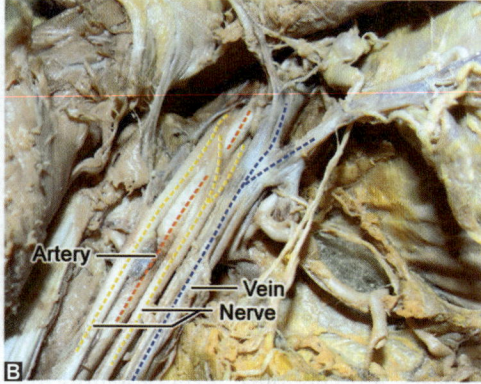

Figs. 13.6A and B: Neurovascular bundle.

The plane (intermuscular) along which they are travelling is known as neurovascular plane.
- They vary in size and do not always have all four elements.
- They often have branches that begin deep and travel superficially—supplying muscles, then subcutaneous tissue, and finally terminating in the skin.
- Neurovascular bundle runs between the deep fascia and superficial fascia.
- Many neurovascular bundles run between adjoining muscle bellies.
- Follow the bundle back to see the main nerve trunk and vessels from which they arise and by blunt dissection one can determine other branches.
- Tributaries of veins can be removed for better visualization of arteries and nerves.
- Variations are more common. So, take every opportunity to look at the other cadavers that are being dissected at the same time.

Cleaning a muscle **(Fig. 13.7)**:
- Cleaning is for the ability to see the basic features of a muscle and not esthetic purpose. The basic features to be observed in a muscle are:
  - Borders
  - Origin
  - Insertion
  - Fiber direction

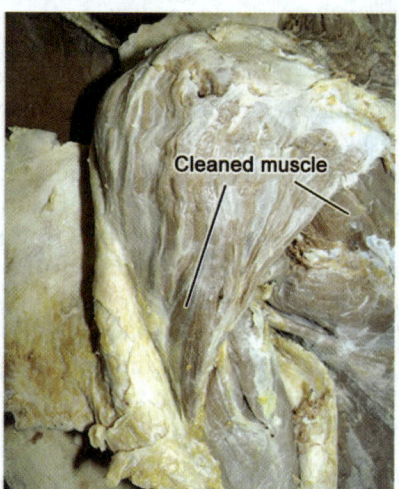

Fig. 13.7: Cleaned muscle.

- Above must be made visible and verified before the muscle is reflected.
- Muscle is reflected by cutting one attachment and folding the muscle on itself.

Identification of vessels and nerves **(Fig. 13.8)**:
- *Arteries*: They have thick wall and a lumen that can be seen.
- *Veins*: These are larger than arteries, dark blue in color, wall is thin and the lumen is collapsed.
- *Nerves*: These feel like a string when lifted up and on cross-section they are fusiform in appearance.
- The course of nerves, arteries, and veins should be cleaned or exposed from the

Chapter 13: Introduction to Dissection of Cadaver

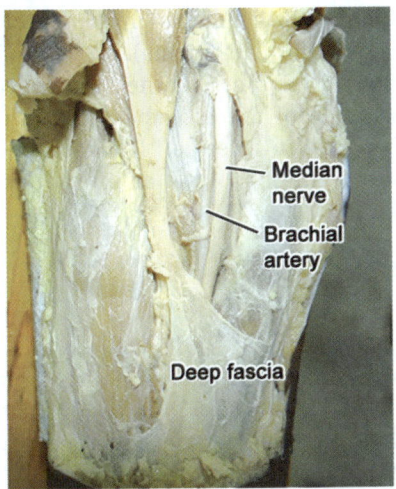

Fig. 13.8: Nerve and artery, deep fascia.

point of origin to termination. Their pattern of branching to be clearly exposed for observation.

- *Venae comitantes*: Deep veins accompany the arteries and they run parallel on either side of the artery like the body guards and are called venae comitantes. They are named after the artery which they are accompanying (radial, ulnar, brachial, anterior tibial and posterior tibial veins) and are more common in extremities. The pulsations of the arteries facilitates venous return and they also act as countercurrent exchange system for conserving body heat. Most often the veins obscure the course of the nerve; hence after identification they can be removed.
- *Do not cut or remove arteries or nerves.*
- *Veins accompanying nerves:* Venae comtantes for nerves are seen accompanying hypoglossal nerve.
- *Arteries accompanying nerves*: These are seen in sciatic nerve (arteria comitans nervi ischiadisi). These are embryological remnants of axis artery of lower limb. Similary in upper limb arteria nervi medianus accompanying median nerve is present (remnant of axis artery of upper limb).
- Cleaning is complete when the *source (origin), course (passing along the regions), and distribution* of the artery, vein, and nerve are visible.

Dissection of a joint (**Figs. 13.9A and B**):
The deepest layer in the limb is the bone. In the trunk the body cavities will be the deepest.

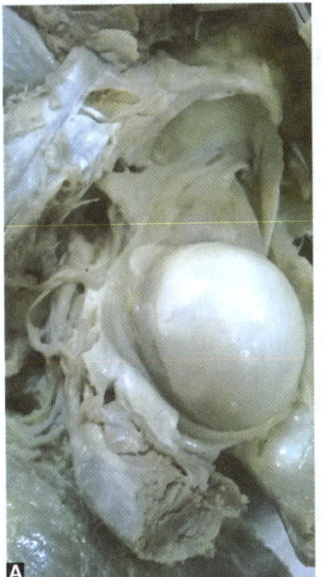
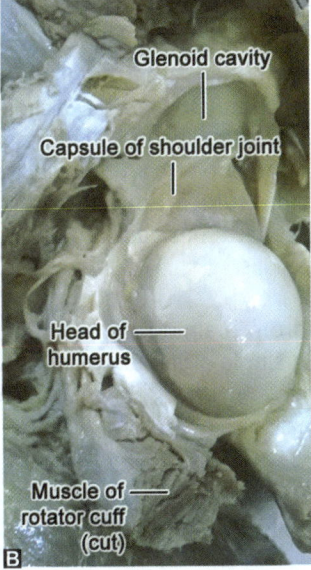

Figs. 13.9A and B: Opened joint.

- Use a scalpel and forceps to dissect the joint.
- Remove all muscles around the joint to expose the joint capsule.
- Opening the joint capsule: The joint capsule and tendons that traverse the capsule will be cut to reveal the articulation.
- Identify the ligaments (thick parts of joint capsule form ligaments).
- Interior of joint: Cut the ligament of the capsule of the dissected joint around its circumference. Incise capsular attachment to look at interior of the joint.

Clinical Application of Dissection of Cadaver

Purpose of Cadaver Dissection in Medicine

Cadaver is used in scientific or medical research by physicians and other scientists for the following purpose:
- Study of anatomy as part of curriculum in the medical, dental, nursing, and allied health sciences. Cadaver is the best teacher you have in this course.
- Identify disease sites as part of pathology.
- Determine cause of death in forensic medicine.
- To provide tissue, to repair a defect in a living human being in cadaveric organ transplantation.
- For practicing surgical skills.

Benefits of Cadaver Dissection

Cadaver can be considered as a single page with all round details with the following advantages:
- A valuable tool for developing observational skills and knowledge of anatomical relations.
- It is nearer to the living in relationship of structures to one another and in their function.
- It facilitates practice of clinical techniques for safe clinical practice, e.g., venesection, site of heart auscultation, surface marking of important viscera, and structures.
- Surgical procedures can be practiced on cadavers for developing safe and innovative surgical skills, e.g., passing a catheter, feeling for hepatorenal pouch, entry to lesser sac, kidney exposure. These procedures boost the confidence of student. It facilitates surgeons.
- Provide tissue to repair a defect in a living human being—cadaveric organ transplantation.
- Enhances coping mechanisms with an involuntary compromise on caring attitude as cadaver is the first patient. Students would be encouraged to examine their own attitudes toward death and learn. It is clinical and emotional preparation for future work.
- *Understanding clinical variations*: Each cadaver is a new source of knowledge with variations. It facilitates understanding of variations and their clinical relevance when compared to a textbook or information from other electronic media.
- In olden days the surgeons used to visit anatomy laboratory and practice their surgical skills. In the recent times cadaver laboratories are used for conducting workshops for practicing the skills.

Organ Donation

Cadaver organs from brain dead person are transplanted into those that require organ transplantation. A single organ donor can save the lives of up to eight people by donation of two kidneys, two lungs, liver, pancreas, heart and intestines. The organs that are used are:
- Brain and spinal cord in research
- Cornea
- Nerve and skin grafting
- Bone marrow transplantation

Contd...

Contd...

- Heart
- Lungs
- Kidneys
- Liver
- Pancreas
- A person can give legal willingness to permit removal of an organ from his/her body for the purpose of transplantation to another person to save the life of one who is dying due to non-availability of that organ. The organ donation can also be done for research.
- This is done by giving consent while the donor is alive or dead with the knowledge of next of kin.
- **Importance of organ donation:**
  - In India nearly 500,000 people die every year because of non-availability of organs for transplantation.
  - This includes 200,000 from liver disease, 150,000 from kidney disease and 50,000 from heart disease.
- **Criteria for organ donation:**
  - There is no age, caste or religion, etc., restriction.
  - The medical condition of the donor is important. Those with cancer, HIV, diabetes, heart or kidney disease cannot be a donor.
  - An individual of less that 18 years can be a donor with the consent of parent.
  - Tissue donation viz. cornea, skin, heart valves and bone marrow can be obtained in case of natural death.
  - Vital organs such as heart, kidneys, liver, pancreas and lungs can be collected as donation in case of brain death.
- **Types of donors:**
  - Living donor: Any person of more than 18 years of age, can voluntarily authorize for removal of any of his/her organ and/or tissue, during his or her lifetime. They will receive donor card that acts like a will for donating the organs.
  - Deceased donor: Anyone, regardless of age, race or gender can become an organ and tissue donor after his/her death (brain dead patient or one with cardiac arrest).
- **Transplantation of Human Organs Act:**
  - This is established for organ donation in brain dead patients.
  - This requires the consent of family members and permission from legal authorities before starting the process.

Voluntary Body Donation

- It is execution of a will during once life time stating the person's wish to donate his whole body or part of it after his death to an institution for its use:
  - In treating patient in need
  - Teaching and training medical and allied health sciences student in anatomy
  - In designing various medical devices
  - In medical research for understanding cardiovascular diseases, neurological (Alzheimer's) disorders, etc.
  - For training surgical skills by practising on the cadavers as in skin suturing techniques shoulder/hip/knee replacement surgeries.

Contd...

Contd…

- A person who wishes to donate his/her body can do so by executing a written will or expressing orally to his kith and kin during terminal illness.
  - The copy of will has to be submitted to the medical institution or body donation program before death with the consent of his kith and kin.
- Instead of whole body one can contribute organ or tissue donation after death.
- The will has to be executed in the presence of two witnesses.
- The factors influencing body donation are social awareness, understanding of importance of body donation in saving the lives of those in need.
- Most donors give willingness for advancement of knowledge and for the usefulness of body parts after death.

Anatomical Basis for Clinical Condition

Case Scenario

Problem: A 35-year male met with a traffic accident and brought to the emergency room of a state government recognized medical college in a critical condition and was kept on ventilator. After thorough examination and investigations he was declared as brain dead. The patient's kith and kin were explained that his chances of becoming normal are nil and were explained about the body and organ donation for consideration.

Questions:

1. Why the kith and kin were informed about body donation and organ donation?
2. Will organ donation be considered if he is declared dead?
3. Whether this hospital can accept body and organ donation?
4. How does the body donation help the medical students?
5. What is cadaver bank?

Anatomical explanation:

1. As the patient is on ventilator if the kith and kin are willing for donating the vital organs, such as kidneys, heart, cornea, skin, liver and bone marrow, these can be retrieved for transplantation into those with failure of one of these vital organs. The purpose of informing kith and kin is to motivate for organ donation.
2. If the victim is declared dead the only organs that can be considered is the cornea, skin, and bone marrow if only they are retrieved within 2 hours of death.
3. Since it is a state government recognized medical institution it can accept body donation. For organ donation if that institute has facilities for organ retrieval, storage, and transport either on its own or in collaboration with a nearby higher medical center can accept.
4. Helps medical students to do cadaveric dissection to understand relations of human anatomical structures. It facilitates the development of psychomotor skills and will motivate them for developing confidence to perform and for improving surgical procedures and skills respectively.
5. Cadaver banks are those that collect and store bone marrow, brain, skin, vessels, etc. for molecular research and cadaver grafting. Cadaveric grafting of bone marrow and skin are useful in burns victims.

Chapter 13: Introduction to Dissection of Cadaver

> ### ☞ Key Concept

Take Home Message—Cadaver Dissection (Mnemonic is DISSECTION)
- **D**oing or performing the task that requires skill.
- **I**nspection or ability to observe the structures exposed.
- **S**eparating or detaching the parts for in-depth observation.
- **S**ense or logic to differentiate the different structural components by feeling with fingers, e.g., artery, vein, and nerve.
- **E**nriching or enhancing the understanding or knowledge of the part.
- **C**utting apart or dividing the part for visualization of deeper structures.
- **T**easing or separating the components of a structure for finer details.
- **I**ntrospection or self-analysis for identification or reasoning the orientation.
- **O**rientation of location of various structures.
- **N**ormal cadaveric location, relations and appearance of structures with clinical application for performing various procedures.

QUESTIONS

1. Name the instruments required for routine cadaver dissection.
2. Name the various structures encountered in the dissection of a limb.
3. What is neurovascular plane?
4. Cadaver respect.
5. Body donation.
6. Organ donation.

MULTIPLE CHOICE QUESTIONS

1. **The organs that are used for transplantation include all, *except*:**
   A. Cornea
   B. Heart
   C. Kidney
   D. Brain

2. **The following statements about use of dissection instruments is correct, *except*:**
   A. Forceps for holding
   B. Scalpel for incisions
   C. Probe for teasing
   D. Chisel for lifting muscles

ANSWERS

1. D   2. D

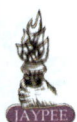

TOP DOC BANE WOHI
JISKA GUIDE HO SAHI

diginerve
A Jaypee Initiative

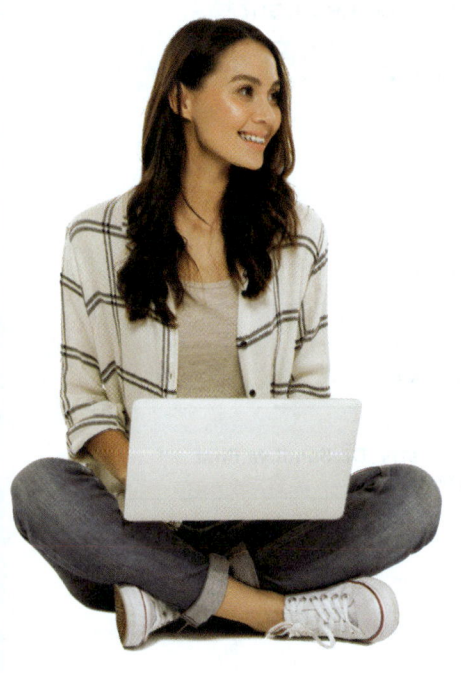

YOUR GUIDE AT EVERY STEP

Expert Knowledge Anytime, Anywhere

SCAN QR CODE
FOR MORE DETAILS

WHY CHOOSE US

Video Lectures

Self-Assessment Questions

Top Faculty

New CBME Curriculum

Clinical Case Based Approach

NEET Preparation

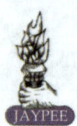

TOP DOC BANE WOHI | JISKA GUIDE HO SAHI

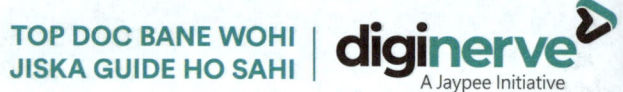

Video Lectures | Notes | Self-Assessment
UnderGrad Courses Available

Community Medicine for UnderGrads — by Dr. Bratati Banerjee

Forensic Medicine & Toxicology for UnderGrads — by Dr. Gautam Biswas

Medicine for UnderGrads — by Dr. Archith Boloor

Microbiology for UnderGrads — by Dr. Apurba S Sastry, Dr. Sandhya Bhat & Dr. Deepashree R

OBGYN for UnderGrads — by Dr. K. Srinivas

Ophthalmology for UnderGrads — by Dr. Parul Ichhpujani & Dr. Talvir Sidhu

Orthopaedics for UnderGrads — by Dr. Vivek Pandey

Pathology for UnderGrads — by Prof. Harsh Mohan, Prof. Ramadas Nayak & Dr. Debasis Gochhait

Pediatrics for UnderGrads — by Dr. Santosh Soans & Dr. Soundarya M

Pharmacology for UnderGrads — by Dr. Sandeep Kaushal & Dr. Nirmal George

Surgery for UnderGrads — by Dr. Sriram Bhat M (SRB)

 Download the App.

*T&C Apply

Contac
+91 8800 418 41
marketing@diginerve.co

INDEX

Page numbers followed by *f* refer to figure, *fc* refer to flowchart, and *t* refer to table

A

Abdomen 10, 152, 220, 223, 225
  anatomical regions of 220
  division of 220
  quadrant of 225*f*, 225*t*
  regions of 224*f*, 224*t*
Abdominal parts 191
Abdominal wall
  anterior 81
  posterior 202
Abdominopelvic cavity 47, 186
Accessory drainage system 145
Achilles reflex 174
Achondroplasia 71, 73*f*
Acini 194
Acne vulgaris 41
Acoustic meatus, external 73
Acromegaly 71, 204
Actin 85
Adam's apple 188
Adductor magnus 88
Adenohypophysis 134
Adenosine triphosphate 85
Adipose cells 27
Adrenal cortex 202
Adrenal medulla 202
Adrenocorticotropic hormone 201
Afferent nerves 158
Agonists 94
Albinism 41
Alimentary canal 193
Alopecia
  areata 41
  totalis 41, 43*f*
  universalis 42
Alveolar ducts 189
Alveolar sacs 189
Alzheimer's disease 215
Alzheimer's disorders 239
Ampulla 199, 200
Anastomoses 135
Anatomic end-artery 137*f*
Anatomical planes 5, 7, 9*t*
  coronal 9
  oblique 10
  sagittal 9
  transverse 9

Anatomical position 5, 6*f*
  description of 6*t*
Anatomical terminology 8
Anatomy 1
  comparative 4
  developmental 1, 2
  evolutionary revolutions in 1
  gross 1, 2
  history of 10
  internal gross 219
  knowledge of 2, 206
  learning of 2
  living 2, 3, 4*f*
  macroscopic 2
  microscopic 1, 2
  radiographic 2
  radiological 206
  regional 5, 5*t*
  subdivisions of 2, 5*t*
  surface 3, 219, 220, 220*t*, 233
  surgical 4
  system-wise 5
    subdivisions of 6*t*
Androgens 202
Aneurysm 139, 212
Angiography 139
Angiology 127
Ankle 116
  jerk 174
Antagonists 94
Antibody 149
  production of 146
Antidiuretic hormone 164, 201
Antigen 149
  presenting cells 149
Aorta 127, 137
Apillary network 130
Aponeurosis 45, 78, 81
Apoptosis 41
Appendicitis 195
Appendicular skeleton 52, 53, 53*f*, 68*t*
Areolar tissue, loose 29
Arterial pulsations, transmitted 134
Arteriogram 211
Arterioles 127, 132
Arteriosclerosis 139
Arteriovenous anastomoses 136, 136*f*
Artery 60, 127, 128, 130*t*, 236

accompanying nerves 237
anastomosis, branches of 61
cerebral 139
elastic 131, 137, 138f
femoral 86
large 128f, 161
medial circumflex 86
medium 132
metaphyseal 60
periosteal 61
pulse, sites for recording 222f
renal 139
splenic 139
structure of 128
thoracodorsal 87
Arthritis 121
Arthrology 100
Arthroplasty 121
Arthroscopy 121
Articular capsule 108
Articular disc 108, 210
Ascites 48
Astrocytes 165, 166
   end feet of 167
   types of 166
Astroglia 165, 166
Atherosclerosis 139
Atmospheric pressure 107
Atrium 125
Atrophy 96
Auscultation 4, 220
Autonomic ganglia 167, 167f
Autonomic nervous system 158, 179
Autonomic reflex arc 174
Axial skeleton 52
   bones of 67t
Axilla 43f, 152
Axillary lines 220, 223f
Axillary nerve 121
Axolemma 161
Axon 160, 161
   collaterals 161
   hillock 160
Axonotmesis 180
Axoplasm 161
Azygos system 134

B

Bacteria killing 41
Balloon angioplasty 212
Barium
   meal 210f
   sulphate 209
Barr body 160
Basal cell carcinoma 42
Basivertebral veins 61
Beaded appearance 147

Biceps
   brachii 78
   femoris 88
Biliary system 211
Biochemistry 1
Biological anthropology 4
Biopsy, tube for 219
Blastocoel 16
Blastocyst cavity 16
Blood
   capillary 145, 147t
   cells 214
      production 53
   circulation, types 131f
   clots 229
   flow, regulation of 137
   pressure 172
   types of 130
Blood vascular system 125, 126, 126t
   clinical application of 138
Blood vessels 20, 211, 212
   classification of 131
   major 220
   types of 127f
Blood-brain barrier 166, 167
B-lymphocytes 149, 151
Body 40, 192, 203
   activities 157
   cavities of 46, 185f
   cell, average 83
   cutting machine 233f
   defense mechanisms of 145, 145fc
   dermatomes of 39f
   description of 6
   growth 200
   movements, terminology of 117
   part of 7
   tissues of 16, 20
   wall, anterolateral 170
Body positions 7t
   Fowler's 8
   left lateral recumbent 7
   lithotomy 8
   prone 7
   reverse Trendelenburg 7
   right lateral recumbent 7
   Sims' 8
   supine 7
   Trendelenburg 7
Bone 55
   appendicular 67
   articulating 107
      parts in 100
   axial 67
   cartilaginous 68
   cells of 62t, 63f
   classification of 65
   compact 65f, 68

composition of 61, 62*fc*, 66*fc*
cutting forceps 231, 233*f*
dense 68
flat 66
formation 68
functions of 53
growing end of 69
irregular 66
lamellae, formation of 63, 64*f*, 69*fc*
long 66, 70*f*, 208*f*
markings on 70
marrow 132, 133, 210
 biopsy 60
 transplant 60, 238
maturation of 210
maxilla 187
membranous 68
microscopic structure of 61
morphological classification of 66*t*, 67*f*
number of 52, 112*t*
parietal 68
parts of long 55, 57*f*
pneumatic 66
postnatal development of 71*t*
sesamoid 66
shape 66
short 66
sphenoid 187
spicule of 63*f*
structure of 61
Bony contour 107
Boutons terminaux 161
Bowels 220
Brachial plexus 170
Brachialis 88
Brachioradialis 78
Brain 20, 52, 157
 ventricles of 211
Brainstem 181
Bromium 209
Bronchial tree 189*f*
Bronchial veins 134
Bronchioles 189
Buerger's disease 139
Bursa 109, 110*t*
 accidental 110
 Achilles 111
 acromial 111
 adventitious 110
 anserine 111
 around knee 109*f*
 deep infrapatellar 111
 housemaids 110
 iliopsoas 110
 interposes 78
 intertubercular 111
 olecranon 110, 111
 prepatellar 110, 111

radial 110
retrocalcaneal 111
subacromial 111
subcoracoid 111
subcutaneous 110
submuscular 110
subpopliteal 110
subtendinous 110
superficial infrapatellar 111
suprapatellar 111
types of 110
ulnar 110

C

Cadaver 1, 230
 dissection 228, 238
 respect 228
Cadaveric oath 229
Calamus scriptorius 10
Calcium phosphate 62
Cancellous bone 57, 68, 210
 microscopic structure of 65
Cancer cells, spread of 154*f*
Capillary endothelial cell 167
Capsule cells 165
Carbon dioxide 145
Cardiac arrest 239
Cardiovascular system 125, 143
Care of cadaver 229
Carpal tunnel 48
Cartilage 53, 188*f*
 articular 107
 arytenoid 188
 calcification of 59, 69
 cells 54
 clinical applications of 54
 detachment of 54
 elastic 54, 56
 growth of 54
 hypertrophied 59
 location of different 55*f*
 remnants of 72*f*
 thinning of 72*f*
 transplantation 55
 tumors of 54
 types of 54, 56*t*
 zone of
  mature 59
  reserve 59
Cartilaginous joint 102, 103*f*, 105
 secondary 106
 symphysis 106*f*
 synchondroses 106*f*
Caval system 134
Celiac ganglia 181
Cell 16, 17, 26, 32, 56, 62
 functions in 18*t*

inner mass of 16
layer of 16
mass of 16
mediated immunity 149
membrane 16, 18, 159
nests 54
organelles 19*f*
osteoblasts 62
osteoclasts 62
osteocytes 62
osteogenic 62
parts of 16
shape of 21
types of 203
Cell body 159
    flask-shaped 163*f*
    shape of 162, 163*f*
    star-shaped 163*f*
Central canal, location of 168
Central lymphoid organs 149
Central nervous system 89, 157, 159, 175*f*, 176
Centrioles 18
Cerebral cortex 162, 163*f*
Cervical region 168
Cervix 200
Chest 189
    X-ray 207*f*
Chisel 231
Cholecystitis 195
Cholelithiasis 195
Chondrocytes 54
Chondrodystrophy 54
Chondrosarcomas 54
Chondrosternal joint 106
Chromatolysis 160
Cilia 21
Cleavage lines 37
Clitoris 128
Colitis 195
Collagen fibers 28
Compact bone 56, 63*f*
    structure of 63
    transverse section of 64*f*
Connective tissue 20, 26, 82, 133
    cells of 27*t*
    classification of 29
    clinical application of 30
    components of 26
    dense regular 29, 78
    fibers of 26, 28*t*
    functions 26
    loose 29
    mucoid 29
    proper 29
    types of 29*t*
Contact lenses 230
Contractile proteins 84
Coronary sinus 134
Cortex 36, 151
Costochondritis 54
Cowper's glands 198
Cranial cavity 157
Cranial nerves 177, 178
Cretinism 204
Crystalloids 145
Cubital fossa, dissection of 234*f*
Cushing's syndrome 204
Cutaneous nerves 235
Cystitis 200
Cytoplasm 16, 18, 160
Cytoplasmic organelle 16, 77*t*
Cytoskeletal framework 18
Cytosol 18

D

Dead body 1
    protect 229
Dead space 129
Deceased donor 239
Decidua 16
Deep fascia 45, 46, 235, 235*f*, 236, 237*f*
    modification of 45, 45*f*
Deep vein thrombosis 139, 212
Dendrites 159, 161
Dense lymphoid tissue 149
Dermatoglyphics 41
Dermatome 38, 170, 171
Dermis 35, 36
Diabetes mellitus 204
Diarthroses 106
Digestive enzymes 194
Digestive system 186, 190, 194
    organs of 190
    parts 190*f*
Digestive tract 20
Diploic bone 65, 65*f*
Dislocation 31, 121, 122
Dissection 228, 230
    beginning 230
    blunt 233
    hall maintenance 229
    instruments for 230
    of cadaver, clinical application of 238
    safety measures 230
    sharp 233
    techniques 233
Dominant pedicle 87
Donors, types of 239
Dorsal venous arch 136*f*
Dove-tail appearance 78, 82*f*
Ducts, pair of 199
Duodenal ulcers 194
Duodenum 192, 193*f*
    part of 223

Index

E

Ear, external 136
Echocardiogram 31
Ectoderm 16
Efferent nerve 158
Effusion 48
Ejaculatory ducts 198
Elbow 70, 115
    movements at 118*f*
Electromyography 96
Elephantiasis 153
Embalming fluids 229
Embryoblast 16
Embryology 1
Emissary veins 134
Encapsulated lymphoid organs 149
Encephalon 157
End-artery 137*f*
    anatomical 137
    functional 137*f*
Endochondral ossification 56, 68
Endocrine 186
Endocrine system 185, 200, 200*f*, 201, 204
    gland of 201
    mechanism of action of 201
Endoderm 16
Endomysium 82, 177
Endoskeleton 65
Endosteum 59
Enteritis 195
Enzymes 22
Eosinophils 28, 149
Ependymal cells 165, 166
Epidermis 35, 36
    layers of 38*f*
Epididymis 197, 198
Epigastric arteries
    inferior 86
    superior 86
Epigastrium 224
Epiglottis 188
Epilepsy 215
Epimysium 82
Epineurium 177
Epiphyseal arteries 61
Epiphyseal cartilage 58, 61, 211*f*
Epiphyseal plate, zones in 58*f*
Epiphyses
    aberrant 58
    atavastic 58
    bony 56
    cartilaginous 56
    pressure 57
    traction 58
    types of 57, 58, 58*f*
    union of various 70
Epitendineum 78

Epithelia 20
    clinical application of 26
    surface 145
    types 21*t*, 23*t*
    simple 21, 22
    stratified 22, 23
Epithelial cells 22, 24*f*, 35
    surface specializations of 24*t*
Epithelial tissue
    classification 20
    layer of 22
Epithelial tumors 26
Epithelium
    simple columnar 21
    simple cuboidal 21
    stratified 22
Eponychium 40
Esophagus 191, 202
    X-ray of 3*f*
Estrogen 199, 203
    functions 203
Exocrine glands, classification of 25
Exoskeleton 65
Extracellular spaces 145
Eye, unaided 16
Eyeball 83, 87

F

Face 115
Facial artery, branches of 135
Facial expression, muscles of 39
Fallopian tubes 199
Fascia 34, 43
    clinical importance of 46
    functions 43
    location 43
    of Gerota 196
    structure 43
    superficial 44, 44*f*, 46, 234, 234*f*, 235, 236
    types 44
Fat 22
    from intestines, absorption of 146
Fatty substances 143
Feeding tubes, insert 212
Femoral vein 130
Femur, adult 57*f*
Fenestrated capillaries 133
Fertilization 197
Fetus
    abnormal 5*f*
    delivery of 197
    development of 197
    in uterus 199*f*
Fibers 26, 32
    elastic 130
    group B 177
    intrafusal 89

myelinated 161, 176
postganglionic 181
preganglionic 181
reticular 28
types of 176
unmyelinated 176
white 28
Fibroblasts 27
Fibrocartilage 56
articular disc of 108
white 54
Fibrosis 30
Fibrous astrocytes 166
Fibrous capsule 45, 108
Fibrous digital flexor sheath 45*f*
Fibrous dysplasia 71
Fibrous flexor sheath 45
Fibrous joint 102, 103*f*, 104*f*
gomphosis 105*f*
subtypes of 103
syndesmosis 104*f*
Fibrous tendon 79
Filaments, thick and thin 84
Fimbriae 199
Finger digit 42*f*
Fissure, anterior median 168
Flexor digitorum profundus 88
Flexor retinaculum 45*f*
Flower spray endings 89
Fluid
balance, maintaining 146
in lung, collection of 4
transportation of 126
types of 125
Fluoroscopy 209, 210
Follicle cells 201
Follicle stimulating hormone 201
Fontanel 52, 105, 105*f*
Foramen 73
Force and movement 79
Forceps 231, 232*f*
Forearm 116
and ankle 119*f*
Foreign substance 151
Fundus 192

G

Gall stones 212
Gallbladder 192, 194
Gametes 197
Ganglia 158, 161, 181
Gastritis 194
Gastrointestinal tract 193, 211
organs of 190
parts of 190
wall of 191, 191*f*
Genes, transmission of 4

Genital organs
external 197, 198
internal 197
Genital system 186
Gigantism 204
Ginglymus 112
Gland 22
accessory digestive 193
adrenal 201, 202
bulbourethral 198
classification of 25
coverings for 45
endocrine 25
holocrine 25, 41
mammary 25, 134, 199
mixed 25
mucus 25
multicellular 25
parotid 193, 194
pea-sized 201
pineal 203
pituitary 201
prostate 198
sebaceous 25, 37, 39, 40*f*, 41
serous 25
submandibular 193, 194
sudoriferous 41
suprarenal 133
unicellular 25
Glandular epithelia 21, 22
Glucocorticoids 202
Gluteus maximus 86
Goblet cell 25, 25*f*
Goiter 204
Golgi apparatus 18, 161
Golgi bodies 160
Golgi tendon organ 89, 89*f*, 172*f*
Gomphosis 104
Gonads 197, 201, 203
Gracilis 86
Gut arteries 139

H

Hair 36, 39, 40, 40*f*
bulb 36, 40
follicle 36, 39, 40
papilla 40
Haversian canals 63
Haversian system 63, 68
Head
region 221
X-ray 209*f*
Heart 20, 52, 125, 126*f*, 179, 220, 239
and blood vascular system 125
and muscles 209
apex beat of 3
left 126
right 126

Index

Hemangioma 139, 140f
Hemiplegia 90
Hepatic portal system 134
Hepatitis 195
Herpes zoster 49
Hidradenitis suppurativa 42, 43f
Hilton's law 120, 121, 121f
Hilum transmits 195
Hip 116
    movements at 118f
Histology 2
Hollow organs 190
Hormones 22, 201
Human being, development of 16, 19f
Human body 16, 206, 228
    organization of 17t
    venous systems in 134
Human chorionic gonadotropin 204
Human endocrine system, major glands of 201
Human genetics 4
Human growth hormone 201
Humoral immunity 149
Hyaline cartilage 54, 56
Hydronephrosis 200
Hydroureter 200
Hyoid 53
Hypochondrium 224
Hypodermic needle 39
Hypodermis 35, 36, 39
Hypogastrium 224
Hyponychium 40
Hypophyseal portal system 134
Hypophysis cerebri 133

I

Iliac fossa 224
Immune system 204
Immunoglobulins 149
Infarction 139
Injury, causes for 179
Interarterial anastomosis 135, 135f
Interatrial septum 126
Intercellular substance 26, 56
Intermuscular septa 235
Intermuscular septum 45f
Interneuron 164, 174
Interosseous membrane 46
Interstitial fluid, excessive 146
Interstitial lamellae 63
Intervertebral disc 100
    herniation of 54
Intervertebral foramen 169
Intestine 179
    large 192
Intracartilaginous 68
Intracellular organelles 19f
Intracranial venous sinuses 134
Intramembranous ossification 68

Intramuscular injection 96
    sites of 97f
Islets of Langerhans 203

J

Joint 100
    ankle 112
    axes of movement in 117f
    ball and socket 113f, 114
    basiocciput 106
    basisphenoid 106
    biaxial 112
    broad classification of 101fc
    cavity 108
    classification of 100, 101fc, 102t, 103f
    clinical application of 121
    condylar 112, 113f
    diaphysis 106
    dissection of 237
    ellipsoid 112, 113f
    epiphysis 106
    gliding 113f
    hinge 112, 113f
    hip 122
    humeroulnar 112
    hyaline cartilaginous 106
    interphalangeal 112
    midline 106
    movements in 114, 117t
    nerve supply of 117
    neuropathic 121
    normal 72f
    number of 100
    of body, types of 115t
    opened 237f
    pivot 113f
    plane 112
    planner 113f
    polyaxial 114
    primary cartilaginous 106
    radiological appearance of 210
    saddle 113f, 114
    shoulder 110
    socket 104
    space, decrease of 72f
    sternoclavicular 108
    temporomandibular 108, 121
    uniaxial 112

K

Kidney 20, 52, 179, 195, 216, 239
    anatomy of
        macroscopic 2f
        microscopic 3f

coverings of 196
right 195
Knee 116
    jerk 174
    joint 110
        osteoarthritis of 72*f*
Knock knee 121

L

Lambdoid sutures 105
Lamina propria 191
Langer's line 37, 38*f*
Langerhans cells 35
    clinical importance of 37
Laryngeal prominence 188
Laryngitis 190
Laryngopharynx 187
Larynx 188, 188*f*
    cavity 188*f*
    muscles of 188
Leg 116
Ligament 46, 59, 107, 208
    accessory 108, 109
    capsular 108
    extracapsular 109
    intracapsular 109
    periodontal 104
    suspensory 31
    sutural 103
    true 108
Limbs 81, 118*f*, 119*f*
    supply of 170
Lining epithelia, classification of 21
Lipofuscin 161
Lipomas 30
Liposarcoma 30
Lips 136
Liver 25, 52, 128, 133, 179, 193, 194, 195*f*, 216, 239
    sinusoids in 133*f*
    topographic anatomy of 3*f*
Living donor 239
Locomotor system 52
Long bone
    blood supply of 60, 60*f*
    diaphysis of 63*f*
Lower limb 67, 152, 223
    bones of 68*t*
    movement of 1
    region 221
Lower motor neurons 163
Lower respiratory tract 186
Lumbar plexus 170
Lumbar region 168
    left 224
    right 224
Lumen size and patency 130
Lung 179, 189, 189*f*, 209, 220, 239
    fissures of 189
    hilum of 189
    lobes of 189
Lunula 40
Luteinizing hormone 201
Lymph 143, 146
    capillaries 147, 147*t*
    flow of 144*f*, 146, 150*f*
    transportation of 143
Lymph node 149, 150*f*
    biopsy 153
    regional 152*t*
    structure of 151
Lymph vessel 143, 146, 152*t*
    medium-sized 147
    walls of 143
Lymphadenitis 153
Lymphangiography 153
Lymphangitis 153
Lymphatic drainage 148*f*
Lymphatic duct, right 148, 148*f*
Lymphatic system 125, 126*t*, 143, 144*f*
    clinical application of 153
    components of 146
    functions of 145
Lymphatic tissue 150*f*
    classification of 149
Lymphatic vessels 147
Lymphedema 153, 154*f*
Lymphocytes 28, 143, 149
    production of 146
    types of 149
Lymphoid organs
    peripheral 149
    secondary 149
Lymphoid tissue
    diffuse 149
    mucosa-associated 149
Lymphoma 153
Lymphoscintigraphy 153
Lysosomes 18, 160

M

Macroglia 165
Macromolecules 17
Macrophages 27, 145, 149, 151
Mammogram machine 216*f*
Mammography 216
Mandible 53, 119*f*
Marfan's syndrome 31
Marrow cavity 56, 59
Mast cells 27, 149
Medulla 36, 151
Medullary cavity 56, 60
Melanocyte 35
    stimulating hormone 202
Melanoma, malignant 42

Index

Meningocele 5f
Meniscus 108
Merkel cells 37
Merocrine 25
Mesaxon 175
Mesenteric artery, origin of inferior 223
Mesoderm 16, 165
Mesogastrium 48
Metabolic functions 194
Metaphyseal arteries 61
Metaphysis 59, 210
Metarterioles 132
Microglia 165, 166
Microvilli 21
Mineral, storage of 53
Mineralocorticoids 202
Mitochondria 18, 77, 160
Mitotic divisions 16
Mitral valve 126
Monosynaptic reflex 174
Morula 16
Motor end plate 88
Motor nerve 158
Motor neuron 163
    efferent 174
    presynaptic 88, 164
    spinal lower 96
Motor unit 87f
Mouth 190, 191f
    parts 191f
Mucocutaneous junction 34
Mucosa 22, 188
Mucus 22
    acinus 26f
    membrane 22
Multiaxial movement 116
Muscle 82, 88, 107
    arrectores pilorum 40f, 41
    attachments 80
    auricular 44
    bellies 236
    biopsy 96
    bundle 83f
    cardiac 78, 79
    classification of 77fc, 92f, 94f
    cleaned 236f
    composite 88
    contraction of 88, 134, 157
    coverings for 45
    description of 91t
    extent of 79
    extraocular 83, 87
    eyeball 178
    fascicles 82
    gluteal 83
    hybrid 88
    intermediate 90
    involuntary 77, 78

    loss of innervation of 90
    naming of 95, 95t
    occipitofrontalis 44
    parts of 81f
    pump 143
    red 90
    sensory innervation of 88
    shunt 93, 94t
    smooth 79
    spindle 89, 89f, 172f
    spurt 93, 94t
    stabilize 94
    striated 78
    subcutaneous 44
    supplied, part of 170
    tendinous portion of 79
    tissue, type of 90
    tongue 178
    types of 77, 79
    vascular pedicle of 85
    white 90
Muscle fiber 76, 77t, 83, 83f, 84, 88, 130
    color of 90
    direction of 92f
Muscular arteries 132
Muscular dystrophy 96
Muscular fascia 235, 235f
Muscular spasm 96
Muscular system 76
Muscular tissue 20, 29, 76
    general features of 76
    types of 79t
Myasthenia gravis 96, 204
Myelin
    composition of 176
    sheath 175, 176, 180
Myelination
    clinical importance of 176
    process of 175, 175f, 176
Myeloma, multiple 30
Mylohyoid raphe 81
Myocyte, cytoplasm of 83
Myofibril 83f, 84
Myofilaments 84, 85f
    bundle of 84
    types of 84
Myology 76
Myosin 85
Myotendinous junction 78, 82f
Myotomes 170
Myxedema 204

N

Nail 36, 39, 40f
    bed 40
    fold 40
    groove 40
    matrix 40
    plate 40

Nasal cavity 186, 187
    floor of 187
Nasopharynx 187
Natural killer cells 149
Neck 115
    region 221
    X-ray 209f
Nerve 61, 236
    and artery 237f
    coverings for 45
    damage to 180
    fibers 157, 168, 175, 176
    ganglia 157, 165
    inflammation 180
    injury 180
        types of 181f
    irritation 180
    pain 180
    plexus, formation of 170, 170f
    supply 120
        loss of 90
Nervous system 157, 183
    divisions of 158f, 158fc
    subdivisions of 157
Nervous tissue 20, 29, 158
    classification of 159fc
Neuralgia 180
Neurilemmal sheath 161, 176
Neuritis 180
Neurofibrils 161
Neuroglia 158, 164, 165, 166, 168
    types of 166t
Neuromuscular junction 87, 88f
Neuron 158, 167
    afferent sensory 173
    autonomic 163, 163f
    bipolar 162
    classification of 162, 163f
    gamma motor 89
    injury 179
    intermediate 164
    multipolar 162, 168
    neurosecretory 164
    number of 174
    postganglionic 164
    postsynaptic 164
    preganglionic 163
    pseudounipolar 162, 165, 173
    regeneration of 159
    sensory 163
    structure of 159, 160f
    types of 162t
    unipolar 162
Neuropraxia 180, 181f
Neurotmesis 180, 181f
Neurovascular bundle 175f, 236f
Neurovascular hilum 85
Neutrophils 145, 149

Nissl bodies 160
Node of Ranvier 161, 176
Nonepithelial cells 35, 164
Nose
    external 186
    skin of 136
Nuclear bag 89
Nuclear chain 89
Nuclear medicine scans 214
Nucleus 16, 18, 160, 161
Nutrient and oxygen 130
Nutrient foramen 70f
    and artery, direction of 70
Nutrient foramina, number of 60

O

Occlusive arterial diseases 139
Oligodendrocytes 165, 166, 176
Oligodendroglia 165
Onychmycosis 42
Onycholysis 42, 43f
Oral cavity 190, 191
Oral fissure 191
Oral mucosa 191
Organ and tissues 206
Organ donation 238, 239
    criteria for 239
Organ systems 4
Organelles 17
    description of 18t
Oropharynx 187
Osseous 187
Ossification
    clinical application of 70
    law of 69, 70
Osteoarthritis 71
Osteoblasts 59
Osteoclasts 59
Osteogenesis imperfecta 31
Osteology 52
Osteomalacia 71
Osteomyelitis 71
Osteon 52, 68
Osteophytes 108
Osteoporosis 71
Osteotomy 121
Ovum 16
Oxytocin 164, 201

P

Pain, referred 49
Palate 191
Palmar aponeurosis 45f
Palmaris brevis 44
Palpable arteries 138
Palpation 3

Index

Pancreas 193, 193f, 194, 201, 203, 239
    head of 192
Pancreatic secretions 192
Panniculus
    adiposus 44
    carnosus 44
Papilla 36
Paracrine 25
Paralysis 96
Paranasal air sinuses 68, 187, 187f
Parasympathetic nervous system 181, 182f
Parathyroid glands 201, 202
    inferior 202
Parathyroid hormone 202
Parkinson's disease 32
Patellar reflex 174
Pectoralis major 88
Pelvic ostium 200
Percussion notes, types of 222t
Pericardial cavity 48f
Perichondrium 54, 56
Pericytes 27
Perikaryon 158, 159
Perimysium 82
Perinephric fat 196
Perineum 10
Periosteum 59, 63, 71
Peripheral nerve 177, 177f, 180
    classification of 177, 178
Peripheral nervous system 157, 159, 175, 175f
Peripheral vascular diseases 212
Perirenal fat 196
Peritoneal cavity 47, 200
Peritoneum 10, 22
Peyer's patches 192
Pharyngeal arches 178
Pharyngitis 190
Pharynx 187, 187f
    part of 191
Phlebitis 139
Phlebotomy 138
Physical anthropology 4
Physiology 1
Pilosebaceous unit 41
Pineal body 201
Pineal gland, tumors of 204
Pituitary gland, part of 201
Placenta 201, 203
Plantar fasciitis 49
Plasma
    cells 28, 149, 151
    membrane 18, 77
Platysma 44
Pleura 186
Pleural effusion 4
Polysynaptic reflex 174
Porta hepatis 194
Portal system 134
Portal vein 130
Postsynaptic membrane 164
Pregnancy 197
Prenatal ossification centers, chronology of 70t
Pressure gradient micromolecules 145
Primitive germ layers 16
    development of 20f
Progesterone 199, 203, 204
Programmed cell death 41
Prolactin 202
Prostate 197
Protoplasm 77
Pseudostratified columnar epithelium 24
Psoriasis 42
Pulmonary circulation 126, 130
Purkinje cells 162, 163f
Pyelonephritis 200
Pyloric part 192
Pylorus 192
Pyrexia of unknown origin 215

R

Radiological procedures, classification of 206
Radiolucent contrast media 209
Radio-opacity 208
Radioulnar joint, inferior 108
Raphe 81
Receptors, classification of 172
Rectus abdominis 86
Reflex
    arc 173, 174f
    types of 174
    withdrawal 174
Renal capsule 196
Renal fascia 196
Renal ganglia 181
Renal portal system 134
Renal stones 212
Reproductive system 197
    female 198, 199f, 211
    male 197, 198f
Resistance vessels 132
Respiration 1
Respiratory bronchioles 189
Respiratory epithelium 187
Respiratory pump 143
Respiratory system 186, 186f, 187, 189f
    subdivisions of 186
Retina, central artery of 139
Retinacula 46
Rhinitis 189
Rhinorrhea 189
Rhomboideus
    major 94
    minor 94
Rib 53
    cage 195

Ribosomes 18
Rickets 71
Rima glottides 188
Rima vestibuli 188
Root sheath
    external 36
    internal 36

S

Sacral region 168
Salivary gland 179, 193, 193f, 211
    pairs of 193
    sublingual 194
Salpingitis 200
Sarcolemma 76, 83
Sarcoma 30
Sarcomere 83f, 84, 85f
Sarcoplasm 83
Satellite cell 165, 167
Scalpel 231
Schwann cells 165, 167, 175-177
Sciatic nerve 237
Scissors 231, 232f
Scleroderma 30
Sclerosis, amyotrophic lateral 90
Scrotum 197
    layers of 198
Sebum 41
Seminal vesicle 197, 198
Sensory 34
    nerve 158
    receptors, types of 173t
    root fibers 168
Sentinel node biopsy 153
Septum 235
    posterior median 168
Serosa 22
Serous acinus 26f
Serous cavities 47, 47f, 49
Serous membrane 22, 47, 186
    clinical importance of 48
    inflammation of 48
    layers of 47
Serous sac 48f
Sesamoid bone, avascular necrosis of 71
Sesamoiditis 71
Sex differences 70
Sex-chromatin 160
Sexual intercourse 197
Shingles 49
Shock
    absorbs 108
    friction 108
Shoulder 100, 115, 120f, 221
    movements at 118f
Shunt, vascular 136
Sigmoid colon 192

Sinusitis 189
Sinusoids 127, 128, 133
Skeletal maturation 210
Skeletal muscle 79, 80f, 82f, 90, 178
    actions of 93
    blood supply of 85
    classification of 86f, 90
    clinical applications of 96
    end plate of 174
    functions 90
    innervation of 87
    mechanism of contraction of 86f
    microscopic appearance of 83
    motor point 87
    motor unit 87
    structure of 78, 83f
Skeletal system 52
Skeleton 53f
    radiological anatomy of 210
Skin 34, 44f, 132, 133
    and appendages 35f
    appendages of 39
    burns classification 42
    functions 34
    incisions 225, 225f, 234, 234f
        thoracoabdominal 225
        thorax 225
    layers of 35
    microscopic structure of 35f
    reflection 234
    structure of 34
    thick and thin 34
    wrinkles in 38
Skull 53
    foramina of 177
    sagittal section of 65f
Small intestine, parts of 192
Small transducer 216
Small vein 133, 235
Smooth endoplasmic reticulum 77, 160
Soft tissue 209, 216
    abnormalities of 208
Somatic nervous system 158
Somatic reflex arc 174
Sounds, abnormal 220
Spermatic cord 198
Spermatozoa 198
Spider veins 139
Spinal cord 53, 157, 162, 163, 163f, 168, 168f, 181
    cross-section of 168
Spinal ganglia 165, 167f
Spinal nerve 169, 177, 179
    pairs of 168, 171
Spinal segment 168, 169f
Spine 70
Splanchnology 185
Spleen 128, 133, 151, 216
    structure of 151

Splenomegaly 153
Spongy bone 65, 68
    microscopic structure of 65
Sprain 121
Squamous cell carcinoma 42
Squamous epithelium, simple 21
Stereocilia 21
Sternotomy 225
Sternum 53
Stomach 52, 179, 186, 192
    barium meal of 209
    parts 192f
Stratified squamous epithelium
    keratinized 23
    nonkeratinized 23
Stratum corneum 35
Stratum granulosum 35
Stratum lucidum 35
Stratum spinosum 35
Students elbow 110
Subcapsular sinus 151
Subcutaneous injection 39
Subcutaneous tissue, removal of 235
Subscapularis 88
Subserous fascia 46
Substance, subdivisions of 151
Sulcus
    anterolateral 168
    posterior intermediate 168
    posterolateral 168
Sun tanning 42
Sweat gland 25, 37, 39, 41, 179
    apocrine 37
Sympathectomy 90
Sympathetic ganglion 181
Sympathetic nervous system 181, 182f
Synapse
    classification of 164, 165f
    structure of 164f
    type of 164
Synaptic cleft 88, 164
Syndesmosis 103
Synergists 94, 103
Synovial fluid, functions of 109
Synovial joint 102, 103f, 106, 107, 107f, 109, 113f, 117
    classification of 112, 112t
    general structure of 107
Synovial membrane 108
Synovial tendon sheath 48

T

T lymphocytes 149
Teeth 191
Telangiectasis 139
Temperature regulation 34
Tendon 78, 208
    sheath 45, 50
        inflammation 48

Tenosynovitis 48
Terminal arterioles 132
Terminal ganglia 181
Testosterone, effects of 203
Thoracic cavity 185
Thoracic duct 148, 148f
    lymph in 148
Thoracic region 168
Thoracolumbar fascia 235
Thoracotomy 225
Thorax 152, 189, 223
    anatomical lines of 220
    negative pressure within 134
Thromboangiitis obliterans 139
Thrombophlebitis 139
Thrombosis 139
Thumb 120f
    muscles of 87
Thymus 151, 201, 203
Thyroid gland 201, 202
    enlarged 4f
    facilitating 214
    movement of 3
Thyroid stimulating hormone 201
Thyroiditis 204
Thyrotoxicosis 204
Thyroxine 202
Tibiofibular joint, inferior 103
Tissue 17
    adipose 30
    body 209
    cavernous 128, 133
    endocrine 194
    exocrine 194
    fibromuscular 188
    fibrous 43
    fluid 143, 145, 146
Tongue 191
Tonsillitis 153
Total hip replacement 121
Total knee replacement 121
Trabeculae 68
Trabecular bone 68
Trabecular sinus 151
Trachea 188, 189f, 202, 209, 211
Tracheostomy 190
Transitional epithelium 23
Transtubercular plane 224
Transplantation of Human Organs Act 239
Traumatic rupture 54
Tricuspid valve 126
Trigeminal nerve, division of 121
Trigeminal neuralgia 180
Trigger finger 50
Trigone 197
Triiodothyronine 202
Trochanteric bursa, greater 110
Trophoblast, cell of 16

Trunk and neck, movements of 120*f*
Trunk region 221
Tunica adventitia 128, 129, 132
Tunica externa 132
Tunica intima 129
    inner 128
    thickness of 132
Tunica media 129
    middle 128
Typical spinal nerve, course of 169, 169*f*
Typical thoracic spinal nerve 169*f*, 170

U

Umbilical region 224
Upper limb 152, 171, 223
    bones of 68*t*
    region 221
Upper motor neurons 163
Upper respiratory tract 186
Ureter 196
Urethra 195, 197
Urethritis 200
Urinary bladder 179, 195, 196, 197*f*
    interior of 197
Urinary system 186, 195, 209, 211
    developmental anatomy of 3*f*
    parts 196*f*
Urogenital system 200
Urothelium 23
Uterine 199
    endometrium 16
    fibroids 212
    tube 199
Uterus 199, 200
    bending of 200

V

Vagina, anterior wall of 200
Vagotomy 90
Valves 129
Varicella zoster 49
Varicose veins 138, 212
Vas deferens 197

Vasa vasorum 137, 138*f*
    capillaries of 128
Vascular diseases 212
Vascular tree, vessels of 131
Vein 61, 127, 129, 130*t*, 236
    large 129*f*, 133, 235
    of Batson 134
    structure of 128
    tributaries of 236
Vena cava 137
    inferior 128, 130
    superior 128, 130
Venae comitantes 133, 134*f*, 237
Venous anastomosis 136, 136*f*
Venous system 145
    types of 134
Venous valves 129*f*, 134
Ventral ramus 169
Vertebra 53
Vesalius 228
Visceral organs 185
Vitamin D 34
Vitiligo 42, 43*f*
Vocal cords, false 188
Vocal folds 188
Voice box 188
Volkmann's canals 61, 63
Voluntary body donation 239
Voluntary muscle, components of 81*fc*
Vulva 198

W

Waldeyer's lymphatic ring 149
Weight-bearing function 1
Wharton's duct 194
Wind pipe 188
Wrist, movements at 118*f*

X

X-ray machine 208*f*

Y

Young bone, plain X-ray 211*f*